Respiratory Medicine

Series Editors

Sharon I. S. Rounds, Brown University, Providence, USA

Anne E. Dixon, University of Vermont, Larner College of Medicine
Burlington, VT, USA

Lynn M. Schnapp, University of Wisconsin - Madison, Madison, USA

Respiratory Medicine offers clinical and research-oriented resources for pulmonologists and other practitioners and researchers interested in respiratory care. Spanning a broad range of clinical and research issues in respiratory medicine, the series covers such topics as COPD, asthma and allergy, pulmonary problems in pregnancy, molecular basis of lung disease, sleep disordered breathing, and others.

The series editors are Sharon Rounds, MD, Professor of Medicine and of Pathology and Laboratory Medicine at the Alpert Medical School at Brown University, Anne Dixon, MD, Professor of Medicine and Director of the Division of Pulmonary and Critical Care at Robert Larner, MD College of Medicine at the University of Vermont, and Lynn M. Schnapp, MD, George R. And Elaine Love Professor and Chair of Medicine at the University of Wisconsin-Madison School of Medicine and Public Health.

Noah Lechtzin

Editor

Pulmonary Complications of Neuromuscular Disease

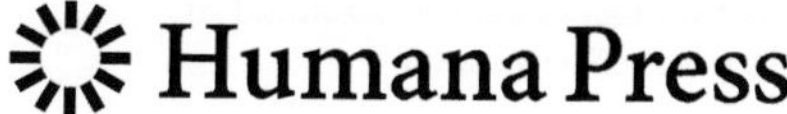 Humana Press

Editor
Noah Lechtzin
Pulmonary and Critical Care Medicine
Johns Hopkins Medicine
Baltimore, MD, USA

ISSN 2197-7372   ISSN 2197-7380   (electronic)
Respiratory Medicine
ISBN 978-3-031-65337-7   ISBN 978-3-031-65335-3   (eBook)
https://doi.org/10.1007/978-3-031-65335-3

This Humana imprint is published by the registered company Springer Nature Switzerland AG
The registered company address is: Gewerbestrasse 11, 6330 Cham, Switzerland

If disposing of this product, please recycle the paper.

Contents

Contributors

Jason Ackrivo Pulmonary, Allergy, and Critical Care Division, Department of Medicine and Neurology, Perelman School of Medicine at the Hospital of the University of Pennsylvania, Philadelphia, PA, USA

Reshma Amin Division of Respiratory Medicine, Department of Pediatrics, The Hospital for Sick Children, University of Toronto, Toronto, ON, Canada

Mirna Attalla Division of Respirology, University of Ottawa, Ottawa, ON, Canada

Joshua Benditt Division of Pulmonary, Critical Care and Sleep Medicine, Department of Medicine, University of Washington, Seattle, WA, USA

Matthew Berlinger LSU Health School of Medicine, Pulmonary and Critical Care Medicine, Baton Rouge, LA, USA

Hugo Carmona Division of Pulmonary, Critical Care and Sleep Medicine, Department of Medicine, University of Washington, Seattle, WA, USA

Andriana Charalampopoulou Neuromuscular Division, Department of Neurology, Johns Hopkins University School of Medicine, The John G. Rangos Sr. Building, Baltimore, MD, USA

Jackie Chiang Division of Respiratory Medicine, Department of Pediatrics, The Hospital for Sick Children, University of Toronto, Toronto, ON, Canada

Philip J. Choi Division of Pulmonary and Critical Care Medicine, NYU Langone Health, New York, NY, USA

Lora L. Clawson Department of Neurology, Johns Hopkins University School of Medicine, Baltimore, MD, USA

Marielena Linda DiBartolo Children's Hospital of Eastern Ontario, Ottawa, ON, Canada

University of Ottawa, Ottawa, ON, Canada

Andrew Graustein Division of Pulmonary, Critical Care and Sleep Medicine, Department of Medicine, University of Washington, Seattle, WA, USA

Division of Pulmonary, Critical Care and Sleep Medicine, Department of Medicine, Veterans Affairs Puget Sound Health Care System, Seattle, WA, USA

Elen Gusman Division of Pulmonary and Critical Care Medicine, Northwestern Medicine, Feinberg School of Medicine, Chicago, IL, USA

Aaron Izenberg Division of Neurology, Department of Medicine, Sunnybrook Health Sciences Center, University of Toronto, Toronto, ON, Canada

Jose Victor Jimenez Department of Internal Medicine, Yale New Haven Hospital, New Haven, CT, USA

Atul A. Kalanuria Division of Neurocritical Care, Department of Neurology, Neurosurgery, Anesthesia and Critical Care, Penn Presbyterian Medical Center, The Hospital of The University of Pennsylvania, Philadelphia, PA, USA

Sherri Lynne Katz Children's Hospital of Eastern Ontario, Ottawa, ON, Canada

Children's Hospital of Eastern Ontario Research Institute, Ottawa, ON, Canada

University of Ottawa, Ottawa, ON, Canada

Noah Lechtzin Pulmonary and Critical Care Medicine, Johns Hopkins Medicine, Baltimore, MD, USA

Jon Maniaci Division of Pulmonary and Sleep Medicine, The Children's Hospital of Philadelphia, Philadelphia, PA, USA

Nicholas John Maragakis Neuromuscular Division, Department of Neurology, Johns Hopkins University School of Medicine, The John G. Rangos Sr. Building, Baltimore, MD, USA

Douglas McKim Department of Medicine, University of Ottawa, Ottawa, ON, Canada

CANVent Respiratory Rehabilitation Services, Ottawa, ON, Canada

Brandon Merical Neurocritical Care, Department of Neurology, The Hospital of The University of Pennsylvania, Philadelphia, PA, USA

Matthew J. Michaels Division of Neurocritical Care, Department of Neurology, Neurosurgery, Anesthesia and Critical Care, Penn Presbyterian Medical Center, The Hospital of The University of Pennsylvania, Philadelphia, PA, USA

Jeremy Orr Department of Pulmonary and Critical Care Medicine, UC San Diego Health, University of California San Diego, La Jolla, CA, USA

Howard B. Panitch Division of Pulmonary and Sleep Medicine, The Children's Hospital of Philadelphia, Philadelphia, PA, USA

14523 HUB for Clinical Collaboration, Philadelphia, PA, USA

David Quintero Shepherd Center, Atlanta, GA, USA

Kathryn Selby Division of Pediatric Neurology, Department of Pediatrics, British Columbia Children's Hospital, University of British Columbia, Vancouver, BC, Canada

Anita K. Simonds Royal Brompton and Harefield Hospital, Guys and St Thomas' NHS Foundation Trust, London, UK

National Heart and Lung Institute, Imperial College, London, UK

Alpa Uchil Department of Neurology, Johns Hopkins University School of Medicine, Johns Hopkins School of Nursing, Baltimore, MD, USA

Philip Wexler Shepherd Center, Atlanta, GA, USA

Lisa F. Wolfe Division of Pulmonary and Critical Care Medicine, Northwestern Medicine, Feinberg School of Medicine, Chicago, IL, USA

Chapter 1
Overview of the Pathophysiology and Epidemiology of Neurologic Disorders Affecting the Respiratory System

Andriana Charalampopoulou and Nicholas John Maragakis

Respiration is a vital physiological process that is responsible for providing oxygen to the body and removing carbon dioxide. Through gas exchange, the respiratory system also contributes to the maintenance of acid-base balance and the support of cellular metabolism [1]. Because of this important role, respiration is highly regulated through a complex and dynamic process that involves the coordination of multiple systems, including the central and peripheral nervous systems, the respiratory muscles, and the cardiovascular system [2]. In this chapter, we will discuss the neural regulation of respiration, focusing on the central and peripheral mechanisms involved in controlling breathing patterns, and how these mechanisms are affected by different neurological diseases.

Brief Overview of the Neural Control of Respiration

The nervous system plays a crucial role in regulating respiration [3]. A complex interplay of neurons, comprising the sensory input, the central neural control of respiration, and the motor output, work together to coordinate the activity of the respiratory muscles and adjust the respiratory mechanics to meet the body's metabolic demands [4]. In addition to the variety of neural circuits forming the main input and output pathways, feedback mechanisms and chemical signals are also part of this process [5]. Figure 1.1 depicts the main neuronal pathways controlling respiration.

A. Charalampopoulou · N. J. Maragakis (✉)
Neuromuscular Division, Department of Neurology, Johns Hopkins University School of Medicine, The John G. Rangos Sr. Building, Baltimore, MD, USA
e-mail: acharal1@jh.edu; nmaragak@jhmi.edu

N. Lechtzin (ed.), *Pulmonary Complications of Neuromuscular Disease*, Respiratory Medicine, https://doi.org/10.1007/978-3-031-65335-3_1

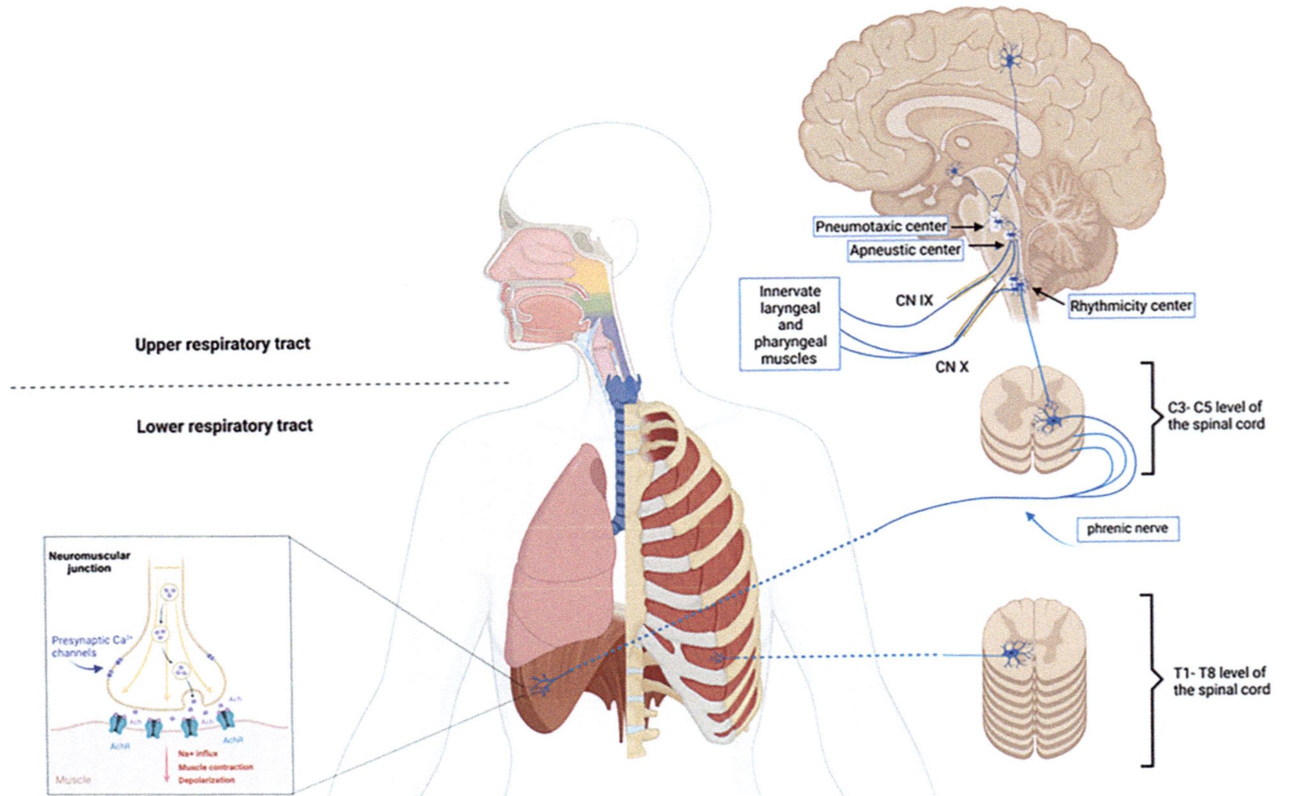

Fig. 1.1 Schematic representation of the main neuronal pathways governing respiration. (BioRender (2022). Human Respiratory System (modified). https://app.biorender.com/biorender-templates/figures/all/t-62ce21d7bac7729d0d03ee40-human-respiratory-system)

Sensory Input

Sensory input in respiration refers to the various sensors and receptors located in the central nervous system, the respiratory system, and the peripheral tissues. These sensors include the chemoreceptors, which detect changes in the levels of carbon dioxide (CO_2), oxygen (O_2), and hydrogen ions in the blood, as well as mechanoreceptors, which detect changes in lung volume/pressure and muscle spindles [6, 7]. Chemoreceptors are further categorized into two separate types: peripheral chemoreceptors and central chemoreceptors specified according to their location in the periphery and the central nervous system, respectively [8].

The process of respiration begins with the detection of changes in blood chemistry by these specialized structures which further trigger signaling of the respiratory centers of the brain. More specifically, two types of chemoreceptors send signals to the respiratory centers in the brainstem, which initiate the regulation of respiration to maintain appropriate levels of oxygen and carbon dioxide in the blood [9]. Peripheral chemoreceptors are located in the carotid arteries and aorta as small clusters of cells, known as the carotid bodies and aortic bodies, respectively. These chemoreceptors are sensitive to changes in the levels of oxygen, carbon dioxide, and pH in the blood [7, 9]. The carotid bodies send sensory signals through the glossopharyngeal nerve (CN IX), traveling to the medulla oblongata and synapsing with the nucleus of the solitary tract (NTS), whereas the aortic bodies' signals are carried via the vagus nerve [7]. On the other hand, central chemoreceptors are located in the brainstem, specifically in the medulla oblongata which is part of the respiratory centers. Central chemoreceptors are sensitive to changes in the levels of carbon dioxide and pH in the cerebrospinal fluid (CSF) [10].

In contrast, mechanoreceptors are mostly found in the bronchial smooth muscle and muscle spindles. As a result of lung overinflation/deflation, neural signals travel to the apneustic center through the vagus nerve and initiate the Hering-Breuer reflex, alternating the depth of breathing [7]. A change in respiration can also be initiated by muscle spindles as signals travel from muscles, tendons, and joints, stimulating inspiratory centers to increase the breathing rate when oxygen demands are higher [7].

Signal Transmission

As mentioned before, chemoreceptors detect changes in blood and CSF chemistry and send signals to the respiratory centers in the brainstem, which are responsible for coordinating breathing. These specialized cells detect changes in these parameters and directly influence the firing rate of neurons in the respiratory center, leading to changes in breathing rate and depth. There are two main respiratory centers in the brainstem processing these signals: the medullary respiratory center and the pontine respiratory center. The medullary respiratory center contains two sets of neurons that control respiration: the dorsal respiratory group (DRG) and the ventral respiratory group (VRG) [2, 10]. The DRG is responsible for generating the basic rhythm of breathing by stimulating the diaphragm and other muscles of inspiration, while the VRG is responsible for both inspiration and expiration, and it is divided into two subgroups: the pre-Bötzinger complex, setting the respiratory rhythm, and the retrotrapezoid nucleus (RTN), detecting changes in carbon dioxide levels and adjusting breathing accordingly [2, 11].

The pontine respiratory center is located in the pons, a region of the brainstem above the medulla, and consists of two regions, the pneumotaxic and the apneustic center that can regulate duration of each breath and prolong inspiration, respectively [7, 12]. The pontine respiratory center is responsible for coordinating the activity of the DRG and VRG and adjusting the breathing patterns (rate and depth) in response to other sensory inputs, such as pain, emotion, and exercise [5].

While the medulla oblongata is the primary brain region responsible for the generation and regulation of breathing, the cortex also plays a role in the modulation of respiration. The cortical regulation of respiration is primarily involved in voluntary breathing, such as during speech or singing, and in the regulation of breathing during certain emotional and cognitive states, such as anxiety, stress, and attention [13]. The cortex can influence the respiratory centers in the medulla oblongata through direct and indirect connections. Studies have shown that certain regions of the cortex, including the prefrontal cortex, insula, and cingulate cortex, are involved in the cortical regulation of respiration [14, 15]. These regions have connections to the medulla oblongata and can modulate the activity of the respiratory centers through various pathways. For example, the prefrontal cortex is involved in the cognitive control of breathing and can modulate the respiratory centers through a pathway that involves the ventral respiratory column (VRC) in the medulla oblongata [15]. The insular cortex is involved in the perception of respiratory sensations, such as breathlessness, and can influence the activity of the respiratory centers through a pathway that involves the NTS in the medulla oblongata. The cingulate cortex is involved in emotional processing and can influence the respiratory centers through a pathway that involves the parabrachial nucleus in the brainstem [16].

Motor Output

Neurons from the medullary respiratory centers project to the phrenic motor neurons located in the ventral horn of the spinal cord [4]. This pathway originates in the medullary respiratory centers, particularly the ventral respiratory group (VRG), and descends to the cervical spinal cord (C3–C5) to synapse directly onto the phrenic motor neurons in the phrenic motor nucleus [4, 7]. The VRG contains both inspiratory and expiratory neurons, and the inspiratory neurons project to the phrenic motor neurons to drive the activity of the diaphragm during inspiration. The activity of the medullary respiratory centers is modulated by input from other regions, such as the pons, which contains the pontine respiratory group (PRG) that influences VRG activity [4, 7].

The respiratory centers send signals to the muscles of respiration, which are responsible for moving the chest cavity and, as a result, air in and out of the lungs. The primary respiratory muscles are the diaphragm and intercostal muscles. In addition, accessory muscles of inspiration also take output from the respiratory centers and refer to scalene, sternocleidomastoid, and external intercostal muscles assisting mostly in labored breathing. The respiratory centers adjust the activity of these muscles to control the rate and depth of breathing [17].

Feedback Loop

The process of respiration is regulated by a feedback loop, in which changes in blood chemistry are detected by chemoreceptors and transmitted to the respiratory centers, which adjust the breathing rate and depth to maintain arterial blood gas homeostasis [18]. The lung stretch reflex, on the other hand, helps to prevent over-inflation of the lungs by inhibiting inspiratory neurons in the brainstem when lung volume reaches a certain threshold [7].

Research and Caveats

Recent research has shed light on some of the neural mechanisms that underlie the neural regulation of respiration. A study published in 2021 used optogenetics to manipulate the activity of specific neurons in the pre-Bötzinger complex of mice, a region of the brainstem that is critical for respiratory rhythm generation. Investigators found that inhibiting a specific type of neuron in this region led to irregular breathing patterns, while activating these neurons led to more regular breathing patterns [19]. Another study published in 2020 investigated the role of the locus coeruleus in mice, a region of the brainstem that is involved in arousal, attention, and stress responses, in the neural regulation of respiration. This group proved that stimulation of the locus coeruleus of mice increased respiratory rate and depth, and that this effect was mediated by a specific type of neuron in the pre-Bötzinger complex [20].

While respiratory studies in animals can provide valuable insights into the underlying neuronal mechanisms of respiratory control, they have inherent limitations that need to be considered when interpreting the results and extrapolating to humans. Translating animal research of the neural control of respiration requires careful consideration of anatomical and physiological differences. Here are some potential caveats to consider:

1. Anatomical differences: First, the anatomical structure of the respiratory system differs among species. For instance, human lungs have a more complex branching

structure than those of rodents, which can affect the distribution of airflow and gas exchange. Similarly, the anatomy of the upper airways, such as the larynx and pharynx, differ among species, which can affect mechanoreceptors' function, breathing mechanics, and airway resistance. Moreover, humans have a larger brainstem and more complex organization and function of the respiratory control centers (e.g., pre-Bötzinger complex) compared to mice so that the mechanisms that control breathing in mice may not be directly applicable to humans [21].

2. Physiological differences: There are differences in the neural pathways that regulate respiration in humans and rodents. The cortical control of breathing is indicative of the diversification between mice and humans. While humans have a well-developed cortex that can modulate breathing in response to various stimuli, the cortical control of breathing in mice is less well understood. The respiratory reflexes that control response to changes in blood/CSF gases, also differ between the two species as mice have a much greater sensitivity to CO_2 than humans [5], which can affect their respiratory responses to changes in CO_2 levels.

Understanding the neural regulation of respiration is also essential for the diagnosis and management of various neurological disorders. Conditions that affect the central nervous system, such as traumatic brain injury, stroke, and neurodegenerative diseases, or the peripheral nervous system, neuromuscular diseases, and peripheral neuropathies, can disrupt the harmonic coordination of sensory inputs, signal transmission, respiratory centers, motor output, and feedback loops leading to respiratory dysfunction. Neurological disorders and the pathophysiological mechanisms by which respiration is affected will be discussed in detail in this chapter.

Epidemiology of Neurological Disorders Affecting the Respiratory System

As described before, the neural control of the respiratory system is extensive and well-orchestrated, explaining why many neurological disorders can affect breathing. However, understanding the epidemiology of neurological disorders affecting the respiratory system is a complex task due to the diverse range of conditions and their unique respiratory characteristics. Consequently, most epidemiological data originate from limited-scale studies, and it is crucial to acknowledge that these estimates can vary depending on the specific population and diagnostic criteria employed in each study. Epidemiological studies highlight the impact of these disorders on respiratory function and some are addressed below.

It is widely accepted that a strong association exists between neuromuscular diseases and respiratory problems, as the involvement of respiratory muscles required for breathing frequently leads to complications [22, 23]. Epidemiological investigations have identified respiratory failure as a common cause of death in these patients, with the incidence and severity of respiratory complications varying according to the specific disease and its progression [24, 25]. For instance, patients with amyotrophic lateral sclerosis (ALS) typically develop respiratory muscle weakness as the disease advances, which eventually becomes a significant contributor to morbidity and mortality [26]. Notably, studies have demonstrated that up to 80% of ALS patients experience respiratory insufficiency at some stage during their illness [27, 28]. Diaphragm weakness, as evidenced by dyspnea at rest/exertion and orthopnea, is a poor prognostic factor and can be the first symptom in about 3% of ALS patients [26]. Another typical example is patients with Duchenne muscular dystrophy (DMD). Respiratory problems are common in DMD, with nearly all individuals developing respiratory muscle weakness as the disease progresses [29, 30]. According to studies, respiratory failure is the leading cause of death in individuals with DMD, usually occurring in the late teens to early 30s [30].

Similarly, individuals with spinal muscular atrophy, myasthenia gravis, and other neuromuscular disorders may encounter respiratory decompensations due to muscle weakness and dysfunction. Studies reveal that it is very common for patients with spinal muscular atrophy (SMA, especially types 1 and 2) to exhibit respiratory dysfunction, and this correlates with more severe disease manifestations and increased hospitalization rates [31, 32]. Moreover, in myasthenia gravis respiratory symptoms can range from mild shortness of breath to severe respiratory failure necessitating mechanical ventilation [33, 34]. Up to 40% of these patients reportedly experience respiratory dysfunction [35], which is associated with more severe disease, higher rates of hospitalization, and decreased respiratory muscle strength compared to healthy individuals [33, 36]. Consequently, respiratory muscle weakness significantly impacts disease severity and quality of life in patients with myasthenia gravis [33].

Respiratory problems are less frequently observed in neuroinflammatory diseases. The respiratory impairments in multiple sclerosis (MS) patients, for instance, have historically been overlooked by clinicians and scientists due to the prominence of other clinical signs [37]. However, studies have revealed altered respiratory function and reduced respiratory muscle strength with increasing disability in MS patients [38]. Surprisingly, respiratory issues account for approximately 47% of total deaths in MS patients [39]. Moreover, Guillain–Barre syndrome (GBS) is another example of a neuroinflammatory disease with respiratory impact. Respiratory complications are observed in up to 30% of GBS patients and range from mild respiratory muscle weakness to severe respiratory failure requiring mechanical ventilation [40, 41]. The risk of respiratory dysfunction in GBS is higher in patients with severe disease and longer illness duration [41].

Respiratory dysfunction frequently arises as a complication of stroke, particularly in patients who experience a severe stroke or have comorbidities such as pneumonia or chronic obstructive pulmonary disease (COPD) [42, 43]. Studies report that stroke patients commonly experience respiratory complications, with pneumonia being the most common [44]. These complications were associated with increased mortality and prolonged hospital stays [44].

These findings underscore the significant impact of respiratory dysfunction on individuals with neurological diseases, highlighting the importance of monitoring and managing respiratory function. Pulmonologists are an essential part of the comprehensive care of patients with neuromuscular disease, particularly in addressing and managing respiratory complications as well as in patient education and support [45]. As respiratory health plays a critical role in the overall well-being of individuals with neurological disorders, it is imperative for healthcare professionals to conduct regular respiratory assessments and establish multidisciplinary teams involving pulmonologists. With their specialized expertise, they can evaluate respiratory function, monitor disease progression, and provide personalized interventions to support optimal respiratory health and enhanced quality of life to patients with neurological diseases.

Respiratory Dysfunction Aspect of Neurological Disorders

After discussing in detail, the intricate relationship between the nervous system and respiration, we will focus on a comprehensive analysis of the pathophysiology of various neurological disorders that can disrupt the respiratory system. By categorizing these disorders based on the anatomical localization of their pathology, we can gain a deeper understanding of the mechanisms contributing to respiratory dysfunction. From disorders affecting the brainstem to motoneuronopathies, phrenic nerve disorders, neuromuscular junction-related disorders, and myopathies, we examine the specific pathophysiology and discuss the current hypotheses in the generation of the disease-related symptoms of patients. By highlighting the underlying mechanisms of these disorders, we aim to summarize the current knowledge and facilitate the development of effective management strategies for individuals experiencing respiratory impairments associated with neurological conditions.

Table 1.1 summarizes the main mechanisms by which a broad list of neurological disorders affect respiration, the most notable of which are described in detail later in this chapter.

Disorders Affecting the Brainstem

As described before, the brainstem serves as a vital control center for respiration, orchestrating the coordination of neural signals that drive the respiratory muscles. In this section, we explore the pathophysiology of disorders such as neuromyelitis optica, multiple sclerosis, and stroke, which can disrupt the respiratory function primarily by affecting the brainstem.

Table 1.1 Primary and secondary mechanisms of respiratory involvement in neurological disorders

Neurological disorder	Primary mechanism of respiratory involvement	Other mechanisms of respiratory involvement (if any)
Disorders affecting respiratory centers of the brain		
Neuromyelitis optica [46–51]	Phrenic nerve demyelination of autoimmune etiology	Inflammation, impaired neural signaling, loss of motor control, reduced respiratory muscle strength
Multiple sclerosis [52–59]	Demyelination (of autoimmune etiology) of nerves in the medulla, pons, and upper cervical spinal cord that are involved in respiration	Inflammation of the brainstem and the spinal cord affecting the phrenic nerve nucleus at the C3–C5 level, loss of neural connections, impaired respiratory muscle coordination
Stroke [60–62]	Brainstem respiratory centers damage due to ischemia or hemorrhage	Cortical stroke causing damage of the neural descending pathway to the brainstem
Parkinson's disease [193, 194]	Neurodegeneration affects movement control and leads to rigidity and weakness of respiratory muscles	
Wilson's disease [195–198]	Copper buildup in various organs, including the brain, which leads to impaired neural control of respiratory muscles	Copper deposition in respiratory muscles, reduced respiratory muscle strength
Spinocerebellar ataxias [199, 200]	Impaired coordination and control of respiratory muscles due to progressive degeneration of the cerebellum and its connections	
Sleep apnea [201–204]	Reduced central neural drive to respiratory muscles, upper airway collapse, impaired respiratory muscle coordination	
Epilepsy [205–207]	Impaired neural control, respiratory muscle dysfunction, disrupted breathing patterns during seizures	
Motoneuronopathies		
Amyotrophic lateral sclerosis [63–70]	Upper (primary motor cortex and corticobulbar tract) and lower (brainstem and spinal cord) motor neuron demyelination and degeneration	Impaired neuromuscular transmission reduces respiratory response. Respiratory muscles' fatigue due to their continuous effort to compensate for weakness can contribute to reduced vital capacity and respiratory infections

(continued)

Table 1.1 (continued)

Neurological disorder	Primary mechanism of respiratory involvement	Other mechanisms of respiratory involvement (if any)
Spinal muscular atrophy [71, 72]	Genetic cause of lower motor neuron degeneration innervating respiratory muscles	
Post-polio syndrome [77–81]	Lower motor neuron loss (spinal cord)	Chest wall deformities leading to compromised breathing. Brainstem respiratory centers involvement
Disorders affecting the phrenic nerve		
Phrenic nerve injury (traumatic, radiation, tumor, surgery) [84–93, 95–104]	Phrenic nerve damage due to traumatic injury, surgical/iatrogenic, radiation, and tumor compression	
Guillain–Barre syndrome [110–116]	Autoimmune damage of the phrenic nerve	Inflammation causing demyelination and impaired neuromuscular transmission
Brachial plexopathies/radiculopathies [105–109]	Damage/inflammation of the nerve roots or plexus contributing to the formation of the phrenic nerve or other peripheral nerves innervating respiratory muscles	
CIDP/AIDP [117–124]	Chronic inflammation and demyelination of peripheral nerves/phrenic nerve	
Peripheral neuropathies: Acquired (e.g., diabetic) and inherited (e.g., Charcot–Marie tooth disease) [208–213]	Disruption of the neural signals from the peripheral nerves (phrenic and nerves innervating the intercostal muscles) to the respiratory muscles, resulting in respiratory weakness or paralysis	
Neuromuscular junction-related disorders		
Myasthenia gravis [128–137]	Respiratory muscles' neuromuscular junction dysfunction (postsynaptic antibodies) leading to muscle weakness	
Lambert–Eaton syndrome [139–146]	Respiratory muscles' neuromuscular junction dysfunction (presynaptic antibodies) leading to muscle weakness	
Botulism [147–153, 155, 156]	Botulinum toxin inhibition of the release of acetylcholine and decreased signaling of the muscle	
Myopathies		

(continued)

Table 1.1 (continued)

Neurological disorder	Primary mechanism of respiratory involvement	Other mechanisms of respiratory involvement (if any)
Muscular dystrophies (DMD, BD, FSHD, LGMD, etc.) and other inherited myopathies (HMERF, Pompe disease, myotonia congenita, etc.) [160–170]	Genetic disorders affecting the structure and/or function of the muscle causing progressive muscle fiber degeneration, impaired neuromuscular transmission, reduced respiratory muscle strength	*Myotonia specific mechanism:* Muscle stiffness or prolonged muscle contractions
Acquired myopathies (IMNM, dermatomyositis, antisynthetase syndrome, drug-induced, critical illness, etc.) [171–192]	Myofiber damage, inflammation, impaired neuromuscular transmission	Scoliosis, kyphoscoliosis causing restricting pattern of lung disease and compromised breathing

Neuromyelitis Optica

Neuromyelitis optica (NMO) is an autoimmune disorder primarily affecting the optic nerves and spinal cord that results from the development of autoantibodies to the Aquaporin 4 protein. It is characterized by recurrent episodes of optic neuritis (inflammation of the optic nerve) and transverse myelitis (inflammation of the spinal cord). While NMO primarily affects the central nervous system, it can lead to respiratory dysfunction through involvement of the brainstem or, less commonly, the cervical spinal cord which are both vital regions of the CNS responsible for controlling respiratory control among other functions [46, 47]. It is reported that up to 22% of NMO patients can develop respiratory dysfunction after the onset of the disease [48]. Moreover, one study reported that respiratory failure attributed to the acute cervical myelitis appeared in 33% of the relapsing patients and in 9% of the monophasic patients [49].

In NMO, inflammation can extend to the brainstem which houses respiratory centers including the medullary respiratory centers and the pontine respiratory group [49]. Damage of these centers is the most common mechanism that can lead to abnormalities in respiratory rhythm generation and control [49]. Moreover, demyelination of neurons projecting to the respiratory centers of the brainstem can disrupt the normal functioning of these centers and the ascending or descending neural pathways involved in breathing regulation. Disruption of the descending pathways that transmit signals from the brainstem to the spinal cord can result in impaired coordination of muscles, decreased respiratory drive, and respiratory muscle weakness or even paralysis [46].

Other possible mechanisms in NMO involved in breathing dysregulation include the inflammation of the spinal cord above T5 (transverse myelitis) [47]. However, damage that leads to severe respiratory dysfunction is rare [49, 50]. Spinal cord lesions can disrupt the transmission of respiratory signals from the brainstem through the autonomic nervous system or the phrenic nerve to the respiratory muscles, contributing to the respiratory symptoms of these patients [49]. When the phrenic nerve is involved due to high cervical spinal cord inflammation, this is manifested by diaphragmatic paralysis [51].

Respiratory dysfunction in NMO can lead to symptoms such as shortness of breath, difficulty breathing, ineffective cough, and decreased respiratory muscle strength. It is important to note that the specific mechanisms of respiratory dysfunction in NMO may vary among individuals, and additional research is needed to fully elucidate these mechanisms.

Multiple Sclerosis

Multiple sclerosis (MS) is a chronic autoimmune disorder that affects the central nervous system, including the brain and spinal cord. While MS primarily manifests as a disease of the white matter, it can also impact the brainstem, leading to respiratory dysfunction [52].

There are several pathophysiological mechanisms through which MS affects respiration. One of them is demyelination of nerves in the CNS involved in respiration. In MS, the immune system mistakenly attacks the myelin sheath, the protective covering of nerve fibers in the central nervous system, causing demyelination. Lesions mainly in the brainstem, as well as in areas such as the medulla, pons, and upper cervical spinal cord, can disrupt the neural pathways responsible for respiratory regulation in these patients [53]. Among other impairments, demyelination can also interrupt the pathway descending from the brainstem all the way to the phrenic and accessory respiratory muscle nerves and, thus, dysregulates the transmission of signals to the respiratory muscles resulting in weakness and compromised breathing [53]. It is also believed that demyelination in the caudal medulla (nucleus tractus solitarius) is associated with sympathetic overstimulation and increased hydrostatic pulmonary pressure causing edema [54].

Another mechanism through which respiration is affected in MS patients is the inflammatory process. Inflammation in MS contributes to the destruction of myelin and the formation of immune cell infiltrates [55]. When extending to the brainstem, it can affect the integrity and function of respiratory centers, leading to abnormalities in ventilatory control. In addition to demyelination and inflammation, MS pathology can lead to axonal damage, which further impairs the transmission of respiratory signals. Axonal loss contributes to the decrease in the motor output to the respiratory muscles compromising their strength and coordination [56, 57].

The combination of these pathophysiological factors in MS can lead to various respiratory dysfunctions, including respiratory muscle weakness, decreased respiratory drive, impaired coordination of breathing muscles, neurogenic pulmonary edema, and sleep-disordered breathing. Consequently, individuals with MS may experience symptoms such as dyspnea, orthopnea, confusion, reduced lung function, ineffective cough, increased susceptibility to respiratory infections, as well as respiratory failure at a late stage of the disease [54]. However, the brain has a remarkable ability to adapt and rewire neural connections and, in response to MS-related damage, neuroplasticity may occur, allowing for compensation and the recruitment of alternative pathways to maintain respiratory function to some extent [58, 59]. Thus, the presence of respiratory pathology varies among individuals.

Stroke

Stroke is a neurological condition characterized by the sudden interruption of blood flow to the brain, leading to brain cell damage and dysfunction. It can be either ischemic or less commonly hemorrhagic [60]. Ischemic stroke can disrupt the function of respiratory centers and neural pathways by obstructing the blood flow to the brainstem or, more rarely, the cortex (close to respiratory centers) due to a blockage or clot in the supporting vasculature, whereas hemorrhagic stroke can directly damage the structure and morphology of these regions due to bleeding. When a stroke affects the brainstem and its respiratory centers (ventral-dorsal medullary respiratory groups and the pontine respiratory group), it causes abnormalities in respiratory rhythm generation and control [61]. Moreover, stroke-related damage to descending neuronal pathways that transmit signals from the cortex (cortical stroke) or the brainstem (brainstem stroke) can result in impaired coordination of respiratory muscle activity [61]. This can lead to respiratory muscle weakness, paralysis, or reduced coordination, affecting the ability of these patients to breathe effectively [61].

Pulmonary complications resulting from a stroke mostly depend on the location and extent of the brainstem involvement. They can range from mild respiratory difficulties (e.g., shortness of breath) in lateral medullary syndrome to more severe respiratory muscle weakness, impaired coordination of breathing muscles, as well as compromised respiratory drive, as reported in three patients with left cingulate cortex, left insula, and right paramedian thalamus stroke [61, 62]. Eventually, such complications can lead to respiratory failure, pneumonia, pleural effusions, acute respiratory distress syndrome, and lung edema, which are among the major causes of death at this group of patients [42].

For a complete overview of the respiratory dysfunction mechanisms, it is important to note that stroke can also impact swallowing function (dysphagia). Dysphagia can increase the risk of aspiration, where food or liquid enters the airway instead of the digestive tract, leading to potential respiratory complications such as aspiration pneumonia [42].

Motor Neuron Diseases

The degeneration and loss of motor neurons affect various nerves and regions involved in the neural control of respiration. In the motor neuron diseases described in this subchapter, respiratory dysfunction typically arises from the degeneration and loss of motor neurons that innervate the muscles involved in breathing. The specific muscles affected and the severity of respiratory impairment may vary depending on the underlying disorder and its progression.

Amyotrophic Lateral Sclerosis

Amyotrophic lateral sclerosis (ALS) is a progressive neurodegenerative disease that primarily affects the motor neurons (upper and lower motor neuron), which are responsible for transmitting signals from the brain to the muscles. Motor neuron degeneration plays an important role in the respiratory decline of ALS patients and, thus, respiratory complications are common in these patients especially as the disease progresses [63]. It is important to note that the exact mechanisms underlying upper motor neuron dysfunction in ALS are not fully understood. The disease is complex and involves multiple pathological processes, including RNA processing defects, defects in protein quality control, neuroinflammation, glutamate excitotoxicity, autophagic pathways, and oxidative stress [64]. The specific sequence of events leading to respiratory symptoms can vary among individuals with ALS, but the disruption of signal transmission from the upper motor neurons to the lower motor neurons and subsequent respiratory muscle weakness are central components [65].

In the context of respiration, upper motor neuron dysfunction refers to the degeneration or damage to the motor neurons located in the cerebral cortex and brainstem, particularly in the primary motor cortex and the corticobulbar tract [66]. The corticobulbar tract carries motor signals from the primary motor cortex to the cranial nerves, including those involved in controlling respiratory muscles [67]. With UMN dysfunction in ALS, the transmission of these signals to the respiratory muscles becomes disrupted. Consequently, the disruption of signal transmission from the UMNs to the LMNs in the brainstem and spinal cord affects the activation of respiratory muscles. This inadequate activation leads to weakened or insufficient contraction of the respiratory muscles, including the diaphragm and intercostal muscles. The combination of UMN dysfunction and respiratory muscle weakness can lead to alterations in the breathing pattern. Thus, individuals with ALS may exhibit shallow or ineffective breathing, reduced lung ventilation, and difficulty generating sufficient respiratory airflow [68].

As expected, lower motor neuron (LMN) lesions also play a significant role in affecting respiration of ALS patients. LMNs are located in the brainstem nuclei and the anterior horn of the spinal cord and directly innervate the respiratory muscles, including the diaphragm, intercostal muscles, and other muscles involved in breathing [69]. With LMN dysfunction and loss in ALS, the transmission of signals from the motor neurons in the spinal cord to the respiratory muscles becomes compromised. This impaired neural input results in suboptimal activation of the respiratory muscles followed by weakness, atrophy, and impaired contraction [69]. The combination of LMN dysfunction and respiratory muscle weakness leads to respiratory compromise. Individuals with ALS may experience shallow, labored, or irregular breathing patterns. They may have difficulty taking deep breaths, clearing secretions, and maintaining adequate ventilation [69]. As the disease progresses, respiratory compromise becomes more severe. Continued loss of LMNs and respiratory muscle weakness can result in respiratory insufficiency, reduced lung function, impaired gas exchange, and decreased ability to effectively cough. Moreover, in some individuals with ALS, the bulbar region of the brainstem, which controls functions like speech, swallowing, and breathing, can be affected [70]. Bulbar involvement can lead to weakness and dysfunction of the muscles involved in swallowing and controlling the airway, increasing the risk of aspiration and respiratory complications [70]. A vast majority of patients eventually experience these complications as bulbar function declines [69, 70].

As ALS progresses, the respiratory muscles experience increasing fatigue due to their continuous effort to compensate for weakness. Respiratory muscle fatigue can contribute to reduced pulmonary vital capacity, impaired cough function, and an increased risk of respiratory infections [63, 69]. The respiratory dysfunction in ALS typically worsens over time, leading to respiratory insufficiency and the need for respiratory support which will be comprehensively discussed in Chap. 10.

Spinal Muscular Atrophy

Spinal muscular atrophy (SMA) is a genetic neuromuscular disorder characterized by the degeneration and loss of motor neurons in the spinal cord and brainstem. In SMA, there is a mutation or deletion in the survival motor neuron 1 or 2 (SMN1, SMN2) gene, which leads to a deficiency of survival motor neuron (SMN) protein. The SMN protein is crucial for the survival and maintenance of motor neurons. Without sufficient levels of SMN protein, the motor neurons degenerate and die over time [31]. As we discuss the common pathophysiology of respiration in SMA, we should appreciate that the appearance and severity of the respiratory complications depend on the SMA subtype and individual factors [71].

The respiratory dysfunction in SMA is primarily caused by the involvement of the lower motor neurons that control the muscles involved in breathing. Respiratory dysfunction in SMA arises due to the progressive degeneration and loss of motor neurons that innervate the muscles responsible for breathing, such as the diaphragm, the intercostal muscles, and other accessory muscles of respiration [72]. Although the involvement of the diaphragm is particularly critical in SMA-related respiratory dysfunction when it occurs, it is reported to be relatively spared in SMA. On the contrary, the intercostal muscles, which aid in expanding and contracting the ribcage during breathing, are the respiratory muscles predominantly impaired in SMA [72]. Unlike in ALS, upper motor neuron loss is not observed in SMA. Due to the continuous demand placed on weakened respiratory muscles in SMA, respiratory muscle fatigue can occur [72]. Prolonged muscle fatigue can further compromise respiratory function and contribute to respiratory distress and respiratory failure [71].

In some individuals with SMA, particularly those with more severe forms of the condition, bulbar muscle weakness can occur. This weakness can affect the ability to effectively cough, swallow, and maintain an open airway, leading to an increased risk of respiratory complications [71].

As the disease progresses, the respiratory dysfunction in SMA can lead to respiratory insufficiency and the development of respiratory complications, such as recurrent infections, atelectasis (collapse of lung tissue), and respiratory failure. Without appropriate interventions, respiratory compromise can become life-threatening in severe cases of SMA [32, 72].

Other Motor Neuronopathies

Primary lateral sclerosis (PLS) is a rare neurodegenerative disorder characterized by the selective degeneration of upper motor neurons responsible for the voluntary control of movement [73]. From reports to date, the specific pathway to respiratory symptoms in PLS is not well-defined, but the involvement of upper motor neurons can lead to certain respiratory manifestations. While the lower motor neurons are generally spared in PLS, respiratory dysfunction can still occur due to weakness in the upper respiratory muscles, such as those involved in coughing and clearing the airways [74, 75]. The UMN lesion in PLS can disrupt the normal conduction of nerve impulses and ultimately affect the transmission of respiratory signals between the brainstem and respiratory muscles. This can result in respiratory symptoms such as reduced respiratory muscle strength, diminished cough reflex, and impaired coordination of respiratory muscles. These symptoms may contribute to difficulty in clearing respiratory secretions and a decreased ability to generate adequate airflow [76].

Poliomyelitis and post-polio syndrome are a consequence of poliovirus infection. Poliovirus perturbs spinal motor neurons (lower motor neurons), ultimately impacting respiratory function. By binding to specific receptors on motor neurons, the virus initiates intracellular entry and neuronal damage, particularly within the context of those controlling respiratory musculature such as the diaphragm and intercostal muscles [77]. The acute phase of infection elicits muscle weakness and, in severe instances, respiratory failure. Although surviving motor neurons attempt compensation, the latent emergence of post-polio syndrome (25–40% of polio survivors) [78] can rekindle muscular debility, frequently including respiratory muscles [79]. The cumulative attrition of motor neurons could impart a chronic state of respiratory insufficiency in post-polio patients [80, 81].

Disorders Affecting the Phrenic Nerve

As described before, the phrenic nerve, arising from the cervical spinal nerves C3–C5, assumes a vital role in the respiratory system by innervating the diaphragm muscle, which is instrumental in breathing. Certain disorders have a particular predilection for affecting the phrenic nerve, leading to significant respiratory dysfunction. It is also essential to acknowledge the existence of the accessory phrenic nerve (APN), which exhibits variable prevalence (about one-third of the population) and origins [82], thereby contributing to the diverse phenotypic expression observed in conditions affecting the phrenic nerve and/or the APN [83]. In cases of phrenic nerve damage, the collateral innervation provided by the APN has the potential to preserve respiratory function and prevent diaphragmatic dysfunction [83]. However, the comprehensive understanding and investigation of the APN's role in these conditions remain limited. Nevertheless, to provide a comprehensive overview, it is important to recognize the potential implications of the APN in contributing to the variable presentation among patients with phrenic nerve damage.

This section focuses on the pathophysiology of disorders that primarily cause respiratory dysfunction by affecting the phrenic nerve such as injury (trauma, radiation, tumor, surgery), Guillain–Barre syndrome (GBS), brachial plexopathies/radiculopathies, chronic inflammatory demyelinating polyneuropathy (CIDP), or acute inflammatory demyelinating polyneuropathy (AIDP).

Phrenic Nerve Injury

There are four main types of injury that can affect the phrenic nerve: traumatic injury, surgical/iatrogenic, radiation, and tumor compression. In all these cases, the injury to the phrenic nerve disrupts the normal transmission of signals from the brain to the diaphragm. This can result in paralysis or weakness of the diaphragm on the affected side, leading to an impaired ability to breathe deeply and efficiently [84–86]. Depending on the severity and extent of the injury, respiratory symptoms may range from mild respiratory distress to significant respiratory compromise [85]. Treatment approaches for phrenic nerve injuries depend on the specific cause and severity and may include conservative management, rehabilitation, and occasionally surgical interventions to restore diaphragmatic function if possible [87].

Among the most common causes of phrenic nerve injury is trauma [85, 88]. Penetrating and blunt trauma to the neck and chest, such as from a severe blow or impact, can cause damage to the phrenic nerve. One study reported that 1–7% of patients with penetrating trauma present with some degree of diaphragmatic dysfunction or paralysis [89]. Although injury of the phrenic nerve in the thoracic cavity is relatively uncommon as the nerve pathway is deeply interpolated between the lung and the pericardium, this can occur in cases of motor vehicle accidents, severe falls, stab wounds, or sports-related injuries. Direct trauma or compression of the nerve can occur directly due to fractured ribs or dislocated shoulder joints [89–91]. The resulting damage disrupts the transmission of signals between the brain and the diaphragm, leading to respiratory dysfunction.

Iatrogenic causes also constitute a significant portion of the phrenic nerve injuries [86]. Surgeries in the neck, chest, or upper abdomen, particularly cardiothoracic surgeries (15% of these patients according to one study) [88], may involve manipulation or inadvertent damage to the phrenic nerve. For example, during procedures like thymectomy, coronary artery bypass grafting (CABG), valve replacements, or lung surgeries, the phrenic nerve can be accidentally injured [88]. Cases of cardiac ablations performed due to underlying atrial fibrillation have also been reported to cause thermal injury to the phrenic nerve in 0.4% of these patients according to a multicenter study [87, 92]. Moreover, interventions like brachial plexus anesthetic block using an interscalene approach can cause swelling and hematoma of the scalenus muscle leading to phrenic nerve compression and palsy [93]. According to a retrospective study, interscalene nerve block caused diaphragmatic dysfunction in 17% of the patients [88]. Other causes of phrenic nerve damage can be surgery for thoracic outlet syndrome, cervical lymphadenopathy, and radiofrequency ablation of tumors [88]. The latter often used in the treatment of thoracic cancers (such as lung cancer or lymphomas), can inadvertently affect the nearby phrenic nerve and lead to inflammation, scarring, or fibrosis, causing impaired conduction of nerve signals and subsequent respiratory dysfunction [88]. Surgical/iatrogenic trauma of any kind to the nerve usually results in paralysis and disruption of its function [85]. Consequently, complications can occur such as dyspnea on exertion, orthopnea, sleeping disorders, easy fatigability as well as gastrointestinal reflux, bloating, and recurring infections [94]. However, it is very important to appreciate that such diaphragmatic weakness may present postoperatively and be falsely attributed to nerve damage during surgery. It is important to recognize that postoperative isolated diaphragmatic paralysis can be myasthenic in origin and may respond to immunosuppressive therapy [95].

Radiation therapy is a common treatment modality for various thoracic malignancies and mediastinal tumors [96]. While it can effectively target and kill cancer cells, it may also affect nearby healthy tissues, like the phrenic nerve, via the production of hydroxyl radicals [97]. The extent of phrenic nerve involvement by radiation depends on several factors, such as the total radiation dose, the fractionation schedule (how the radiation is delivered in divided doses), the specific target area, and the patient's individual anatomy. Phrenic nerve radiation can lead to phrenic nerve dysfunction or palsy, resulting in weakness or paralysis of the diaphragm as reported in Hodgkin lymphoma and breast cancer patients [96, 97]. As with any medical treatment, patients receiving radiation therapy should be closely monitored for potential side effects, including those related to the phrenic nerve. Timely recognition and appropriate management of phrenic nerve dysfunction are essential to address respiratory challenges effectively and optimize outcomes for individuals undergoing radiation therapy [98].

Tumor compression is another very important cause of phrenic nerve injury. Tumors in the chest or mediastinum (the central compartment of the chest) can exert pressure on the phrenic nerve, leading to its compression or infiltration [99, 100]. This compression can impair the nerve's function, resulting in diaphragmatic paralysis or weakness and respiratory dysfunction [99]. Tumors that commonly affect the phrenic nerve include lung tumors (e.g., small-cell and non-small-cell lung carcinoma) [101, 102], mediastinal tumors (e.g., thymoma) [103], or tumors that have metastasized to the chest (e.g., breast) [104].

Brachial Plexopathies/Radiculopathies

Brachial radiculopathies and plexopathies refer to conditions that affect the nerve roots and the brachial plexus originating from the cervical spinal nerves. These conditions can potentially affect the phrenic nerve when forming from the spinal roots C3–C5, leading to respiratory dysfunction [105].

Radiculopathies involve the compression or inflammation of individual nerve roots as they exit the spinal column. When the cervical spinal nerve roots (C3–C5) that contribute to the phrenic nerve are affected, it can lead to respiratory dysfunction [106]. Radiculopathies can occur due to various factors, including herniated disks, degenerative changes in the spine (such as spondylosis), spinal stenosis, or nerve root compression caused by tumors or infections [106]. When the nerve roots that give rise to the phrenic nerve are affected, it can disrupt the transmission of signals from the brain to the diaphragm. This results in impaired diaphragmatic movement and respiratory dysfunction. For example, chronic cervical spinal stenosis can lead to subclinical pulmonary dysfunction due to the involvement of the phrenic nerve with $FEV_1\%$ predicted to be the most sensitive parameter in the detection of this disorder according to one study [84]. It is worth noting that although radiculopathies affecting the phrenic nerve can occur, they are relatively uncommon compared to other causes of phrenic nerve dysfunction [84, 106].

The brachial plexus is a network of nerves originating from the spinal nerves C5–T1. It supplies the motor and sensory innervation to the upper extremities [105]. Brachial plexopathies refer to injuries or disorders that affect this network of nerves and can result from various causes, including trauma (such as subclavian vein catheterization, shoulder injuries, or traction injuries during childbirth), compression (such as thoracic outlet syndrome), inflammation (such as in autoimmune conditions like brachial neuritis), or tumors in the region (such as Pancoast tumors) [107]. If the nerve roots or segments of the brachial plexus that give rise to the phrenic nerve are affected, it can disrupt the normal conduction of signals to the diaphragm and result in reduced diaphragmatic movement and respiratory dysfunction. Phrenic nerve injury is reported to be relatively frequent in cases of brachial plexopathies, with an estimated incidence ranging from 10% to 20% [107]. However, it is worth noting that unilateral diaphragmatic paralysis often remains asymptomatic at rest, leading to a considerable number of undetected phrenic nerve injuries in the context of brachial plexus injury [107, 108].

Management of brachial plexopathies and radiculopathies involves addressing the underlying cause. Treatment approaches may include pain management, physical therapy, rehabilitation exercises, and, in some cases, surgical intervention to relieve nerve compression [109]. In instances where the phrenic nerve is affected, respiratory support may be necessary to assist with breathing until nerve function improves. The specific treatment plan will depend on the underlying cause, severity, and individual patient characteristics.

Guillain–Barre Syndrome

Guillain–Barre syndrome (GBS), also called acute inflammatory demyelinating polyradiculopathy (AIDP), is an autoimmune disorder characterized by the immune system mistakenly attacking the peripheral nerves and has an annual incidence of 1/100,000 people worldwide [110]. The exact cause of GBS is not fully understood, but it is often preceded by a bacterial or viral infection, such as respiratory or gastrointestinal infections [110]. The immune response triggered by the infection leads to an inflammatory response that mostly damages the myelin sheath (the protective covering) of the peripheral nerves, including the phrenic nerve [110, 111]. Additionally, GBS can also cause damage to the nerve fibers themselves, known as axonal degeneration [112]. This can disrupt the conduction of nerve impulses along the phrenic nerve, resulting in respiratory muscle weakness or paralysis.

Studies suggest that 30% of GBS patients will develop respiratory failure [41] and electrophysiological examination of the phrenic nerve is a promising method for the anticipation of those patients at risk [113]. Prolonged phrenic nerve latency, which indicates either axonal degeneration or mild segmental demyelination in the early stages of the disease, is among the electrophysiological findings observed when the phrenic nerve is affected [112, 114, 115].

In GBS, immune-mediated damage to the phrenic nerve can result in paralysis or weakness of the diaphragm muscle on one or both sides indicating the important role of the impaired conduction of the signals along the phrenic nerve in the pathology and mortality of GBS [116]. Consequently, reduced diaphragmatic movement and respiratory dysfunction occur, typically presenting as a restrictive pattern [111]. The degree of respiratory dysfunction depends on the extent of phrenic nerve involvement. In severe cases, patients may experience respiratory failure and require mechanical ventilation to support breathing until the nerve damage resolves and recovery occurs [40, 111].

It is important to note that while respiratory involvement is a significant concern in GBS, the majority of patients with GBS have good potential for recovery with appropriate medical care and supportive interventions. However, the recovery process can vary and may take weeks to months, with some individuals requiring ongoing rehabilitation and respiratory support during the recovery period [40].

Chronic Inflammatory Demyelinating Polyneuropathy

CIDP (chronic inflammatory demyelinating polyneuropathy) is an acquired immune-mediated disorder affecting the peripheral nerves. While CIDP and GBS are both immune-mediated disorders that affect the peripheral nerves and share some similarities, they are easily distinguished due to different disease duration, progression, symptom duration, and distribution [117]. CIDP is characterized by chronic inflammation and demyelination, resulting in the damage of the protective myelin sheath surrounding the nerves. Although the precise cause of CIDP remains unclear, it is believed to involve an aberrant immune response targeting the peripheral nerves. The condition typically progresses gradually over months or years, and while respiratory dysfunction is rare, it has been observed in a small percentage of cases (approximately 1–9%) [118].

Among individuals with CIDP, up to 80% have reported demyelination of the phrenic nerve [118]. However, this phrenic nerve damage often presents without noticeable clinical symptoms and can be reversed with appropriate treatment [119, 120]. In cases where respiratory failure does occur, it is attributed to phrenic neuropathy and the subsequent denervation of respiratory muscles [111]. This denervation can manifest as either unilateral or bilateral impairment [121, 122].

Similar to Guillain–Barre syndrome, CIDP involves an autoimmune response whereby the immune system erroneously recognizes components of the peripheral nerves as foreign and launches an immune attack against them. This immune response leads to chronic inflammation and demyelination, which disrupts the conduction of nerve impulses [123]. One suggested mechanism for respiratory failure in CIDP involves chronic conduction blocks in the phrenic nerves, as evidenced by the absence of phrenic motor responses [124]. However, it is important to note that phrenic nerve palsy in CIDP remains uncommon [125].

The severity of respiratory involvement in CIDP varies among individuals, ranging from mild breathing difficulties to respiratory failure [126]. It is crucial to monitor and manage respiratory function carefully in individuals with CIDP, particularly in cases where phrenic nerve damage is present. By employing appropriate therapeutic interventions, the progression of respiratory dysfunction can be mitigated, and the prognosis for individuals with CIDP can be improved [125, 126].

Neuromuscular Junction-Related Disorders

The neuromuscular junction is a critical interface between the peripheral nerves and skeletal muscles, playing a crucial role in the transmission of signals that allow for voluntary muscle movement. Disorders affecting the neuromuscular junction can disrupt this essential communication, leading to various impairments, including respiratory dysfunction [127]. This chapter explores a range of neuromuscular junction-related disorders and their pathophysiology contributing to respiratory compromise.

Myasthenia Gravis

Myasthenia gravis (MG) is a neuromuscular junction-related disorder characterized by muscle weakness and fatigue, including the respiratory muscles. The commonly implicated proteins in the neuromuscular junction against which autoantibodies are produced, include the *nicotinic acetylcholine receptors (n-AChR's), muscle-specific kinase (MuSK),* and *lipoprotein-related protein 4 (LRP4).* Formation and maintenance of the neuromuscular junction is based upon the Agrin–LRP4–MuSK protein complex, including the distribution and clustering of the nicotinic AChR [128].

Although respiratory pathology is rare at presentation in myasthenia gravis, it is not uncommon throughout the course of disease, with an estimated 30% of these patients displaying respiratory symptoms [129]. More specifically, around 5–20% of patients with AChR-MG are reported to develop respiratory symptoms that require support with mechanical ventilation (myasthenic crisis) [130]. Moreover, MuSK-MG is reported to affect predominantly young adults and over 40% of these patients present with bulbar weakness, usually associated with respiratory involvement [131, 132]. To our knowledge, the mechanism by which the patients classified into different subgroups of MG (e.g., Ach-R MG compared to seronegative MG patients) present variable respiratory involvement is not known.

However, there are some common pathways that can explain respiratory involvement in the pathophysiology of myasthenia gravis. More specifically, in MG, the autoimmune response targets the nicotinic acetylcholine receptors at the neuromuscular junction, leading to impaired neuromuscular transmission. These receptors are responsible for binding the neurotransmitter acetylcholine and initiating an influx of ions responsible for the cascade of muscle contraction. The antibodies in myasthenia gravis bind to and block the nAChR or cause their internalization and degradation, reducing the density of functional receptors at the neuromuscular junction. The impaired neuromuscular transmission is characterized by compromised nerve impulse transmission from motor neurons to muscle fibers leading to reduced generation of muscle contractions [133]. When the target muscles are innervated primary and accessory phrenic nerves, the impaired signaling causes diaphragm and intercostal muscle weakness which clinically translates as dyspnea [134]. Respiratory failure resulting to myasthenia gravis crisis (MC) remains a significant concern and poses a substantial threat to the overall well-being of individuals with myasthenia gravis [135]. Moreover, phrenic nerve damage may occur in MG patients that undergo thymectomy as a complication of the surgery [95].

The combined effects of impaired neuromuscular transmission, reduced response of respiratory muscles to neural stimulation, and weakness in the phrenic and intercostal nerves contribute to respiratory dysfunction in myasthenia gravis. Patients may experience symptoms such as shortness of breath, and respiratory failure, particularly during episodes of increased muscle use or exacerbation of the autoimmune response [133, 136]. The management of myasthenia gravis involves treatment approaches aimed at improving neuromuscular transmission, such as medications to enhance acetylcholine availability or inhibit acetylcholinesterase. Immunosuppressive therapies may also be used to modulate the autoimmune response. In severe cases, respiratory support may be necessary to assist with breathing [137].

Lambert–Eaton Myasthenic Syndrome

Lambert–Eaton myasthenic syndrome (LEMS) is a neuromuscular junction-related disorder that can contribute to respiratory dysfunction [138]. It is characterized by muscle weakness, with a predilection for affecting proximal muscles, including the respiratory muscles [139]. LEMS can manifest either as a paraneoplastic syndrome connected to cancer (referred as cancer-associated LEMS) or as an autoimmune phenomenon in the absence of malignancy (referred as nontumor LEMS) [140]. Approximately, 50–60% of all LEMS cases are linked to a preexisting malignancy, specifically small-cell lung carcinoma (SCLC) [140]. Respiratory involvement occurs in about 16% of LEMS patients [141] and is usually mild with a restrictive functional pattern, but when complicated by COPD, respiratory failure can eventually occur [139]. Although respiratory failure is uncommon in LEMS, it can occasionally occur due to the administration of paralytic agents or coinciding pulmonary disorders [142]. Artificial ventilation was documented in up to 11% of LEMS cases [143]. In rare cases, respiratory failure is the presenting symptom of LEMS patients [144].

Lambert–Eaton myasthenic syndrome causes impairment of the NMJ that can lead to respiratory dysfunction of these patients through another pathophysiological mechanism than myasthenia gravis. It involves an autoimmune response during which the immune system produces antibodies that target the voltage-gated calcium channels (VGCCs) at the neuromuscular junction. More specifically, these antibodies bind to the VGCCs on the presynaptic membrane of motor neurons and interfere with the influx of calcium ions into the nerve terminal, leading to a reduced release of acetylcholine and impaired signaling from motor neurons to muscle fibers. The motor neurons that innervate the respiratory muscles, including the diaphragm and intercostal muscles, can be involved in the autoimmune response and the disrupted neural signaling causing respiratory muscle weakness [139]. When the damage at the NMJ is extensive, usually in later stages of the disease, this weakness can lead to compromised breathing [145].

It is important to note that Lambert–Eaton myasthenic syndrome , also known as "myasthenic syndrome," is often associated with muscle weakness that improves with muscle use or repetitive nerve stimulation [145]. This is in contrast to myasthenia gravis, where muscle weakness worsens with muscle use. However, respiratory involvement in LEMS can still lead to respiratory compromise and require appropriate management.

Treatment for LEMS typically involves addressing the underlying autoimmune disorder and managing the symptoms. This may include immunosuppressive therapies, plasmapheresis, symptomatic treatment with cholinesterase inhibitors to enhance acetylcholine availability, and occasionally intravenous immunoglobulin (IVIG) therapy [146]. Close monitoring and collaboration with healthcare professionals are essential to optimize respiratory function and overall management of LEMS.

Botulism

Botulism is a neuromuscular junction-related disorder that can contribute to respiratory dysfunction. It is caused by the presence of botulinum toxin, which inhibits the release of acetylcholine, the neurotransmitter responsible for transmitting signals from motor neurons to muscle fibers [147]. Botulism occurs when an individual ingests food contaminated with the botulinum toxin, which is produced by the bacterium *Clostridium botulinum.* The toxin can also be acquired through wounds or inhaled in rare cases. Patients with botulism commonly experience the involvement of cranial nerves, as well as muscles in the axial, limb, and respiratory regions [148].

Once internalized, the neurotoxin is delivered by the lymphatic and blood circulation to the nerve terminals where it specifically targets and affects the neuromuscular junction [148]. It acts by blocking the release of acetylcholine from the presynaptic nerve terminal. The botulinum toxin binds to and interferes with the proteins involved in the fusion of acetylcholine-containing vesicles with the presynaptic membrane. This prevents the release of acetylcholine into the synaptic cleft [148]. Through this mechanism, botulism affects the motor neurons that innervate the skeletal muscles, including the respiratory muscles. The reduced availability of acetylcholine impairs the transmission of signals from motor neurons to the respiratory muscles. The nerves involved in the mechanisms of respiratory dysfunction of botulism patients include those that innervate the intercostal muscles, the diaphragm, and other muscles responsible for breathing [149]. This weakness can lead to respiratory difficulties and compromised breathing [148, 150].

It is important to note that the severity of respiratory involvement in botulism can vary due to different inoculum sizes, host susceptibilities, and time to presentation [147]. In severe cases, respiratory paralysis may occur, requiring immediate medical intervention and respiratory support to ensure adequate oxygenation and ventilation in the affected individuals. A study reported a reduced mortality from 60% to approximately 3% [151–156], highlighting that prompt medical attention with timely administration of antitoxins and supportive care, particularly respiratory support, is crucial in botulism cases, and early intervention can improve outcomes [140].

From the above, we can appreciate that treatment options for botulism involve a combination of supportive care and administration of botulinum antitoxin. The antitoxin helps to neutralize any unbound botulinum toxin and prevent further damage. Respiratory support, such as mechanical ventilation or noninvasive ventilation, may be necessary to manage respiratory failure [147].

Myopathies

Myopathies are a group of disorders characterized by the dysfunction or damage to skeletal muscles. They can be broadly classified into two categories: the inherited myopathies and the acquired myopathies. Many myopathies, either inherited or acquired, can significantly contribute to respiratory dysfunction [157]. In general, the progressive muscle weakness and atrophy in these disorders impair the function of respiratory muscles, including the diaphragm and intercostal muscles. This compromises the ability to generate sufficient respiratory force and consequently breathing [158]. Moreover, in particular myopathies, kyphoscoliosis and chest wall deformities are present, which are associated with restrictive lung disease. Additionally, weakness of the laryngeal and pharyngeal muscles can further compromise airway clearance and predispose patients to pneumonia [159]. Understanding the impact of myopathies on respiratory function through the underlying pathophysiological mechanisms is crucial for early detection, appropriate management, and optimizing respiratory support in individuals affected by these disorders. In this chapter, we will discuss the main myopathies that impact respiratory dysfunction and the pathophysiological mechanism through which this occurs.

Muscular Dystrophies and Other Inherited Myopathies

Muscular dystrophies are a group of genetic disorders that primarily affect the muscles, including respiratory muscles. The most common muscular dystrophy is Duchenne muscular dystrophy (DMD). The disease mostly affects boys, typically presenting with progressive limb weakness, difficulty rising from a lying position, frequent falls. Around the age of 10–12, they experience respiratory muscle weakness, which progresses to respiratory failure and death in this population [160]. DMD is caused by mutations in the dystrophin gene, leading to the absence or deficiency of the dystrophin protein. The impairment of dystrophin results in increased susceptibility of muscle fibers to damage during muscle contraction [161]. As the disease progresses, muscle fibers are replaced by fibrotic and adipose tissue, leading to atrophy of muscles. The diaphragm that loses its contractile strength, and the intercostal muscles degenerate, leading to reduced expansion of the chest cavity [160]. This phenomenon further contributes to the inability to generate sufficient negative pressure during inhalation [160]. Moreover, individuals affected by myopathies like DMD might encounter reduced mobility and weakened axial muscles, contributing to the progression of scoliosis and lung collapse [161]. This condition tends to advance, especially during growth spurts, and can disrupt rib mechanics during respiration, potentially leading to decreased lung capacity [161]. According to studies, the administration of steroid therapy has demonstrated a correlation with a decreased incidence of scoliosis in certain cases of myopathies. Managing scoliosis and kyphosis in individuals with myopathies necessitates the implementation of physical therapy, orthotic devices, and, when required, surgical interventions to address severe curvature of the spine and sustain an improved quality of life [161].

More muscular dystrophies, such as Becker muscular dystrophy, facioscapulohumeral dystrophy (FSHD), limb–girdle muscular dystrophies (LGMD), and myotonic dystrophy, also contribute to respiratory dysfunction through similar mechanisms. Generally, progressive muscle weakness and atrophy affect the respiratory muscles, impairing their ability to support efficient breathing [158]. In Becker muscular dystrophy, there is a partial deficiency of dystrophin, resulting in a milder form of the disease compared to DMD. However, a significant but mild respiratory decline can still occur, leading to respiratory compromise [162]. In FSHD, respiratory complications due to diaphragm weakness or skeletal deformities like scoliosis are the most commonly reported. A study suggested that most of FSHD patients will develop a restrictive pattern of lung disease, with approximately 10–20% of individuals experiencing pulmonary complications [163]. In limb–girdle muscular dystrophy, respiratory muscles can also be affected and, as the disease progresses, insufficiency requiring noninvasive ventilation occurs in up to 20% of these patients depending on the type of LGMD [164]. Lastly, in myotonic dystrophy, a disorder mainly characterized by muscle stiffness and prolonged muscle contractions (myotonia), respiratory involvement has a complex etiology [165]. Apart from the respiratory muscle weakness and myotonia, patients also experience upper airway muscle dysfunction which frequently leads to obstructive sleep apnea and aspiration [159]. Moreover, there are indications for central respiratory dysregulation in these individuals, although this is still a subject of debate and consensus has yet to be reached [165]. Respiratory insufficiency is among the leading causes of death for these patients [166].

Other inherited myopathies that can result in respiratory compromise are hereditary myopathy with early respiratory failure (HMERF) and late onset Pompe disease (LOP). Regarding HMERF, the *TTN* gene (encoding the sarcomere protein titin) carries a mutation [167]. The disease is characterized by early diaphragmatic weakness that progresses over time, eventually leading to respiratory failure, making respiratory care a significant part of the management of these patients [168]. Similarly, most of late-onset Pompe disease patients, about 75% according to studies, also develop respiratory dysfunction during the course of the disease. The cause is a mutation in a gene encoding acid alpha glycosidase responsible for the breakdown of glycogen—especially at the muscle level. Respiratory failure is a major cause of death for these patients [169].

The progressive weakening of the respiratory muscles in inherited myopathies results in respiratory insufficiency manifesting as shortness of breath, decreased exercise tolerance, and an increased risk of respiratory infections [170]. In advanced stages, individuals may require ventilatory support, such as noninvasive ventilation or tracheostomy, to maintain sufficient ventilation and prevent respiratory failure [158].

Acquired Myopathies

Acquired myopathies are muscle disorders that can arise from various causes, including autoimmune diseases, infections, medications, metabolic abnormalities, and critical illness. The variability in etiologies reveals that they constitute a diverse group of muscle disorders, and they can lead to respiratory dysfunction by compromising the ability of the respiratory muscles to support efficient respiratory mechanics. Although these diseases are mostly associated with subclinical respiratory muscle dysfunction, the consequences can be severe. Since treatment options are available, it is particularly important for healthcare providers to monitor these changes [159].

Idiopathic inflammatory myopathies, such as immune-mediated necrotizing myopathy (IMNM) and antisynthetase syndrome, can cause the development of respiratory dysfunction. More specifically, IMNM is an autoimmune myopathy associated with certain medications (e.g., statins), antibodies (anti-HMGCR, anti-SRP), cancer, viral infections, and other connective tissue diseases [171]. It is believed that the immune system mistakenly targets and attacks muscle fibers, leading to phagocytosis, necrosis, and subsequent muscle damage [172, 173]. Although uncommon, respiratory muscles can be involved in IMNM patients. Up to 38% of SRP-positive IMNM patients develop interstitial lung disease visible on CT but with no apparent clinical symptoms [174]. On the contrary, antisynthetase syndrome (AS) is a condition highly associated with respiratory impairment as it mainly manifests as interstitial lung disease, myositis, and arthritis [175]. Patients with AS develop autoantibodies, and the severity of the disease is believed to be associated with the presence of these antibodies [176, 177]. Although the syndrome is rare, the prevalence of a respiratory component, which ranges between 67% and 100%, makes it an important component of the differential diagnosis of interstitial lung disease [177]. Individuals with idiopathic inflammatory myopathies, such as IMNM and AS, may experience shortness of breath and coughing [178]. Immunosuppressive agents and corticosteroids are usually required for the management of these diseases [179].

Dermatomyositis is another autoimmune myopathy characterized by muscle inflammation and skin involvement. The pathogenesis of dermatomyositis is not fully understood, but involves an autoimmune reaction targeting both muscle and skin tissues [180]. In dermatomyositis, the immune system attacks blood vessels, leading to vasculopathy and subsequent muscle and skin damage with inflammatory infiltrates consisting mostly of T lymphocytes and B lymphocytes [181]. Besides muscle weakness and inflammation, individuals with dermatomyositis may develop interstitial lung disease (ILD) [180]. ILD involves inflammation and fibrosis in the lung tissue, impairing lung function and gas exchange [182]. The exact mechanisms underlying the development of ILD in dermatomyositis are not fully understood, but immune-mediated processes such as antisynthetase antibodies [180], and microvascular abnormalities likely play a role. Respiratory involvement in dermatomyositis is reported from 10% to 45% of the patients [180] and can manifest as dyspnea, cough, and decreased exercise tolerance. The severity of respiratory dysfunction can vary, ranging from mild impairment to significant respiratory compromise requiring respiratory support [183].

Other acquired myopathies can also affect respiratory function. For example, critical illness myopathy is a common complication in individuals admitted to intensive care units for a prolonged period and presents with the highest frequency of respiratory involvement among all acquired myopathies [184, 185]. It is characterized by generalized muscle weakness and atrophy, primarily affecting the limb and respiratory muscles. The exact mechanisms are not fully understood, but factors such as systemic inflammation, metabolic derangements, immobilization, and corticosteroid use may contribute to muscle fiber dysfunction [185]. Another example is drug-induced myopathy caused as a side effect by certain medications, such as corticosteroids, statins, and certain antiretroviral drugs [186]. These medications may disrupt muscle cell metabolism, mitochondrial function, or induce direct toxic effects on muscle fibers [186]. Depending on the severity, drug-induced myopathies can lead to compromised respiratory function [186, 187]. One more example is viral myositis in which viral infections directly affect the muscles leading to weakness. Infections such as influenza, Coxsackievirus, and certain viral hepatitis strains have been associated with myositis, and in severe cases respiratory muscles can be affected [188]. Some individuals with COVID-19, caused by the SARS-CoV-2 virus, may also develop myositis [189]. Although respiratory muscle involvement in COVID-19 myositis is not as common as other forms of respiratory complications seen in severe COVID-19 cases, it can contribute to respiratory dysfunction in some patients [190]. Lastly, overlap myositis or myositis in the context of an underlying rheumatologic disease (systemic lupus erythematosus, scleroderma) can cause respiratory dysfunction due to respiratory muscle pathogenesis [191, 192].

References

1. West JB. Respiratory physiology: the essentials. Baltimore: Lippincott Williams & Wilkins; 2012.
2. Hall JE. Guyton and Hall textbook of medical physiology, Jordanian edition e-book. London: Elsevier Health Sciences; 2016.
3. Ramirez J-M, Richter DW. The neuronal mechanisms of respiratory rhythm generation. Curr Opin Neurobiol. 1996;6(6):817–25.
4. Feldman JL, Del Negro CA. Looking for inspiration: new perspectives on respiratory rhythm. Nat Rev Neurosci. 2006;7(3):232–41.
5. Guyenet PG, Bayliss DA. Neural control of breathing and CO_2 homeostasis. Neuron. 2015;87(5):946–61.
6. Sheel AW, Romer LM. Ventilation and respiratory mechanics. Compr Physiol. 2011;2(2):1093–142.
7. Moutlana H. Physiological control of respiration. South Afr J Anaesth Analg. 2020;26(6):S128–32.
8. Feather A, Randall D, Waterhouse M. Kumar and Clark's clinical medicine e-book. Elsevier Health Sciences; 2020.
9. Dempsey JA, Smith CA. Pathophysiology of human ventilatory control. Eur Respir J. 2014;44(2):495–512.
10. Nattie E. CO_2, brainstem chemoreceptors and breathing. Prog Neurobiol. 1999;59(4):299–331.
11. Smith JC, et al. Structural and functional architecture of respiratory networks in the mammalian brainstem. Philos Trans R Soc B Biol Sci. 2009;364(1529):2577–87.
12. Loewy AD, Spyer KM. Central regulation of autonomic functions. New York: Oxford University Press; 1990.
13. Lumb AB, Thomas CR. Nunn's applied respiratory physiology eBook. Elsevier Health Sciences; 2020.
14. Critchley HD. Neural mechanisms of autonomic, affective, and cognitive integration. J Comp Neurol. 2005;493(1):154–66.

15. Moreira TS, Mulkey DK. New advances in the neural control of breathing. J Physiol. 2015;593(Pt 5):1065.
16. von Leupoldt A, et al. The unpleasantness of perceived dyspnea is processed in the anterior insula and amygdala. Am J Respir Crit Care Med. 2008;177(9):1026–32.
17. Kumar V, Abbas AK, Aster JC. Robbins basic pathology e-book. Elsevier Health Sciences; 2017.
18. Del Negro CA, Wilson CG. Anatomy of the respiratory neural network. In: Control of breathing during sleep. CRC Press; 2022. p. 2–23.
19. Yackle K, et al. Breathing control center neurons that promote arousal in mice. Science. 2017;355(6332):1411–5.
20. Li P, et al. The peptidergic control circuit for sighing. Nature. 2016;530(7590):293–7.
21. Feldman JL, Del Negro CA, Gray PA. Understanding the rhythm of breathing: so near, yet so far. Annu Rev Physiol. 2013;75:423–52.
22. Watson K, et al. Respiratory muscle training in neuromuscular disease: a systematic review and meta-analysis. Eur Respir Rev. 2022;31(166):220065.
23. Graustein A, Carmona H, Benditt JO. Noninvasive respiratory assistance as aid for respiratory care in neuromuscular disorders. Front Rehabil Sci. 2023;4:1152043.
24. Racca F, et al. Practical approach to respiratory emergencies in neurological diseases. Neurol Sci. 2020;41:497–508.
25. Voulgaris A, et al. Respiratory involvement in patients with neuromuscular diseases: a narrative review. Pulm Med. 2019;2019:2734054.
26. Masrori P, Van Damme P. Amyotrophic lateral sclerosis: a clinical review. Eur J Neurol. 2020;27(10):1918–29.
27. Martinez NP, et al. How our amyotrophic lateral sclerosis patients die. Eur Respiratory Soc; 2020.
28. Pisa FE, Logroscino G, Battiston PG, Barbone F. Hospitalizations due to respiratory failure in patients with amyotrophic lateral sclerosis and their impact on survival: a population-based cohort study. BMC Pulm Med. 2016;16:136.
29. Sergew A, Wolfe L. Noninvasive ventilation, an issue of sleep medicine clinics, e-book, vol. 15. Elsevier Health Sciences; 2020.
30. Garegnani L, et al. Antioxidants to prevent respiratory decline in people with Duchenne muscular dystrophy and progressive respiratory decline. Cochrane Database Syst Rev. 2021;12(12):CD013720.
31. Prior TW, Leach ME, Finanger E. Spinal Muscular Atrophy. In: Literature Cited. University of Washington, Seattle, Seattle (WA); 1993. PMID: 20301526.
32. Fauroux B, et al. Respiratory management of children with spinal muscular atrophy (SMA). Arch Pédiatr. 2020;27(7):7S29–34.
33. Gilhus NE. Myasthenia gravis, respiratory function, and respiratory tract disease. J Neurol. 2023;270:1–12.
34. Deters D, Patel DI. Myasthenia gravis presentation and treatment variations: a case study approach. J Am Assoc Nurse Pract. 2019;31(5):319–23.
35. Farrugia ME, Goodfellow JA. A practical approach to managing patients with myasthenia gravis—opinions and a review of the literature. Front Neurol. 2020;11:604.
36. Hehir MK, Silvestri NJ. Generalized myasthenia gravis: classification, clinical presentation, natural history, and epidemiology. Neurol Clin. 2018;36(2):253–60.
37. Razi O, et al. Respiratory issues in patients with multiple sclerosis as a risk factor during SARS-CoV-2 infection: a potential role for exercise. Mol Cell Biochem. 2022;478(7):1533–59.
38. Rietberg MB, et al. Respiratory muscle training for multiple sclerosis. Cochrane Database Syst Rev. 2017;12(12):CD009424.
39. Hirst C, et al. Survival and cause of death in multiple sclerosis: a prospective population-based study. J Neurol Neurosurg Psychiatry. 2008;79(9):1016–21.
40. Garg M. Respiratory involvement in Guillain–Barre syndrome: the uncharted road to recovery. J Neurosci Rural Pract. 2017;8(03):325–6.

41. Willison HJ, Jacobs BC, van Doorn PA. Guillain-barre syndrome. Lancet. 2016;388(10045):717–27.
42. Rochester CL, Mohsenin V. Respiratory complications of stroke. In: Seminars in respiratory and critical care medicine. New York: Thieme Medical Publishers, Inc.; 2002.
43. Kumar S, Selim MH, Caplan LR. Medical complications after stroke. Lancet Neurol. 2010;9(1):105–18.
44. Robba C, et al. Mechanical ventilation in patients with acute ischaemic stroke: from pathophysiology to clinical practice. Crit Care. 2019;23:1–14.
45. Ackrivo J. Pulmonary care for ALS: progress, gaps, and paths forward. Muscle Nerve. 2023;67(5):341–53.
46. Jarius S, et al. Neuromyelitis optica. Nat Rev Dis Prim. 2020;6(1):85.
47. Jarius S, et al. MOG-IgG in NMO and related disorders: a multicenter study of 50 patients. Part 2: epidemiology, clinical presentation, radiological and laboratory features, treatment responses, and long-term outcome. J Neuroinflammation. 2016;13:1–45.
48. Zantah M, Coyle TB, Datta D. Acute respiratory failure due to neuromyelitis optica treated successfully with plasmapheresis. Case Rep Pulmonol. 2016;2016:1287690.
49. Nardone R, et al. Seronegative neuromyelitis optica presenting with life-threatening respiratory failure. J Spinal Cord Med. 2016;39(6):734–6.
50. Otake K, et al. Neuromyelitis optica with rapid respiratory failure: a case report. Acute Med Surg. 2021;8(1):e655.
51. Bennji S, et al. Neuromyelitis optica with unilateral diaphragmatic paralysis. Case Rep. 2018;2018:bcr-2018-225984.
52. Mutluay F, Gürses H, Saip S. Effects of multiple sclerosis on respiratory functions. Clin Rehabil. 2005;19(4):426–32.
53. Gosselink R, Kovacs L, Decramer M. Respiratory muscle involvement in multiple sclerosis. Eur Respir J. 1999;13(2):449–54.
54. Tzelepis GE, McCool FD. Respiratory dysfunction in multiple sclerosis. Respir Med. 2015;109(6):671–9.
55. Campbell G, Mahad DJ. Mitochondrial dysfunction and axon degeneration in progressive multiple sclerosis. FEBS Lett. 2018;592(7):1113–21.
56. De Stefano N, et al. Evidence of axonal damage in the early stages of multiple sclerosis and its relevance to disability. Arch Neurol. 2001;58(1):65–70.
57. Su KG, et al. Axonal degeneration in multiple sclerosis: the mitochondrial hypothesis. Curr Neurol Neurosci Rep. 2009;9(5):411–7.
58. Tomassini V, et al. Neuroplasticity and functional recovery in multiple sclerosis. Nat Rev Neurol. 2012;8(11):635–46.
59. Flachenecker P. Clinical implications of neuroplasticity—the role of rehabilitation in multiple sclerosis. Front Neurol. 2015;6:36.
60. Ilkhomovna KM, Eriyigitovich IS, Kadyrovich KN. Morphological features of microvascular tissue of the brain at hemorrhagic stroke. Am J Med Sci Pharm Res. 2020;2(10):53–9.
61. Barnett HM, Davis AP, Khot SP. Stroke and breathing. In: Handbook of clinical neurology. Elsevier; 2022. p. 201–22.
62. Hermann DM, et al. Central periodic breathing during sleep in acute ischemic stroke. Stroke. 2007;38(3):1082–4.
63. De Carvalho M, Swash M, Pinto S. Diaphragmatic neurophysiology and respiratory markers in ALS. Front Neurol. 2019;10:143.
64. López-Pingarrón L, et al. Role of oxidative stress on the etiology and pathophysiology of amyotrophic lateral sclerosis (ALS) and its relation with the enteric nervous system. Curr Issues Mol Biol. 2023;45(4):3315–32.
65. Hardiman O. Management of respiratory symptoms in ALS. J Neurol. 2011;258(3):359–65.
66. Naumann JP. Amyotrophic lateral sclerosis, the primary motor neuron disease. Downtown Rev. 2015;1(2):5.

67. Maramattom BV, Wijdicks EF. Neurology of pulmonology and acidbase disturbance. In: Neurology and clinical neuroscience. Elsevier; 2007. p. 1569–76.
68. Singh D, et al. Assessment of respiratory functions by spirometry and phrenic nerve studies in patients of amyotrophic lateral sclerosis. J Neurol Sci. 2011;306(1–2):76–81.
69. Singh TD, Wijdicks EF. Neuromuscular respiratory failure. Neurol Clin. 2021;39(2):333–53.
70. Niedermeyer S, Murn M, Choi PJ. Respiratory failure in amyotrophic lateral sclerosis. Chest. 2019;155(2):401–8.
71. Kolb SJ, Kissel JT. Spinal muscular atrophy. Neurol Clin. 2015;33(4):831–46.
72. Veldhoen ES, et al. Natural history of respiratory muscle strength in spinal muscular atrophy. Respiratory morbidity in neuromuscular diseases, with focus on spinal muscular atrophy. 2022;17:51.
73. Wijesekera LC, Nigel Leigh P. Amyotrophic lateral sclerosis. Orphanet J Rare Dis. 2009;4:1–22.
74. Gouveia RG, et al. Evidence for central abnormality in respiratory control in primary lateral sclerosis. Amyotroph Lateral Scler. 2006;7(1):57–60.
75. Almeida V, et al. Primary lateral sclerosis: predicting functional outcome. Amyotroph Lateral Scler Frontotemporal Degener. 2013;14(2):141–5.
76. Servera E, Mari J, Sancho J. Neuromuscular disease. Upper motor neuron. In: Encyclopedia of respiratory medicine. Academic Press; 2006. p. 118–124.
77. Racaniello VR. One hundred years of poliovirus pathogenesis. Virology. 2006;344(1):9–16.
78. Hirani S, Spinner D. Post-polio syndrome. Pain: a review guide; 2019. p. 1231–3.
79. Trojan DA, Cashman NR. Post-poliomyelitis syndrome. Muscle Nerve. 2005;31(1):6–19.
80. Punsoni M, et al. Post-polio syndrome revisited. Neurol Int. 2023;15(2):569–79.
81. Craighead JE. Enteroviruses. Pathology and pathogenesis of human viral disease. 2000. Chapter 1. p. 1–28.
82. Banneheka S. Morphological study of the ansa cervicalis and the phrenic nerve. Anat Sci Int. 2008;83:31–44.
83. Graves MJ, et al. Origin and prevalence of the accessory phrenic nerve: a meta-analysis and clinical appraisal. Clin Anat. 2017;30(8):1077–82.
84. Fahad EM, Hashm ZM, Nema IM. Cervical spinal stenosis and risk of pulmonary dysfunction. Int J Crit Illn Inj Sci. 2020;10(1):16.
85. Mandoorah, S. and T. Mead, Phrenic nerve injury. 2018.
86. Kaufman MR, Bauer T, Brown D. Surgical treatment of phrenic nerve injury. UpToDate. Waltham, MA; 2019.
87. Kaufman MR, Ferro N, Paulin E. Phrenic nerve paralysis and phrenic nerve reconstruction surgery. In: Handbook of clinical neurology. Elsevier; 2022. p. 271–92.
88. Kaufman MR, et al. Phrenic nerve reconstruction for effective surgical treatment of diaphragmatic paralysis. Ann Plast Surg. 2021;87(3):310–5.
89. Al-Thani H, et al. Descriptive analysis of right and left-sided traumatic diaphragmatic injuries; case series from a single institution. Bull Emerg Trauma. 2018;6(1):16.
90. Ulkü R, et al. Phrenic nerve injury after blunt trauma. Int Surg. 2005;90(2):93–5.
91. Nhan NH, et al. Blunt traumatic left atrial appendage rupture and cardiac herniation. Asian Cardiovasc Thorac Ann. 2014;22(5):598–600.
92. Whiteley J, Shoeib M, Bilancia R. Iatrogenic phrenic nerve palsy. Shanghai Chest. 2021;5:27.
93. Koogler A, Kushelev M. Review of persistent phrenic nerve palsy. Int J Neurorehabil. 2018;5(319):2376-0281.1000319.
94. Kaufman MR, Bauer TL, Brown DP. Surgical treatment of phrenic nerve injury. Waltham, MA: Up To Date. 2018.
95. Howard RS. Respiratory failure because of neuromuscular disease. Curr Opin Neurol. 2016;29(5):592–601.
96. Avila EK, Goenka A, Fontenla S. Bilateral phrenic nerve dysfunction: a late complication of mantle radiation. J Neuro-Oncol. 2011;103:393–5.

97. Stubblefield MD. Radiation fibrosis syndrome: neuromuscular and musculoskeletal complications in cancer survivors. PM&R. 2011;3(11):1041–54.
98. Pham HH, Newman N, Osmundson EC. Radiation-induced peripheral neuropathy after thoracic stereotactic ablative radiotherapy: case report. JTO Clin Res Rep. 2022;3(8):100370.
99. Reed JC. Chapter 6—Elevated diaphragm. In: Chest radiology. 7th ed. Elsevier; 2019. p. 63–70.
100. Schoeller T, et al. Successful immediate phrenic nerve reconstruction during mediastinal tumor resection. J Thorac Cardiovasc Surg. 2001;122(6):1235–7.
101. Bernhardt EB, Jalal SI. Small cell lung cancer. Cancer treatment and research; vol 170. Springer, Cham. 2016. p. 301–22.
102. Akhurst T. Staging of non-small-cell lung cancer. PET Clin. 2018;13(1):1–10.
103. Quint LE. Thoracic complications and emergencies in oncologic patients. Cancer Imaging. 2009;9(Special issue A):S75.
104. Yamashita T, Watahiki M, Asai K. Mediastinal metastasis of breast cancer mimicking a primary mediastinal tumor. Am J Case Rep. 2020;21:e925275-1.
105. Prabhakar S, Dhatt S, Hooda A. Examination of the peripheral nervous system. Handbook of clinical examination in orthopedics: an illustrated guide. Springer, Singapore. 2019. p. 5–25.
106. Yekzaman BR, et al. Phrenic nerve dysfunction secondary to cervical neuroforaminal stenosis: a literature review. World Neurosurg. 2022;167:74.
107. Franko OI, Khalpey Z, Gates J. Brachial plexus trauma: the morbidity of hemidiaphragmatic paralysis. Emerg Med J. 2008;25(9):614–5.
108. Crowe CS, et al. The diagnostic utility of inspiratory-expiratory radiography for the assessment of phrenic nerve palsy associated with brachial plexus injury. Acta Neurochir. 2023;165:1–8.
109. Rubin DI. Brachial and lumbosacral plexopathies: a review. Clin Neurophysiol Pract. 2020;5:173–93.
110. Papri N, et al. Guillain–Barré syndrome in low-income and middle-income countries: challenges and prospects. Nat Rev Neurol. 2021;17(5):285–96.
111. Orlikowski D, et al. Respiratory dysfunction in Guillain-Barré syndrome. Neurocrit Care. 2004;1:415–22.
112. Zifko U, et al. Respiratory electrophysiological studies in Guillain-Barre syndrome. J Neurol Neurosurg Psychiatry. 1996;60(2):191–4.
113. Naresh K, et al. Sensitivity and specificity of phrenic nerve electrophysiology to predict mechanical ventilation in the Guillain-Barré syndrome. Muscle Nerve. 2023;68(2):191–7.
114. Ajith M. Utility of multiple segment stimulation and serial nerve conduction studies in Guillain Barre Syndrome. Vellore: Christian Medical College; 2011.
115. Shiva Kumar R. Phrenic nerve conduction in Guillian Barre syndrome. 2008.
116. van den Berg B, et al. Mortality in guillain-Barre syndrome. Neurology. 2013;80(18):1650–4.
117. Reynolds J, George Sachs M, Stavros K. Chronic inflammatory demyelinating polyradiculoneuropathy (CIDP): clinical features, diagnosis, and current treatment strategies. R I Med J. 2016;99(12):32.
118. Cocito D, et al. Subclinical electrophysiological alterations of phrenic nerve in chronic inflammatory demyelinating polyneuropathy. J Neurol. 2005;252:916–20.
119. Sen BK, Pandit A. Phrenic nerve conduction study in the early stage of Guillain–Barre syndrome as a predictor of respiratory failure. Ann Indian Acad Neurol. 2018;21(1):57.
120. Tataroglu C, Ozkul A, Sair A. Chronic inflammatory demyelinating polyneuropathy and respiratory failure due to phrenic nerve involvement. J Clin Neuromuscul Dis. 2010;12(1):42–6.
121. Ripellino P, et al. Bilateral phrenic neuropathy responsive to intravenous immunoglobulin treatment. Clin Transl Neurosci. 2019;3(2):2514183X19891606.
122. Haji K, Butler E, Royse C. A case of chronic inflammatory demyelinating polyneuropathy with reversible alternating diaphragmatic paralysis: case study. Crit Ultrasound J. 2015;7(1):1–3.

123. Vallat J-M, Sommer C, Magy L. Chronic inflammatory demyelinating polyradiculoneuropathy: diagnostic and therapeutic challenges for a treatable condition. Lancet Neurol. 2010;9(4):402–12.
124. Stojkovic T, et al. Phrenic nerve palsy as a feature of chronic inflammatory demyelinating polyradiculoneuropathy. Muscle Nerve. 2003;27(4):497–9.
125. Jha S, et al. Unusual features in chronic inflammatory demyelinating polyneuropathy: good outcome after prolonged ventilatory support. J Neurosci Rural Pract. 2011;2(02):171–3.
126. Ridenour L, et al. CIDP: a rare but treatable cause of respiratory failure. In: D79. SRN: curious cases in sleep and respiratory medicine. American Thoracic Society; 2020. p. A7622.
127. Iyer SR, Shah SB, Lovering RM. The neuromuscular junction: roles in aging and neuromuscular disease. Int J Mol Sci. 2021;22(15):8058.
128. Beloor Suresh A. Myasthenia gravis. Treasure Island, FL: StatPearls Publishing LLC; 2022.
129. Katzberg HD, et al. Respiratory dysfunction and sleep-disordered breathing in children with myasthenia gravis. J Child Neurol. 2020;35(9):600–6.
130. Dresser L, et al. Myasthenia gravis: epidemiology, pathophysiology and clinical manifestations. J Clin Med. 2021;10(11):2235.
131. Sanders DB, et al. Clinical aspects of MuSK antibody positive seronegative MG. Neurology. 2003;60(12):1978–80.
132. Pasnoor M, et al. Clinical findings in MuSK-antibody positive myasthenia gravis: a US experience. Muscle Nerve. 2010;41(3):370–4.
133. Binu A, et al. Pathophysiological basis in the management of myasthenia gravis: a mini review. Inflammopharmacology. 2022;30(1):61–71.
134. Benditt JO. Pathophysiology of neuromuscular respiratory diseases. Clin Chest Med. 2018;39(2):297–308.
135. Huang X, et al. The systemic inflammation markers as possible indices for predicting respiratory failure and outcome in patients with myasthenia gravis. Ann Clin Transl Neurol. 2023;10(1):98–110.
136. Gilhus NE, et al. Myasthenia gravis and infectious disease. J Neurol. 2018;265:1251–8.
137. Peragallo JH. Pediatric myasthenia gravis. Semin Pediatr Neurol. 2017;24:116.
138. Matsumoto H, Ugawa Y. Lambert-Eaton myasthenic syndrome: a review. J Gen Fam Med. 2016;17(2):138–43.
139. Harper CM, Lennon VA. Lambert-Eaton syndrome. In: Myasthenia gravis and related disorders; Current Clinical Neurology. Humana Press, Cham. 2018. p. 221–37.
140. Raja SM. Lambert-Eaton myasthenic syndrome and botulism. Continuum. 2022;28(6):1596–614.
141. Wirtz PW, et al. Differences in clinical features between the Lambert-Eaton myasthenic syndrome with and without cancer: an analysis of 227 published cases. Clin Neurol Neurosurg. 2002;104(4):359–63.
142. Smith AG. Acute ventilatory failure in Lambert-Eaton myasthenic syndrome and its response to 3, 4-diaminopyridine. Neurology. 1996;46(4):1143–5.
143. Kesner VG, et al. Lambert-Eaton myasthenic syndrome. Neurol Clin. 2018;36(2):379–94.
144. William C, et al. Primary respiratory failure as the presenting symptom in Lambert–Eaton myasthenic syndrome. Muscle Nerve. 1993;16(7):712–5.
145. Jayarangaiah A, Kariyanna T. Lambert Eaton myasthenic syndrome. 2018.
146. Bodkin C, Pascuzzi RM. Update in the management of myasthenia gravis and Lambert-Eaton myasthenic syndrome. Neurol Clin. 2021;39(1):133–46.
147. Jeffery IA, Karim S. Botulism. In StatPearls. 2017. StatPearls Publishing.
148. Pirazzini M, Montecucco C, Rossetto O. Toxicology and pharmacology of botulinum and tetanus neurotoxins: an update. Arch Toxicol. 2022;96(6):1521–39.
149. Sobel J. Botulism. Clin Infect Dis. 2005;41(8):1167–73.
150. Popoff MR, Mazuet C, Poulain B. Botulism and tetanus. In: Rosenberg E, et al., editors. The prokaryotes: human microbiology. Berlin: Springer; 2013. p. 247–90.

151. Kiyokawa M, Haning W. A case report of wound botulism—rare disease on the rise with the opioid crisis. Hawaii J Health Soc Welf. 2021;80(4):88.
152. Moron H, et al. Contribution of single-fiber evaluation on monitoring outcomes following injection of botulinum toxin-a: a narrative review of the literature. Toxins. 2021;13(5):356.
153. Yu PA, et al. Safety and improved clinical outcomes in patients treated with new equine-derived heptavalent botulinum antitoxin. Clin Infect Dis. 2018;66(Suppl_1):S57–64.
154. Sobel J, Rao AK. Making the best of the evidence: toward national clinical guidelines for botulism. Clin Infect Dis. 2018;66(Suppl_1):S1–3.
155. Jackson KA, et al. Botulism mortality in the USA, 1975-2009. Botulinum J. 2015;3(1):6–17.
156. Shapiro RL, Hatheway C, Swerdlow DL. Botulism in the United States: a clinical and epidemiologic review. Ann Intern Med. 1998;129(3):221–8.
157. Nagy H, Veerapaneni KD. Myopathy. In: StatPearls. Treasure Island, FL: StatPearls Publishing; 2022.
158. Shahrizaila N, Kinnear W, Wills A. Respiratory involvement in inherited primary muscle conditions. J Neurol Neurosurg Psychiatry. 2006;77(10):1108–15.
159. Pfeffer G, et al. Diagnosis of muscle diseases presenting with early respiratory failure. J Neurol. 2015;262:1101–14.
160. Mhandire DZ, et al. Breathing in Duchenne muscular dystrophy: translation to therapy. J Physiol. 2022;600(15):3465–82.
161. Domingos J, et al. Dystrophinopathies and limb-girdle muscular dystrophies. Neuropediatrics. 2017;48(04):262–72.
162. De Wel B, et al. Respiratory decline in adult patients with Becker muscular dystrophy: a longitudinal study. Neuromuscul Disord. 2021;31(3):174–82.
163. Hazenberg A, et al. Facioscapulohumeral muscular dystrophy and respiratory failure; what about the diaphragm? Respir Med Case Rep. 2015;14:37–9.
164. Bockhorst J, Wicklund M. Limb girdle muscular dystrophies. Neurol Clin. 2020;38(3):493–504.
165. Hawkins A, et al. Respiratory dysfunction in myotonic dystrophy type 1: a systematic review. Neuromuscul Disord. 2019;29(3):198–212.
166. Henke C, et al. Characteristics of respiratory muscle involvement in myotonic dystrophy type 1. Neuromuscul Disord. 2020;30(1):17–27.
167. Pfeffer G, Chinnery PF. Hereditary myopathy with early respiratory failure synonyms: HMERF, MFM-titinopathy, myofibrillar myopathy with early respiratory failure. 2024.
168. Petrovic M, et al. Hereditary myopathy with early respiratory failure: case report. Egypt J Neurol Psychiatry Neurosurg. 2023;59(1):36.
169. Sixel BS, et al. Respiratory manifestations in late-onset Pompe disease: a case series conducted in Brazil. J Bras Pneumol. 2017;43:54–9.
170. Cardamone M, Darras BT, Ryan MM. Inherited myopathies and muscular dystrophies. Semin Neurol. 2008;28(2):250–9.
171. Khan NAJ, et al. Necrotizing autoimmune myopathy: a rare variant of idiopathic inflammatory myopathies. J Investig Med High Impact Case Rep. 2017;5(2):2324709617709031.
172. DeRon NG, et al. Immune-mediated necrotizing myopathy manifesting after five years of statin therapy. Case Rep Rheumatol. 2023;2023:1178035.
173. Sehgal R, et al. Immune mediated necrotizing myopathy: a cause of isolated myopathy of neck extensor muscle. Clin Med Res. 2016;14(3–4):145–50.
174. Allenbach Y, et al. Immune-mediated necrotizing myopathy: clinical features and pathogenesis. Nat Rev Rheumatol. 2020;16(12):689–701.
175. Korsten P, et al. Antisynthetase syndrome-associated interstitial lung disease: monitoring of immunosuppressive treatment effects by chest computed tomography. Front Med. 2021;7:609595.
176. Johnson C, et al. Clinical and pathologic differences in interstitial lung disease based on antisynthetase antibody type. Respir Med. 2014;108(10):1542–8.

177. Gasparotto M, et al. Pulmonary involvement in antisynthetase syndrome. Curr Opin Rheumatol. 2019;31(6):603–10.
178. Lee C-S, et al. Idiopathic inflammatory myopathy with diffuse alveolar damage. Clin Rheumatol. 2002;21:391–6.
179. Lundberg IE, et al. Idiopathic inflammatory myopathies. Nat Rev Dis Prim. 2021;7(1):86.
180. Bogdanov I, et al. Dermatomyositis: current concepts. Clin Dermatol. 2018;36(4):450–8.
181. Thompson C, Piguet V, Choy E. The pathogenesis of dermatomyositis. Br J Dermatol. 2018;179(6):1256–62.
182. Berend N. Respiratory disease and respiratory physiology: putting lung function into perspective interstitial lung disease. Respirology. 2014;19(7):952–9.
183. Ravi D, Prabhu S. Dermatomyositis: a dermatological perspective. Clin Dermatol Rev. 2019;3(1):18–22.
184. Latronico N, Peli E, Botteri M. Critical illness myopathy and neuropathy. Curr Opin Crit Care. 2005;11(2):126–32.
185. Cheung K, et al. Pathophysiology and management of critical illness polyneuropathy and myopathy. J Appl Physiol. 2021;130(5):1479–89.
186. Jain KK, Jain KK. Drug-induced myopathies. In: Drug-induced neurological disorders; Springer, Cham. 2021. p. 493–509.
187. Manoj M, et al. Drug-induced myopathy. Indian J Rheumatol. 2019;14(Suppl 1):S27–36.
188. Finsterer J, et al. Secondary myopathy due to systemic diseases. Acta Neurol Scand. 2016;134(6):388–402.
189. Kumar D, et al. Neurological manifestation of SARS-CoV-2 induced inflammation and possible therapeutic strategies against COVID-19. Mol Neurobiol. 2021;58(7):3417–34.
190. Paliwal VK, et al. Neuromuscular presentations in patients with COVID-19. Neurol Sci. 2020;41:3039–56.
191. Di Bartolomeo S, Alunno A, Carubbi F. Respiratory manifestations in systemic lupus erythematosus. Pharmaceuticals. 2021;14(3):276.
192. Popescu NA, et al. Respiratory failure in a rare case of juvenile dermatomyositis–systemic scleroderma overlap syndrome. Maedica. 2020;15(3):394.
193. Torsney K, Forsyth D. Respiratory dysfunction in Parkinson's disease. J R Coll Physicians Edinb. 2017;47(1):35–9.
194. Docu Axelerad A, et al. Respiratory dysfunctions in Parkinson's disease patients. Brain Sci. 2021;11(5):595.
195. Aravindan A, et al. Challenges in anesthesia in Wilson's disease: a systematic review of the existing literature. Cureus. 2023;15(1):e33334.
196. Mahajan O, et al. Rapid and slow, twist and turn wing beating: think of Wilson's disease. Int J Nutr Pharmacol Neurol Dis. 2023;13(1):77–9.
197. Crone NE, Jinnah H, Reich SG. Wilson's disease presenting with an unusual cough. Mov Disord. 2005;20(7):891–3.
198. Shribman S, Warner TT, Dooley JS. Clinical presentations of Wilson disease. Ann Transl Med. 2019;7(Suppl 2):S60.
199. Sriranjini S, et al. Subclinical pulmonary dysfunction in spinocerebellar ataxias 1, 2 and 3. Acta Neurol Scand. 2010;122(5):323–8.
200. Biswas DD, et al. Neuro-respiratory pathology in spinocerebellar ataxia: a review. J Neurol Sci. 2022;443:120493.
201. Daulatzai MA. Pathogenesis of cognitive dysfunction in patients with obstructive sleep apnea: a hypothesis with emphasis on the nucleus tractus solitarius. Sleep Disord. 2012;2012:251096.
202. Eckert DJ, et al. Central sleep apnea: pathophysiology and treatment. Chest. 2007;131(2):595–607.
203. Yang Q, et al. Intermittent hypoxia from obstructive sleep apnea may cause neuronal impairment and dysfunction in central nervous system: the potential roles played by microglia. Neuropsychiatr Dis Treat. 2013;9:1077–86.

204. Aihara K, et al. Measurement of dyspnea in patients with obstructive sleep apnea. Sleep Breath. 2013;17:753–61.
205. Kanth K, Park K, Seyal M. Severity of peri-ictal respiratory dysfunction with epilepsy duration and patient age at epilepsy onset. Front Neurol. 2020;11:618841.
206. Barot N, Nei M. Autonomic aspects of sudden unexpected death in epilepsy (SUDEP). Clin Auton Res. 2019;29:151–60.
207. Seyal M, et al. Respiratory changes with seizures in localization-related epilepsy: analysis of periictal hypercapnia and airflow patterns. Epilepsia. 2010;51(8):1359–64.
208. Tang EW, et al. Respiratory failure secondary to diabetic neuropathy affecting the phrenic nerve. Diabet Med. 2003;20(7):599–601.
209. Brannagan TH, et al. Proximal diabetic neuropathy presenting with respiratory weakness. J Neurol Neurosurg Psychiatry. 1999;67(4):539–41.
210. Burakgazi AZ, Höke A. Respiratory muscle weakness in peripheral neuropathies. J Peripher Nerv Syst. 2010;15(4):307–13.
211. Da Costa R, et al. Bilateral phrenic nerve palsy in a diabetic causing respiratory failure. Indian J Crit Care Med. 2018;22(10):737.
212. Spiesshoefer J, et al. Phrenic nerve involvement and respiratory muscle weakness in patients with Charcot-Marie-Tooth disease 1A. J Peripher Nerv Syst. 2019;24(3):283–93.
213. Junior WM, et al. Respiratory dysfunction in Charcot–Marie–Tooth disease type 1A. J Neurol. 2015;262:1164–71.

Chapter 2
Assessing Respiratory Function in the Patient with Neuromuscular Disease

Jose Victor Jimenez and Philip J. Choi

Introduction

The assessment of respiratory function in the patient with neuromuscular disease can be challenging for even seasoned clinicians, particularly in the presence of symptoms prior to a formal diagnosis. Clinicians must understand the common clinical presentations of patients with neuromuscular disease, effectively obtain a complete history and perform a detailed physical examination, as well as understand the available testing to adequately assess and monitor respiratory function in patients with neuromuscular diseases. The following chapter will provide a framework for clinicians to perform a comprehensive assessment of patients with diagnosed or suspected neuromuscular conditions.

Physiology of Respiratory Pump Failure

Respiratory failure is a frequent complication of all forms of neuromuscular disease and a leading cause of death [1]. The concept of respiratory pump failure describes the limited ability of the respiratory musculature (primarily the diaphragm and intercostal muscles) to generate a pressure gradient between the atmosphere and the thoracic cavity and mobilize air in and out the lungs. The respiratory pump fails

J. V. Jimenez
Department of Internal Medicine, Yale New Haven Hospital, New Haven, CT, USA
e-mail: josevictor.jimenezceja@yale.edu

P. J. Choi (✉)
Division of Pulmonary and Critical Care Medicine, NYU Langone Health,
New York, NY, USA
e-mail: philip.choi@nyulangone.org

N. Lechtzin (ed.), *Pulmonary Complications of Neuromuscular Disease*,
Respiratory Medicine, https://doi.org/10.1007/978-3-031-65335-3_2

when there is an increase in the workload (obesity, decreased chest, or lung compliance), a decrease in the contractile force against the workload (decreased central drive, impaired neural transmission to the respiratory muscles, or primary muscle weakness), or a mixture of both. Inspiratory pump failure (diaphragmatic weakness) leads to diminished power to generate pressure gradients to produce adequate airflow with each muscle contraction. Consequently, there is a decrease in vital capacity, total lung capacity, and functional residual capacity (particularly when lying flat). These changes may eventually lead to alveolar hypoventilation, impaired gas exchange, and carbon dioxide (CO_2) accumulation. In patients with an intact respiratory center, the normal physiological response to hypercapnia will be an increase in minute ventilation. However, with a weak inspiratory pump, incapable of generating significant intrathoracic pressure gradients, the increase in minute ventilation will be predominantly driven by respiratory rate as opposed to tidal volume, leading to increased dead space ventilation. The ultimate consequence will be persistent hypercapnia and higher risk of acute decompensations. The timing and clinical course of these events will be dependent on the etiology of the pump failure and the interventions, including noninvasive ventilation, applied throughout the natural history of the disease [2]. Although the concept of pump failure focuses on respiratory muscles such as the diaphragm and intercostal muscles, patients with neuromuscular diseases may present with involvement of other muscle groups that can also contribute to hypoventilation. Involvement of upper airway muscles can produce oropharyngeal dysphagia and aspiration, leading to chronic parenchymal abnormalities, recurrent infections, and bronchiectasis. In addition, upper airway collapse, particularly during sleep, can lead to obstructive sleep apnea that may worsen hypoventilation related to respiratory muscle weakness. Similarly, involvement of expiratory muscles (in conjunction with upper airway and diaphragmatic dysfunction) impairs the efficiency of cough. Throughout this chapter, we will review the clinical manifestations of respiratory failure in patients with neuromuscular disease and tools available to diagnose, assess, and follow-up patients throughout the course of their disease.

Clinical Manifestations of Neuromuscular Respiratory Failure

Dyspnea and Respiratory Muscle Weakness

In neuromuscular disorders, dyspnea is thought to result from an input-output mismatch. Reduced tidal volumes secondary to muscular weakness are sensed by mechanoreceptors in the pulmonary parenchyma, leading to an increased central respiratory effort to increase ventilation. The impaired muscular output cannot match the signal. Therefore, feedback from the sensory receptors does not match the intended effort, leading to dyspnea [3]. Due to the reduced physical mobility of patients with neuromuscular disorders, dyspnea is often a late presenting symptom.

Therefore, an appropriate clinical history is of utmost importance. An early symptom of respiratory muscle weakness is frequently orthopnea. Weakness may be unmasked when lying flat or during water immersion [4], as when the abdominal cavity is displaced, the diaphragm cannot overcome the increased load. As general weakness progresses, simply inquiring about dyspnea as a general symptom may be inadequate. Understanding perceived symptoms based on level of activity can help clinicians understand the patient's respiratory reserve. Transfers in and out of a bed or wheelchair may elicit symptoms for patients with limited ambulation, while patients with severe respiratory muscle dysfunction may become short of breath with talking or eating. On physical examination, accessory muscle use may be evident when sitting upright or during forced exhalation. Patients with preserved diaphragmatic function but intercostal muscle weakness develop bell-chest deformity and chest paradox, a classic pattern in children with spinal muscular atrophy.

As neuromuscular weakness progresses, dyspnea becomes a major determinant of quality of life and the driver of psychiatric comorbidities, such as anxiety and depression. In neuromuscular disorders, dyspnea is often underestimated as it lacks correlation with pulmonary function tests (PFTs) and gas exchange alterations [5, 6]. Nonetheless, treating dyspnea, regardless of objective signs of respiratory dysfunction, is associated with improved quality of life [7, 8] and is the main consideration for NIV initiation in Europe [9]. Therefore, assessing breathlessness is a key component during history taking in all neuromuscular patients.

While many patients with neuromuscular disorders develop dyspnea due to respiratory pump failure, clinicians must also recognize that many conditions are multisystem in nature and should consider a broad differential diagnosis initially and with unexpected clinical changes. Respiratory muscle weakness can coexist with interstitial lung disease (particularly in inflammatory myopathies), heart failure (a hallmark of muscular dystrophy), intrathoracic masses (thymoma in patients with myasthenia gravis), pulmonary arterial hypertension (particularly group III in long-standing disease), and restrictive thoracic cage abnormalities. In addition, pulmonary embolism should be considered in cases of acute dyspnea that may be related to prolonged immobility. A thorough examination and history taking are essential for diagnostic accuracy.

Sleep Disturbances

Nocturnal hypoventilation might be the presenting feature of respiratory dysfunction in patients with neuromuscular disorders. It usually presents with daytime somnolence, morning headaches, fatigue, and cognitive impairment. Snoring and witnessed apneas may be reported by patient's family. Atypical symptoms such as nocturia and nocturnal cramps are frequently reported [10].

In patients with neuromuscular disorders, nocturnal hypoventilation may occur due to diaphragmatic weakness (diaphragmatic/pseudo-central sleep disorder breathing) [11], a decrease in the ventilatory response to hypercapnia, obstructive sleep apnea (either due to pharyngeal muscle weakness, pharyngeal neuropathy, or bulbar palsy) [12], or central hypoventilation (e.g., in patients with muscular dystrophy and cardiomyopathy) [13].

Bulbar Signs and Symptoms

Bulbar dysfunction refers to the motor unit involvement of the cranial nerves (either the nuclei, nerve, neuromuscular junction, or the muscle itself) localized to the hindbrain (glossopharyngeal, vagus, accessory, or hypoglossal nerve) and is typically manifested by dysphagia, dysarthria, nasal speech, drooling, impaired cough reflex, and airway collapse during inspiration [14]. Speech impairment results from the flaccid or spastic paresis of the oropharyngeal musculature and is clinically manifested as changes in voice tone (especially nasal speech), slurring, inappropriate pauses (especially in long phrases), and changes in pitch (either too low in flaccid paralysis or too high in spastic) [15]. Involvement of the oropharyngeal musculature in neuromuscular disorders has important implications for the pulmonologist as it can bias the interpretation of pulmonary function tests due to inadequate seal and upper airway collapse [16]. Classical signs of bulbar involvement are tongue atrophy, protruding tongue, orofacial fasciculations, drooling, soft palate drop, and facial weakness.

Laryngospasm is the rapid and sudden contraction of the laryngeal sphincter, leading to partial or complete airway occlusion. Although it was originally described in the setting of weaning from mechanical ventilation, laryngospasm can occur spontaneously in up to 50% of patients with spinobulbar muscular atrophy [17] and 20% of patients with ALS [18]. Laryngospasm is thought to be secondary to an irritant stimulus (such as reflux) with an inhibitory neuron loss of the laryngeal sphincter [15]. Laryngospasm is manifested as an acute, sudden sensation of choking and audible stridor. The clinician should consider this condition in the differential diagnosis of intermittent unexplained dyspnea, as the management options are different from the usual management of chronic hypercapnic respiratory failure.

Perhaps the most important implication of bulbar involvement in NMD is the pharyngeal musculature impairment for swallowing coordination and inefficient cough, which predispose to bronchial aspiration and choking. It is usually manifested as oropharyngeal dysphagia with difficulty in the initial phase of swallowing with or without cough. Some patients may describe prolonged eating time, severe weight loss, and recurrent respiratory infections as opposed to difficulty swallowing [19]. A poor cough effort, especially in the inspiratory phase should raise concern for pharyngeal weakness. Bulbar involvement may contribute to the sensation of breathlessness even with intact diaphragmatic function [20].

Pulmonary Function Tests in Neuromuscular Respiratory Failure

Basic Pulmonary Function Testing (PFTs): Spirometry and Lung Volumes

Pulmonary function tests are summarized in Table 2.1. Failure of the respiratory pump impairs the mobilization of air (the respiratory stroke volume) both on inspiration and expiration which results in a restrictive pattern. Spirometry reveals a reduced forced expiratory volume in the first second (FEV_1) proportional to the reduction in forced vital capacity (FVC), resulting in a normal FEV_1/FVC ratio on spirometry. Total lung capacity is reduced on plethysmography and diffusion of CO_2 ($DLCO_2$) is usually preserved unless concomitant pulmonary disease is present (e.g., interstitial lung disease in inflammatory myopathies or pulmonary hypertension in long-standing hypoxemia secondary to restriction).

Early in the course of neuromuscular disease, lung volumes and flows may remain unaffected in the upright position, leading to normal PFTs despite clinically significant weakness and dyspnea [21]. Respiratory pump weakness can be

Table 2.1 Commonly used pulmonary function tests in neuromuscular disease

Test	Benefits	Limitations
Forced vital capacity	• Readily performed in the outpatient setting • Clear guidelines for interpretation • A qualifying criterion for NIV initiation • Can be performed in the supine position if normal upright	• Technical limitations in patients with bulbar dysfunction
Slow vital capacity	• Improved accuracy for patients with bulbar dysfunction compared to FVC	• Not as standardized as FVC • No criteria for NIV initiation
Maximum inspiratory pressure	• Sensitive test for inspiratory muscle strength • May detect early respiratory muscle weakness • A qualifying criterion for NIV initiation	• Not as readily performed as spirometry • Highly dependent on effort and technique • Technical limitations in patients with bulbar dysfunction • Limits of normal not as robust as FVC
Maximum expiratory pressure	• Tests for expiratory muscle strength • May be helpful in detecting ineffective cough due to expiratory muscles	• Not as readily performed as spirometry • Highly dependent on effort and technique • Unclear limits of normal
Sniff nasal inspiratory pressure	• Technically easier for patients with bulbar dysfunction than MIP • May detect early muscle weakness	• Not readily performed • No accepted NIV qualification criteria

unmasked by performing PFTs in the supine position, where the abdominal contents displace the diaphragm, thus increasing the contractile load. A decrease of >10% in FVC or FEV1 in the supine position compared to the upright is abnormal, and a >20% decrease has a 90% sensitivity for diagnosing respiratory weakness [22–25]. In patients with predominant expiratory muscle weakness, residual volumes may be increased [2].

Spirometry measurements may grossly underestimate true lung function in patients with bulbar or facial muscle weakness due to the inability to generate an adequate seal with the mouthpiece, leading to leaks in the circuit or intermittent upper airway collapse [26]. In advanced NMD, a slow VC (SVC) maneuver can overcome the limitations of FVC by reducing the influence of bulbar and oral muscle weakness during forced exhalation. SVC has been used in randomized controlled trials as it strongly correlates with meaningful clinical events [27].

Following initial baseline pulmonary function tests, spirometry should be monitored at regular intervals, as reductions in FVC serve as a prognostic indicator for pulmonary infections [28], need for tracheostomy [29], and overall survival [30, 31]. In addition, in the United States, FVC values serve as one of the qualifying criteria for NIV in neuromuscular disease. Currently, Medicare guidelines use an FVC cutoff <50% to qualify for non-invasive ventilation (NIV). However, in patients with ALS, emerging evidence suggest a survival benefit with early NIV initiation, even with FVC ≥80% [32].

Testing for Respiratory Muscle Strength: MIP, MEP, and SNIP

While PFTs are regularly used in the evaluation of patients with neuromuscular disease, it is important to remember that lung volumes serve as a surrogate for muscle strength but are not a measurement of muscle strength itself. A reduced TLC or FVC can arise from interstitial lung disease or impaired inspiratory muscle contraction that does not permit full lung expansion. Similarly, an increased RV can signify air trapping from increased airway resistance or impaired expiratory muscle function that does not permit full exhalation. Direct measurements of respiratory muscle strength through maximal inspiratory (MIP) and maximal expiratory pressure (MEP) maneuvers can help confirm that neuromuscular weakness is the driver for abnormal PFTs [33]. MIP and MEP maneuvers are performed by inhaling through a flanged mouthpiece until reaching total lung capacity (MIP) and exhaling to residual volume (MEP). The mouthpiece is attached to a small chamber specifically designed to have a controlled leak (a 2 mm hole), which prevents glottis closure and the use of facial muscles during forced maneuvers. The use of a closed mouthpiece allows minimal lung volume change during the maneuvers. Therefore, the resulting pressures reflect muscular strength rather than lung mechanics. MIP is primarily determined by the diaphragm and the accessory chest wall muscles, whereas MEP is determined by both the accessory chest wall and abdominal muscles. MIP and MEP are effort-dependent and prone to error if not properly performed [21, 22]. Multiple measurements should be performed and averaged before reporting a value [34]. For the maneuver to be reliable and replicable, the patient needs to properly form a seal around the mouthpiece to avoid leaks and underestimation of pressures. This is often a limitation in patients with bulbar weakness. Similarly, as MIP is measured at FRC, significant air trapping or restriction (especially with severe impairment in chest wall recoil) may skew the measurement of inspiratory pressures independently of respiratory muscular strength.

MIP is a more sensitive marker of diaphragmatic weakness than FVC [35], and it may be considered a screening tool for individuals at risk for respiratory weakness [34]. It correlates with breathlessness (particularly exertional dyspnea) [36], nocturnal hypoventilation, and overall quality of life [22]. MIP decrements usually precede changes in FVC and is currently considered an indication for NIV initiation in patients with ALS [19]. Although MIP has been shown to be a predictor of mortality and deterioration of FVC, the cutoff points for clinically meaningful ventilatory impairment are unclear [31]. According to the ATS/ERS standards, a MIP of $-80\,cmH_2O$ in men and $-70\,cmH_2O$ in woman excludes clinically significant inspiratory muscle weakness [37]. However, multiple factors should be considered when interpreting these numbers. Sex is one of the main determinants of respiratory muscle pressures (30% more in males) and is usually considered in the cutoffs for the percentages of predictive values [38]. However, age is associated with a linear decline of MIP, and weight is positively correlated with increased predictive MIP [39]. Both factors are not typically considered in MIP limits of normality but should be considered when interpreting abnormal values in patients with NMD. Currently, a MIP lower than $-60\,cmH_2O$ is one criterion to qualify for NIV initiation by Medicare and Medicaid guidelines. However, a significant decline from baseline should alert the clinician for the potential of ongoing respiratory pump failure and consider NIV initiation based on symptomatology.

Data supporting the use of MEP as a predictor for clinically meaningful outcomes is less robust than for MIP. The values for normality are usually wide and inconsistent among observational studies (typically above $130\,cmH_2O$ in men and above $100\,cmH_2O$ in women). MEP measures expiratory muscle strength, particularly abdominal muscles. However, given the high positive pressures elicited by this maneuver, patients with facial weakness are usually unable to perform this maneuver without leak. Normal values are particularly good negative predictor for expiratory muscle impairment and may indicate good cough strength, with the caveat that the strength of cough is also influenced by maximal inspiration, which is limited in diaphragmatic weakness.

The sniff nasal inspiratory pressure (SNIP) is a feasible alternative for assessing respiratory muscle weakness in patients with bulbar weakness who have significant leaks through the mouthpiece during MIP measurement. During SNIP testing, inspiratory pressures are measured through a plug occluding one nostril while sniff maneuvers are performed from FRC through the unconcluded one [40]. SNIP correlates with esophageal pressures and is a good surrogate for diaphragmatic force when compared with transdiaphragmatic pressure measurements. A decline in SNIP predicts nocturnal desaturations, respiratory failure, need for tracheostomy and gastrostomy, [41] and death [42]. When compared to MIP, the limits of agreement between these two tests are wide, which likely represent different components of respiratory muscle weakness depicted by each test. As it is simpler to perform and more reproducible, it is thought that SNIP reflects a more complete activation of the inspiratory muscles [43]. Currently, SNIP is not considered in NIV qualification criteria by Medicare. NIV should be considered well before patients reach a SNIP lower than 40 cmH_2O, as reaching this threshold is associated with a median survival of 6 months. In patient with ALS, SNIP declines predict the need for NIV better than MIP or FVC [44]. Important limitations for a reliable SNIP measurement are nasal conditions that diminishes the diameter of the nostrils such as congestion, prior surgery, or masses [45]. In addition, increased airway airflow resistance reduces the transmission of rapid pressures changes (e.g., sniffing) between the alveoli and the airway and underestimate SNIP. Therefore, SNIP may underestimate muscle strength in patients with coexisting airways disease [46–48].

PFTs in Patients with Tracheostomy

With improvements in NIV technology, ventilator dependence is no longer considered an absolute indication for tracheostomy placement in patients with neuromuscular disease [49, 50]. However, those patients who develop an acute life-threatening decompensation have severe bulbar dysfunction and associated laryngeal spasm, or cannot achieve adequate alveolar ventilation with NIV might benefit from tracheostomy placement [51]. Once a tracheostomy is placed, clinicians must decide whether further assessments of lung function are valuable, reliable, or necessary. For patients requiring continuous invasive ventilation, ongoing PFT measurements may not change clinical management. However, for patients who initially undergo tracheostomy for severe bulbar dysfunction, as opposed to respiratory muscle weakness may benefit from future assessments to determine the need for mechanical ventilation support. However, there is controversy regarding whether respiratory function can be adequately assessed with pulmonary function tests, which are deemed unreliable and difficult to perform in this population. In a retrospective analysis, Sheshadri and colleagues described a technique for performing pulmonary function tests in tracheostomized patients [52]. By removing the tracheostomy cannula and sealing potential leaks with an adhesive baseplate, the authors were able to obtain acceptable (according to ATS acceptability criteria) FEV1 and FVC measures in 43 of the 50 subjects studied. However, end-of-test criteria (exhalation time greater than 6 s and plateau criteria) were met in a minority of the subjects. To be noted, most of the patients studied in this cohort had a tracheostomy placed for obstructive anatomic reasons (such as laryngectomy or tumor obstruction), and only a minority had pulmonary pathology. Although this data supports the feasibility of performing PFTs in patients with tracheostomy, patients should be selected appropriately and tests should be performed for clinically meaningful information that may impact decision making.

Ancillary Tests Assessing Respiratory Muscle Weakness

Fluoroscopic Sniff Test

The fluoroscopic sniff test consists of a noninvasive fluoroscopic evaluation of diaphragmatic cephalocaudal excursion during a sniff maneuver. It is typically used for the diagnosis of unilateral diaphragmatic palsy. An abnormal test consists of a normal physiological descent of the unaffected diaphragm and a paradoxical ascent (more than 2 cm) of the paralyzed diaphragm [53]. For the test to be accurate, the patient must be disconnected from positive pressure ventilation. The fluoroscopic sniff test has 90% sensitivity for the diagnosis of unilateral diaphragmatic paralysis [54] and is considered the gold standard for its diagnosis. A positive test predicts improved pulmonary function after surgical diaphragmatic plication, particularly in symptomatic patients [55]. However, its specificity is poor [56], as up to 6% of healthy adults have paradoxical motion of the diaphragm [57].

When bilateral diaphragmatic weakness is suspected, the role of the fluoroscopic sniff test is less clear. During inspiration, the abdominal muscles relax, allowing for diaphragmatic descent unrelated to its contraction, secondary to the outward recoil of the abdominal wall. This could be misinterpreted as normal physiologic descent. Similarly, the cephalad movement of the ribcage secondary to the contraction of the accessory muscles can create a visual illusion of diaphragmatic motion. In a small case series, only 20% of patients with bilateral diaphragmatic weakness had a positive fluoroscopic sniff test [58]. Therefore, fluoroscopic evaluation of the diaphragm should be reserved for patients in whom unilateral dysfunction is suspected, such as patients with dyspnea and history of blunt cervical trauma, thoracic surgery, radiation to the chest, neck manipulation, or cases of suspected brachial plexus neuropathy [54]. In patients with systemic neuromuscular disease, the fluoroscopic sniff test might falsely reassure the physician. If used, it should be interpreted in conjunction with other physiological testing.

Diaphragmatic Electromyography

Needle diaphragmatic electromyography (EMG) and phrenic nerve conduction testing can aid in the diagnosis of diaphragmatic weakness, with the advantage of providing information regarding the etiology of diaphragm dysfunction. EMG can help differentiate muscular and neuropathic causes of diaphragmatic weakness, and conduction studies permit to distinguish nerve conduction blocks versus demyelination [59]. Although these tests have a high sensitivity and specificity for the diagnosis of diaphragmatic weakness, they require advanced technical expertise for its adequate execution and interpretation [60, 61]. Needle electromyography is uncomfortable and carries the risk of muscular injury and pneumothorax, which limits its use in daily clinical practice except in highly specialized centers [62].

Diaphragmatic Ultrasonography

The use of ultrasound (US) for diaphragmatic assessment is an emerging, noninvasive technique that allows the clinician to obtain real-time anatomic and functional assessments of the diaphragm (see Figs. 2.1 and 2.2). Diaphragmatic US has been extensively studied in the intensive care unit [63–66], particularly for weaning from mechanical ventilation, where it has demonstrated a sensitivity and specificity of 80% for predicting successful weaning from mechanical ventilation [67]. Most recently, diaphragmatic US has been used in neuromuscular disease to diagnose respiratory muscle weakness [68].

Compared to diaphragmatic fluoroscopy, diaphragmatic US has a higher diagnostic accuracy for detecting diaphragmatic weakness [69], probably due to the multimodal components it assesses. Diaphragmatic US evaluates both the excursion of the muscle throughout the thoracic-abdominal space (at end inspiration and end expiration) as well as the thickening of the diaphragm muscle fibers during the respiratory cycle [70]. In addition, the use of ultrasonography may provide additional clues regarding less common contributing factors to impaired diaphragm movement, including pleural fluid or masses [59]. When the etiology of diaphragmatic dysfunction is unclear, concomitant use of phrenic nerve stimulation and visual assessment of diaphragmatic excursion/thickness with US helps distinguish upper from lower motor neuron disease [71].

In patients with ALS, changes in diaphragmatic thickening fraction throughout time predict NIV initiation [68] and pulmonary function test decline [72], whereas improvements in thickening fraction predict reinnervation and recovery in patients with diaphragmatic paralysis [73]. Interestingly, in patients with Duchenne muscular dystrophy, early in the disease the diaphragm can undergo pseudohypertrophy (analogous to the gastrocnemius muscles) followed by progressive atrophy throughout the years [74]. Although diaphragmatic ultrasonography is a promising technique for the diagnosis and follow-up of patients with diaphragmatic weakness, the

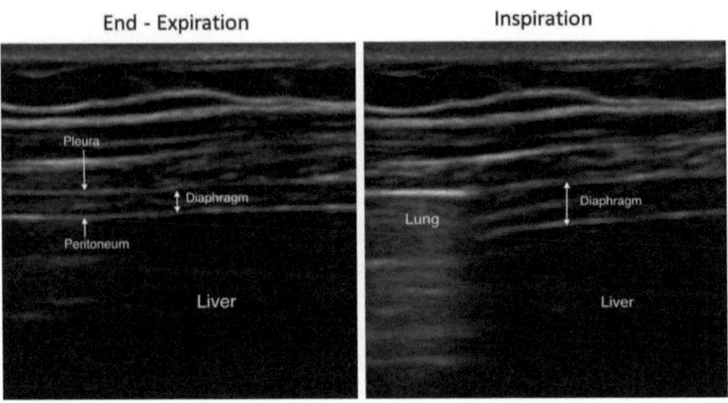

Fig. 2.1 Diaphragm ultrasound on end expiration and end inspiration (Images courtesy of Dr. F. Dennis McCool)

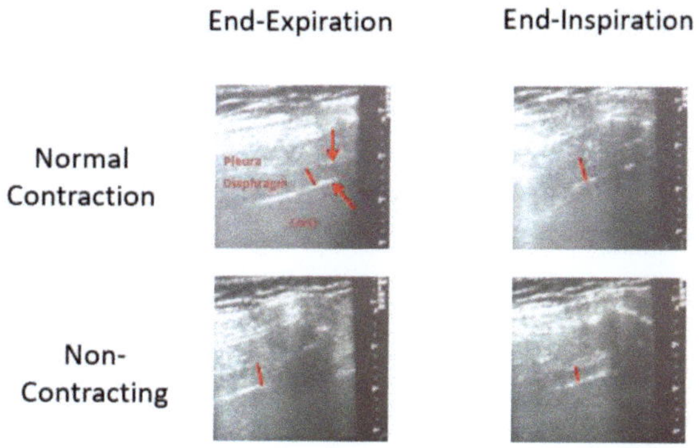

End-Expiration   End-Inspiration

Normal Contraction

Pleura
Diaphragm

Non-Contracting

Fig. 2.2 Diaphragm ultrasound comparing normal contraction and noncontracting diaphragm

requirement for prior training and interobserver variability (mostly dependent on the skills of the operator) limits its widespread current use.

Assessing Alveolar Ventilation in Neuromuscular Disease

Implications and Detection of Hypercapnia in Neuromuscular Disease

While some neuromuscular conditions such as myasthenia gravis and Guillain–Barre syndrome can present with acute hypercapnic respiratory failure, most are chronic conditions, putting patients at risk of developing chronic hypercapnic respiratory failure if not appropriately managed with NIV. There is growing evidence that hypercapnia in both acute and chronic states is associated with increased morbidity and mortality [75, 76]. Hypercapnia impairs alveolar fluid reabsorption [77], neutrophil phagocytosis [78], cytokine expression, epithelial regeneration, and other immune response against bacteria [79] and viruses [80], independent from extracellular pH. In addition to its effects on host defenses, elevated CO_2 has direct effects on skeletal muscle function, inducing catabolic muscle wasting and impairing muscle regeneration [81] in both respiratory and nonrespiratory skeletal muscles [82]. Saturated total body CO_2 stores, in the setting of persistent hypoventilation, leads to rapid rises in blood CO_2 levels with minor changes in ventilation [83]. This growing data suggesting the harmful direct effects of elevated blood CO_2 supports the monitoring of $PaCO_2$ as an important initial and longitudinal assessment of patients with neuromuscular disease. An elevated $PaCO_2$ >45 is an indication for the initiation of NIV in neuromuscular disease. NIV is associated with improved survival in numerous conditions including neuromuscular disease, and studies suggest that reductions in $PaCO_2$ or maintenance of normocapnia may be potential mechanisms for this survival benefit [84–87]. Unfortunately, other assessments of respiratory function including imaging and PFTs correlate poorly with the development of hypercapnia [88]. Therefore, it is important that clinicians have the appropriate tools to assess for the development of hypercapnia secondary to alveolar hypoventilation. Table 2.2 summarizes methods for measuring PCO_2.

Blood Gas Analysis

Arterial blood gas testing remains the gold standard for the detection of hypercapnia [89]. However, in the outpatient setting there are several barriers impeding its routine use, such as the access to a blood gas analyzer, patient discomfort, hyperventilation before and during the procedure (which can skew the results) [90], and the inability to continuously monitor changes in CO_2 while on mechanical ventilation. Arterialized capillary blood gas analysis represents an alternative technique, which is less invasive and time-consuming [91]. It has shown to have a good correlation with arterial blood gases when it is sampled from the earlobe [92]. To be noted, in order to obtain an adequate sample, vasodilation of the earlobe capillaries should be achieved with heat prior to obtaining the sample. Although it is an attractive, less-invasive alternative to arterial blood sampling, capillary blood gas analyzers are not widely available. Venous blood gases are increasingly utilized in the hospital

Table 2.2 Methods of assessing PCO_2 in the outpatient setting

	Benefits	Limitations
Arterial blood gas	• Gold standard for PCO_2 • Assesses pH	• Patient discomfort • Access to blood gas lab • Single time point • No continuous monitoring of $PaCO_2$
Arterialized capillary blood	• Less invasive than ABG • Good correlation with arterial blood	• Access to blood gas lab • Not widely available • Single time point • No continuous monitoring of $PaCO_2$
Venous blood gas	• Less invasive than ABG • Assesses pH	• Wide confidence interval when comparing to ABG • Access to blood gas lab
End-tidal CO_2	• Real-time estimation of $PaCO_2$ • Relatively inexpensive • Can be used for continuous monitoring	• Accuracy diminishes with increased dead space and age • Cannot be used for patients on continuous NIV
Transcutaneous CO_2	• Real-time estimation of $PaCO_2$ • Can be used for continuous monitoring, including with continuous NIV • Minimal bias • Narrow confidence interval when comparing to ABG	• Expensive • Accuracy diminishes at higher $PaCO_2$ • Technical maintenance of devices

setting. However, the limits of agreement between arterial and venous blood CO_2 are wide [93, 94], and therefore should be used with caution.

Noninvasive PCO_2 Measurement

End-Tidal Pressure of Expired CO_2 ($PetCO_2$)

Given the limitations of obtaining ABG samples on a regular basis, noninvasive techniques that can be performed simply and rapidly are important in the management of respiratory failure in neuromuscular disease. $PetCO_2$ or capnography uses quantitative infrared absorption spectroscopy to measure a wavelength of 4.3 mm, which corresponds with CO_2 absorption of light [89]. Capnography has been extensively studied in mechanically ventilated patients using the infrared sensor inside the ventilator circuit (mainstream capnography) or a small gas sample from the circuit (sidestream capnography) [95]. The sensor detects the wavelength of CO_2 which is processed and displayed on a monitor as a function of time or end-tidal volume. $PetCO_2$ measures the partial pressure of CO_2 at the end of exhalation in the alveoli, and while it provides an estimation of $PaCO_2$ with mean differences of 3–5 mmHg between $PetCO_2$ and $PaCO_2$ [96], accuracy of $PetCO_2$ worsens in patients with increased physiologic dead space, altered cardiac output, and increased age. In addition, $PetCO_2$ cannot be accurately measured for patients on continuous NIV due to the intentional mask leak, which limits its use in the setting of NIV titrations. $PetCO_2$ values can be obtained quickly and compared to transcutaneous CO_2 is relatively inexpensive. Therefore, if used in the clinical setting for patients with neuromuscular disease, clinicians must keep these limitations in mind when interpreting the results.

Transcutaneous CO_2

Transcutaneous carbon dioxide monitoring ($PtcCO_2$) is a noninvasive technique in which the skin is gently warmed by a small sensor to vasodilate the skin capillaries, and an electrolyte solution is applied between the skin and the sensor (Fig. 2.3). Capillary vasodilation allows carbon dioxide levels to equilibrate with those of the arterial bed, a process commonly referred to as arterialization. The change in temperature on the skin promotes gas exchange between the skin and the electrolyte solution overlying it, which generates a pH change that is detected by the sensor [97]. The device then uses the Henderson–Hesselbach formula to calculate CO_2 and an algorithm to account for body temperature and metabolic correction factors before displaying an estimated $PaCO_2$. This process requires 5–10 min from sensor placement until a stable reading is provided by the device. Once the reading of an estimated CO_2 is displayed, the clinician obtains real-time monitoring of CO_2 levels,

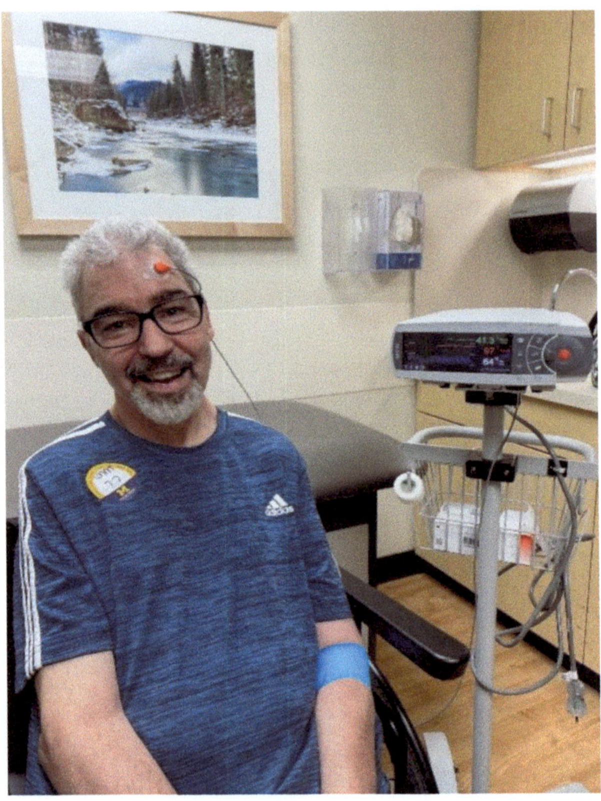

Fig. 2.3 Transcutaneous CO_2 monitoring with a Sentec device

with a lag of about 2 min between real-time serum changes in CO_2 [98]. $PtcCO_2$ provides an alternative, noninvasive method for longitudinal monitoring of alveolar ventilation.

In the acute setting, studies regarding the reliability of $PtcCO_2$ compared with $PaCO_2$ show mixed results [99–101], with some variability possibly related to the specific $PtcCO_2$ device used for measurements [102–107]. In addition, the correlation with $PaCO_2$ is dependent on the degree of hypercapnia with lower agreement between $PtcCO_2$ and $PaCO_2$ at higher $PaCO_2$ values [108–110]. $PtcCO_2$ also has limitations when used in the setting of critical illness and shock [111–113]. However, in the setting of stable outpatient neuromuscular disease, $PtcCO_2$ has been shown to have good correlation with $PaCO_2$ [114, 115], and has been used as an effective tool in decision making for inpatient initiation of NIV [116]. Because $PtcCO_2$ is a measurement of arterial CO_2, it can be used in the setting of continuous NIV titration. Currently, several home ventilators offer integrated $PtcCO_2$ monitoring that can be correlated with NIV download data. The caveat of prolonged $PtcCO_2$ monitoring is that decalibration of the sensors during the study might lead to artificial drifts in $PtcCO_2$ levels, a phenomenon known as calibration drift. Although frequently described in the literature, recent studies using modern monitors have minimal drifts in $PtcCO_2$ levels when compared with arterial blood gases.

At the current time, high cost likely hinders wide dissemination of $PtcCO_2$ monitors. In addition, several technical factors should be considered when using $PtcCO_2$ sensor: improper application of the sensor, presence of bubbles within the interface of the sensor and skin, improper calibration, and conditions such as edema or increased thickness of the skin, which might result in imprecise measurements.

Serum Bicarbonate

Serum bicarbonate is a surrogate for blood CO_2 levels and rises concomitantly with CO_2 levels in the setting of chronic hypercapnia. In patients with obesity, levels higher than 27 mEq/L predict daytime hypercapnia with a sensitivity of 92% [117]. Manuel and colleagues recently proposed that eucapnic elevations in serum bicarbonate levels predict nocturnal hypoventilation in patients with obesity hypoventilation syndrome [118]. The implications and correlation to patients with neuromuscular disease is unclear, but there is no rationale for suspecting that the physiological response to chronically elevated CO_2 should be different in this population [119]. Although serum HCO_3 can be useful to detect patients with chronic hypercapnia and may give a general sense of responses to NIV, multiple cofounders of acid-base homeostasis such as concomitant diuretic, mineralocorticoids use, chronic kidney disease, or renal tubular disorders may limit its practical use for the monitoring of alveolar ventilation [120].

Conclusion

Assessing the respiratory function of patients with neuromuscular disease involves thorough history taking, keen physical examination skills, and knowledge of the appropriate testing necessary to have a full understanding of an individual patient's physiology. Given the limitations of each individual test, as well as the variability in presentation and progressive nature of neuromuscular diseases, multiple modalities of testing should be used and repeated over time to optimally manage patients through the course of their illness. Spirometric evaluation, imaging techniques, and longitudinal measurements of blood CO_2 can all assist in the initiation of appropriate home ventilation as well as proper management once on therapy.

References

1. Perrin C, Unterborn JN, Ambrosio CD, Hill NS. Pulmonary complications of chronic neuromuscular diseases and their management. Muscle Nerve. 2004;29(1):5–27.

2. Voulgaris A, Antoniadou M, Agrafiotis M, Steiropoulos P. Respiratory involvement in patients with neuromuscular diseases: a narrative review. Pulm Med. 2019;2019:2734054.

3. Lanini B, Misuri G, Gigliotti F, et al. Perception of dyspnea in patients with neuromuscular disease. Chest. 2001;120(2):402–8.

4. Schoenhofer B, Koehler D, Polkey MI. Influence of immersion in water on muscle function and breathing pattern in patients with severe diaphragm weakness. Chest. 2004;125(6):2069–74.

5. Vogt S, Schreiber S, Kollewe K, et al. Dyspnea in amyotrophic lateral sclerosis: the Dyspnea-ALS-Scale (DALS-15) essentially contributes to the diagnosis of respiratory impairment. Respir Med. 2019;154:116–21.

6. Bourke SC. Respiratory involvement in neuromuscular disease. Clin Med (Lond). 2014;14(1):72–5.

7. Bourke SC, Tomlinson M, Williams TL, Bullock RE, Shaw PJ, Gibson GJ. Effects of non-invasive ventilation on survival and quality of life in patients with amyotrophic lateral sclerosis: a randomised controlled trial. Lancet Neurol. 2006;5(2):140–7.

8. AlBalawi MM, Castro-Codesal M, Featherstone R, et al. Outcomes of long-term noninvasive ventilation use in children with neuromuscular disease: systematic review and meta-analysis. Ann Am Thorac Soc. 2022;19(1):109–19.

9. Heiman-Patterson TD, Cudkowicz ME, De Carvalho M, et al. Understanding the use of NIV in ALS: results of an international ALS specialist survey. Amyotroph Lateral Scler Frontotemporal Degener. 2018;19(5–6):331–41.

10. Lo Coco D, Mattaliano P, Spataro R, Mattaliano A, La Bella V. Sleep-wake disturbances in patients with amyotrophic lateral sclerosis. J Neurol Neurosurg Psychiatry. 2011;82(8):839–42.

11. Fermin AM, Afzal U, Culebras A. Sleep in neuromuscular diseases. Sleep Med Clin. 2016;11(1):53–64.

12. Aboussouan LS. Sleep-disordered breathing in neuromuscular disease. Am J Respir Crit Care Med. 2015;191(9):979–89.

13. Kryger MH, Steljes DG, Yee WC, Mate E, Smith SA, Mahowald M. Central sleep apnoea in congenital muscular dystrophy. J Neurol Neurosurg Psychiatry. 1991;54(8):710–2.

14. Andersen T, Sandnes A, Brekka AK, et al. Laryngeal response patterns influence the efficacy of mechanical assisted cough in amyotrophic lateral sclerosis. Thorax. 2017;72(3):221–9.

15. Kuhnlein P, Gdynia HJ, Sperfeld AD, et al. Diagnosis and treatment of bulbar symptoms in amyotrophic lateral sclerosis. Nat Clin Pract Neurol. 2008;4(7):366–74.

16. Banerjee SK, Davies M, Sharples L, Smith I. The role of facemask spirometry in motor neuron disease. Thorax. 2013;68(4):385–6.

17. Sperfeld AD, Hanemann CO, Ludolph AC, Kassubek J. Laryngospasm: an underdiagnosed symptom of X-linked spinobulbar muscular atrophy. Neurology. 2005;64(4):753–4.

18. Forshew DA, Bromberg MB. A survey of clinicians' practice in the symptomatic treatment of ALS. Amyotroph Lateral Scler Other Motor Neuron Disord. 2003;4(4):258–63.

19. Niedermeyer S, Murn M, Choi PJ. Respiratory failure in amyotrophic lateral sclerosis. Chest. 2019;155(2):401–8.

20. Lo Mauro A, Aliverti A. Physiology of respiratory disturbances in muscular dystrophies. Breathe (Sheff). 2016;12(4):318–27.

21. Oliveira MJP, Rodrigues F, Firmino-Machado J, et al. Assessment of respiratory muscle weakness in subjects with neuromuscular disease. Respir Care. 2018;63(10):1223–30.

22. Schoser B, Fong E, Geberhiwot T, et al. Maximum inspiratory pressure as a clinically meaningful trial endpoint for neuromuscular diseases: a comprehensive review of the literature. Orphanet J Rare Dis. 2017;12(1):52.

23. Allen SM, Hunt B, Green M. Fall in vital capacity with posture. Br J Dis Chest. 1985;79(3):267–71.

24. Fromageot C, Lofaso F, Annane D, et al. Supine fall in lung volumes in the assessment of diaphragmatic weakness in neuromuscular disorders. Arch Phys Med Rehabil. 2001;82(1):123–8.

25. Lechtzin N, Wiener CM, Shade DM, Clawson L, Diette GB. Spirometry in the supine position improves the detection of diaphragmatic weakness in patients with amyotrophic lateral sclerosis. Chest. 2002;121(2):436–42.
26. Pfeffer G, Povitz M. Respiratory management of patients with neuromuscular disease: current perspectives. Degener Neurol Neuromuscul Dis. 2016;6:111–8.
27. Andrews JA, Meng L, Kulke SF, et al. Association between decline in slow vital capacity and respiratory insufficiency, use of assisted ventilation, tracheostomy, or death in patients with amyotrophic lateral sclerosis. JAMA Neurol. 2018;75(1):58–64.
28. Dohna-Schwake C, Ragette R, Teschler H, Voit T, Mellies U. Predictors of severe chest infections in pediatric neuromuscular disorders. Neuromuscul Disord. 2006;16(5):325–8.
29. Phillips MF, Quinlivan RC, Edwards RH, Calverley PM. Changes in spirometry over time as a prognostic marker in patients with Duchenne muscular dystrophy. Am J Respir Crit Care Med. 2001;164(12):2191–4.
30. Czaplinski A, Yen AA, Appel SH. Forced vital capacity (FVC) as an indicator of survival and disease progression in an ALS clinic population. J Neurol Neurosurg Psychiatry. 2006;77(3):390–2.
31. Schmidt EP, Drachman DB, Wiener CM, Clawson L, Kimball R, Lechtzin N. Pulmonary predictors of survival in amyotrophic lateral sclerosis: use in clinical trial design. Muscle Nerve. 2006;33(1):127–32.
32. Vitacca M, Montini A, Lunetta C, et al. Impact of an early respiratory care programme with non-invasive ventilation adaptation in patients with amyotrophic lateral sclerosis. Eur J Neurol. 2018;25(3):556–e533.
33. Evans JA, Whitelaw WA. The assessment of maximal respiratory mouth pressures in adults. Respir Care. 2009;54(10):1348–59.
34. Laveneziana P, Albuquerque A, Aliverti A, et al. ERS statement on respiratory muscle testing at rest and during exercise. Eur Respir J. 2019;53(6):1801214.
35. Mendoza M, Gelinas DF, Moore DH, Miller RG. A comparison of maximal inspiratory pressure and forced vital capacity as potential criteria for initiating non-invasive ventilation in amyotrophic lateral sclerosis. Amyotroph Lateral Scler. 2007;8(2):106–11.
36. Killian KJ, Jones NL. Respiratory muscles and dyspnea. Clin Chest Med. 1988;9(2):237–48.
37. American Thoracic Society/European Respiratory Society. ATS/ERS statement on respiratory muscle testing. Am J Respir Crit Care Med. 2002;166(4):518–624.
38. Hautmann H, Hefele S, Schotten K, Huber RM. Maximal inspiratory mouth pressures (PIMAX) in healthy subjects—what is the lower limit of normal? Respir Med. 2000;94(7):689–93.
39. Harik-Khan RI, Wise RA, Fozard JL. Determinants of maximal inspiratory pressure. The Baltimore Longitudinal Study of Aging. Am J Respir Crit Care Med. 1998;158(5 Pt 1):1459–64.
40. Heritier F, Rahm F, Pasche P, Fitting JW. Sniff nasal inspiratory pressure. A noninvasive assessment of inspiratory muscle strength. Am J Respir Crit Care Med. 1994;150(6 Pt 1):1678–83.
41. Zoccolella S, Capozzo R, Quaranta VN, et al. Reduction of sniff nasal inspiratory pressure (SNIP) as an early indicator of the need of enteral nutrition in patients with amyotrophic lateral sclerosis. Brain Sci. 2021;11(8):1091.
42. Capozzo R, Quaranta VN, Pellegrini F, et al. Sniff nasal inspiratory pressure as a prognostic factor of tracheostomy or death in amyotrophic lateral sclerosis. J Neurol. 2015;262(3):593–603.
43. Fitting JW. Sniff nasal inspiratory pressure: simple or too simple? Eur Respir J. 2006;27(5):881–3.
44. Tilanus TBM, Groothuis JT, TenBroek-Pastoor JMC, et al. The predictive value of respiratory function tests for non-invasive ventilation in amyotrophic lateral sclerosis. Respir Res. 2017;18(1):144.
45. Hart N, Polkey MI, Sharshar T, et al. Limitations of sniff nasal pressure in patients with severe neuromuscular weakness. J Neurol Neurosurg Psychiatry. 2003;74(12):1685–7.

46. Stell IM, Polkey MI, Rees PJ, Green M, Moxham J. Inspiratory muscle strength in acute asthma. Chest. 2001;120(3):757–64.
47. Uldry C, Janssens JP, de Muralt B, Fitting JW. Sniff nasal inspiratory pressure in patients with chronic obstructive pulmonary disease. Eur Respir J. 1997;10(6):1292–6.
48. Teschler H, Stamatis G, el-Raouf Farhat AA, Meyer FJ, Costabel U, Konietzko N. Effect of surgical lung volume reduction on respiratory muscle function in pulmonary emphysema. Eur Respir J. 1996;9(9):1779–84.
49. Prigent H, Fauroux B, Attarian S, Annane D, Lofaso F. Tracheostomy in ventilator-dependent patients with slowly progressive neuromuscular disease. Lancet Respir Med. 2023;11(5):410–1.
50. Birnkrant DJ, Bushby K, Bann CM, et al. Diagnosis and management of Duchenne muscular dystrophy, part 2: respiratory, cardiac, bone health, and orthopaedic management. Lancet Neurol. 2018;17(4):347–61.
51. Spataro R, Bono V, Marchese S, La Bella V. Tracheostomy mechanical ventilation in patients with amyotrophic lateral sclerosis: clinical features and survival analysis. J Neurol Sci. 2012;323(1–2):66–70.
52. Sheshadri A, Keus L, Blanco D, et al. Pulmonary function testing in patients with tracheostomies: feasibility and technical considerations. Lung. 2021;199(3):307–10.
53. Laghi FA Jr, Saad M, Shaikh H. Ultrasound and non-ultrasound imaging techniques in the assessment of diaphragmatic dysfunction. BMC Pulm Med. 2021;21(1):85.
54. Billings ME, Aitken ML, Benditt JO. Bilateral diaphragm paralysis: a challenging diagnosis. Respir Care. 2008;53(10):1368–71.
55. Patel DC, Berry MF, Bhandari P, et al. Paradoxical motion on sniff test predicts greater improvement following diaphragm plication. Ann Thorac Surg. 2021;111(6):1820–6.
56. Nafisa S, Messer B, Downie B, et al. A retrospective cohort study of idiopathic diaphragmatic palsy: a diagnostic triad, natural history and prognosis. ERJ Open Res. 2021;7(3):00953.
57. Alexander C. Diaphragm movements and the diagnosis of diaphragmatic paralysis. Clin Radiol. 1966;17(1):79–83.
58. Davis J, Goldman M, Loh L, Casson M. Diaphragm function and alveolar hypoventilation. Q J Med. 1976;45(177):87–100.
59. Sarwal A, Walker FO, Cartwright MS. Neuromuscular ultrasound for evaluation of the diaphragm. Muscle Nerve. 2013;47(3):319–29.
60. Bolton CF, Grand'Maison F, Parkes A, Shkrum M. Needle electromyography of the diaphragm. Muscle Nerve. 1992;15(6):678–81.
61. Mertens L. Diaphragmatic paralysis after cardiac surgery: how to look at it? Pediatr Crit Care Med. 2006;7(5):491–2.
62. Luo YM, Harris ML, Lyall RA, Watson A, Polkey MI, Moxham J. Assessment of diaphragm paralysis with oesophageal electromyography and unilateral magnetic phrenic nerve stimulation. Eur Respir J. 2000;15(3):596–9.
63. DiNino E, Gartman EJ, Sethi JM, McCool FD. Diaphragm ultrasound as a predictor of successful extubation from mechanical ventilation. Thorax. 2014;69(5):423–7.
64. Blumhof S, Wheeler D, Thomas K, McCool FD, Mora J. Change in diaphragmatic thickness during the respiratory cycle predicts extubation success at various levels of pressure support ventilation. Lung. 2016;194(4):519–25.
65. Farghaly S, Hasan AA. Diaphragm ultrasound as a new method to predict extubation outcome in mechanically ventilated patients. Aust Crit Care. 2017;30(1):37–43.
66. Palkar A, Narasimhan M, Greenberg H, et al. Diaphragm excursion-time index: a new parameter using ultrasonography to predict extubation outcome. Chest. 2018;153(5):1213–20.
67. Parada-Gereda HM, Tibaduiza AL, Rico-Mendoza A, et al. Effectiveness of diaphragmatic ultrasound as a predictor of successful weaning from mechanical ventilation: a systematic review and meta-analysis. Crit Care. 2023;27(1):174.
68. Fantini R, Mandrioli J, Zona S, et al. Ultrasound assessment of diaphragmatic function in patients with amyotrophic lateral sclerosis. Respirology. 2016;21(5):932–8.

69. Houston JG, Fleet M, Cowan MD, McMillan NC. Comparison of ultrasound with fluoroscopy in the assessment of suspected hemidiaphragmatic movement abnormality. Clin Radiol. 1995;50(2):95–8.
70. Kilaru D, Panebianco N, Baston C. Diaphragm ultrasound in weaning from mechanical ventilation. Chest. 2021;159(3):1166–72.
71. McCauley RG, Labib KB. Diaphragmatic paralysis evaluated by phrenic nerve stimulation during fluoroscopy or real-time ultrasound. Radiology. 1984;153(1):33–6.
72. Rajula RR, Saini J, Unnikrishnan G, et al. Diaphragmatic ultrasound: prospects as a tool to assess respiratory muscle involvement in amyotrophic lateral sclerosis. J Clin Ultrasound. 2022;50(1):131–5.
73. Summerhill EM, El-Sameed YA, Glidden TJ, McCool FD. Monitoring recovery from diaphragm paralysis with ultrasound. Chest. 2008;133(3):737–43.
74. Laviola M, Priori R, D'Angelo MG, Aliverti A. Assessment of diaphragmatic thickness by ultrasonography in Duchenne muscular dystrophy (DMD) patients. PLoS One. 2018;13(7):e0200582.
75. Vonderbank S, Gibis N, Schulz A, et al. Hypercapnia at hospital admission as a predictor of mortality. Open Access Emerg Med. 2020;12:173–80.
76. Wilson MW, Labaki WW, Choi PJ. Mortality and healthcare use of patients with compensated hypercapnia. Ann Am Thorac Soc. 2021;18(12):2027–32.
77. Shigemura M, Lecuona E, Sznajder JI. Effects of hypercapnia on the lung. J Physiol. 2017;595(8):2431–7.
78. Wang N, Gates KL, Trejo H, et al. Elevated CO_2 selectively inhibits interleukin-6 and tumor necrosis factor expression and decreases phagocytosis in the macrophage. FASEB J. 2010;24(7):2178–90.
79. Gates KL, Howell HA, Nair A, et al. Hypercapnia impairs lung neutrophil function and increases mortality in murine pseudomonas pneumonia. Am J Respir Cell Mol Biol. 2013;49(5):821–8.
80. Casalino-Matsuda SM, Chen F, Gonzalez-Gonzalez FJ, et al. Hypercapnia suppresses macrophage antiviral activity and increases mortality of influenza A infection via Akt1. J Immunol. 2020;205(2):489–501.
81. Korponay TC, Balnis J, Vincent CE, et al. High CO_2 downregulates skeletal muscle protein anabolism via AMP-activated protein kinase alpha2-mediated depressed ribosomal biogenesis. Am J Respir Cell Mol Biol. 2020;62(1):74–86.
82. Shiota S, Okada T, Naitoh H, Ochi R, Fukuchi Y. Hypoxia and hypercapnia affect contractile and histological properties of rat diaphragm and hind limb muscles. Pathophysiology. 2004;11(1):23–30.
83. Giosa L, Busana M, Bonifazi M, et al. Mobilizing carbon dioxide stores. An experimental study. Am J Respir Crit Care Med. 2021;203(3):318–27.
84. Kohnlein T, Windisch W, Kohler D, et al. Non-invasive positive pressure ventilation for the treatment of severe stable chronic obstructive pulmonary disease: a prospective, multicentre, randomised, controlled clinical trial. Lancet Respir Med. 2014;2(9):698–705.
85. Mokhlesi B, Masa JF, Afshar M, et al. The effect of hospital discharge with empiric noninvasive ventilation on mortality in hospitalized patients with obesity hypoventilation syndrome. An individual patient data meta-analysis. Ann Am Thorac Soc. 2020;17(5):627–37.
86. Ackrivo J, Hsu JY, Hansen-Flaschen J, Elman L, Kawut SM. Noninvasive ventilation use is associated with better survival in amyotrophic lateral sclerosis. Ann Am Thorac Soc. 2021;18(3):486–94.
87. Jimenez JV, Ackrivo J, Hsu JY, et al. Lowering PCO_2 with non-invasive ventilation is associated with improved survival in chronic hypercapnic respiratory failure. Respir Care. 2023;68:1613.
88. Boentert M, Glatz C, Helmle C, Okegwo A, Young P. Prevalence of sleep apnoea and capnographic detection of nocturnal hypoventilation in amyotrophic lateral sclerosis. J Neurol Neurosurg Psychiatry. 2018;89(4):418–24.

89. Huttmann SE, Windisch W, Storre JH. Techniques for the measurement and monitoring of carbon dioxide in the blood. Ann Am Thorac Soc. 2014;11(4):645–52.
90. Mallat J, Mohammad U, Lemyze M, et al. Acute hyperventilation increases the central venous-to-arterial PCO_2 difference in stable septic shock patients. Ann Intensive Care. 2017;7(1):31.
91. Dar K, Williams T, Aitken R, Woods KL, Fletcher S. Arterial versus capillary sampling for analysing blood gas pressures. BMJ. 1995;310(6971):24–5.
92. Pitkin AD, Roberts CM, Wedzicha JA. Arterialised earlobe blood gas analysis: an underused technique. Thorax. 1994;49(4):364–6.
93. Byrne AL, Bennett M, Chatterji R, Symons R, Pace NL, Thomas PS. Peripheral venous and arterial blood gas analysis in adults: are they comparable? A systematic review and meta-analysis. Respirology. 2014;19(2):168–75.
94. Byrne AL, Bennett MH, Chatterji R, Symons R, Thomas PS. Arterial and venous blood gases in exacerbations of chronic obstructive pulmonary disease. Intern Med J. 2020;50(1):133–4.
95. Nassar BS, Schmidt GA. Estimating arterial partial pressure of carbon dioxide in ventilated patients: how valid are surrogate measures? Ann Am Thorac Soc. 2017;14(6):1005–14.
96. Wang J, Zhang J, Liu Y, Shang H, Peng L, Cui Z. Relationship between end-tidal carbon dioxide and arterial carbon dioxide in critically ill patients on mechanical ventilation: a cross-sectional study. Medicine (Baltimore). 2021;100(33):e26973.
97. Ackrivo J, Geronimo A. Transcutaneous carbon dioxide monitoring in ALS: assessment of hypoventilation heats up. Muscle Nerve. 2022;65(4):371–3.
98. Storre JH, Steurer B, Kabitz HJ, Dreher M, Windisch W. Transcutaneous PCO_2 monitoring during initiation of noninvasive ventilation. Chest. 2007;132(6):1810–6.
99. Bendjelid K, Schutz N, Stotz M, Gerard I, Suter PM, Romand JA. Transcutaneous PCO_2 monitoring in critically ill adults: clinical evaluation of a new sensor. Crit Care Med. 2005;33(10):2203–6.
100. Mari A, Nougue H, Mateo J, Vallet B, Vallee F. Transcutaneous PCO_2 monitoring in critically ill patients: update and perspectives. J Thorac Dis. 2019;11(Suppl 11):S1558–67.
101. Conway A, Tipton E, Liu WH, et al. Accuracy and precision of transcutaneous carbon dioxide monitoring: a systematic review and meta-analysis. Thorax. 2019;74(2):157–63.
102. Delerme S, Montout V, Goulet H, et al. Concordance between transcutaneous and arterial measurements of carbon dioxide in an ED. Am J Emerg Med. 2012;30(9):1872–6.
103. Gancel PE, Roupie E, Guittet L, Laplume S, Terzi N. Accuracy of a transcutaneous carbon dioxide pressure monitoring device in emergency room patients with acute respiratory failure. Intensive Care Med. 2011;37(2):348–51.
104. Nicolini A, Ferrari MB. Evaluation of a transcutaneous carbon dioxide monitor in patients with acute respiratory failure. Ann Thorac Med. 2011;6(4):217–20.
105. McVicar J, Eager R. Validation study of a transcutaneous carbon dioxide monitor in patients in the emergency department. Emerg Med J. 2009;26(5):344–6.
106. Peschanski N, Garcia L, Delasalle E, et al. Can transcutaneous carbon dioxide pressure be a surrogate of blood gas samples for spontaneously breathing emergency patients? The ERNESTO experience. Emerg Med J. 2016;33(5):325–8.
107. Kelly AM, Klim S. Agreement between arterial and venous pH and pCO_2 in patients undergoing non-invasive ventilation in the emergency department. Emerg Med Australas. 2013;25(3):203–6.
108. Ruiz Y, Farrero E, Cordoba A, Gonzalez N, Dorca J, Prats E. Transcutaneous carbon dioxide monitoring in subjects with acute respiratory failure and severe hypercapnia. Respir Care. 2016;61(4):428–33.
109. Cuvelier A, Grigoriu B, Molano LC, Muir JF. Limitations of transcutaneous carbon dioxide measurements for assessing long-term mechanical ventilation. Chest. 2005;127(5):1744–8.
110. Bobbia X, Claret PG, Palmier L, et al. Concordance and limits between transcutaneous and arterial carbon dioxide pressure in emergency department patients with acute respiratory

failure: a single-center prospective observational study. Scand J Trauma Resusc Emerg Med. 2015;23:40.

111. Rodriguez P, Lellouche F, Aboab J, Buisson CB, Brochard L. Transcutaneous arterial carbon dioxide pressure monitoring in critically ill adult patients. Intensive Care Med. 2006;32(2):309–12.

112. Sorensen KM, Leicht RV, Carlsson CJ, et al. Agreement between transcutaneous monitoring and arterial blood gases during COPD exacerbation. Respir Care. 2021;66(10):1560–6.

113. Barneck M, Papa L, Cozart A, et al. The utility of transcutaneous carbon dioxide measurements in the emergency department: a prospective cohort study. J Am Coll Emerg Physicians Open. 2021;2(4):e12513.

114. Georges M, Nguyen-Baranoff D, Griffon L, et al. Usefulness of transcutaneous PCO_2 to assess nocturnal hypoventilation in restrictive lung disorders. Respirology. 2016;21(7):1300–6.

115. Rafiq MK, Bradburn M, Proctor AR, et al. Using transcutaneous carbon dioxide monitor (TOSCA 500) to detect respiratory failure in patients with amyotrophic lateral sclerosis: a validation study. Amyotroph Lateral Scler. 2012;13(6):528–32.

116. Quigg KH, Wilson MW, Choi PJ. Transcutaneous CO_2 monitoring as indication for inpatient non-invasive ventilation initiation in patients with amyotrophic lateral sclerosis. Muscle Nerve. 2022;65(4):444–7.

117. Mokhlesi B, Tulaimat A, Faibussowitsch I, Wang Y, Evans AT. Obesity hypoventilation syndrome: prevalence and predictors in patients with obstructive sleep apnea. Sleep Breath. 2007;11(2):117–24.

118. Manuel ARG, Hart N, Stradling JR. Is a raised bicarbonate, without hypercapnia, part of the physiologic spectrum of obesity-related hypoventilation? Chest. 2015;147(2):362–8.

119. Adrogue HJ, Madias NE. Secondary responses to altered acid-base status: the rules of engagement. J Am Soc Nephrol. 2010;21(6):920–3.

120. Gonzalez SB, Menga G, Raimondi GA, Tighiouart H, Adrogue HJ, Madias NE. Secondary response to chronic respiratory acidosis in humans: a prospective study. Kidney Int Rep. 2018;3(5):1163–70.

Chapter 3
Sleep-Disordered Breathing in Neuromuscular Disease

Elen Gusman and Lisa F. Wolfe

Abbreviations

AASM	American Academy of Sleep Medicine
ALS	Amyotrophic lateral sclerosis
bpm	Breaths per minute
BUR	Backup rate (set respiratory rate)
cwp	cm H_2O pressure
DMD	Duchenne muscular dystrophy
EPAP	Expiratory positive airway pressure
ESS	Epworth Sleepiness Scale
ETCO$_2$	End-tidal pCO_2
HMV	Home mechanical ventilation
IBW	Ideal body weight
IPAP	Inspiratory positive airway pressure
ms	Milliseconds
NIV	Non-invasive ventilation
NMD	Neuromuscular disease
NREM	Non-rapid eye movement
OHS	Obesity hypoventilation syndrome
OSA	Obstructive sleep apnea
PaCO$_2$	Arterial partial pressure of carbon dioxide
PS	Pressure support
PSG	Polysomnography
PVA	Patient-ventilator asynchrony
RAD	Respiratory Assist Device
REM	Rapid eye movement

E. Gusman (✉) · L. F. Wolfe
Division of Pulmonary and Critical Care Medicine, Northwestern Medicine,
Feinberg School of Medicine, Chicago, IL, USA
e-mail: elen.gusman@northwestern.edu; lwolfe@northwestern.edu

N. Lechtzin (ed.), *Pulmonary Complications of Neuromuscular Disease*,
Respiratory Medicine, https://doi.org/10.1007/978-3-031-65335-3_3

RR	Respiratory rate
S/T	Spontaneous/timed
SCI	Spinal cord injury
SDB	Sleep-disordered breathing
SiNQ-5	Sleep-Disordered Breathing in Neuromuscular Disease Questionnaire
$TcCO_2$	Transcutaneous pCO_2
Ti	Inspiratory time
VA	Alveolar ventilation
VAPS	Volume-assured pressure support
VC	Vital capacity
Vt	Tidal volume

Natural History of Hypoventilation in Neuromuscular Disease-Related Sleep

Respiratory failure in patients with NMD occurs due to respiratory muscle weakness accompanied by an increased respiratory load leading to ineffective ventilation [1]. This can occur acutely as in the case of Guillain–Barre syndrome or myasthenia gravis crisis, or it can develop over time—starting over night during sleep and then progressing throughout the day—as in muscular dystrophies or progressive motor neuron disease. This chapter will focus primarily on the latter, with a specific focus on Duchenne muscular dystrophy (DMD) and amyotrophic lateral sclerosis (ALS). However, the topics described are applicable to many forms of NMD. Table 3.1 provides a list of NMD that are at the greatest risk for developing SDB [2, 3].

Night-Time Symptoms Precede Daytime Symptoms

The most common form of sleep-disordered breathing in neuromuscular disease (NMD) is alveolar hypoventilation. Nocturnal hypoventilation and night-time symptoms precede the development of daytime symptoms and subsequent hypercapnic respiratory failure.

In healthy individuals, respiratory physiology during sleep is markedly different compared to respiratory physiology during wakefulness. Firstly, positional changes that occur during supine sleep affect respiratory mechanics in several distinct ways. Functional residual capacity (FRC, or the volume that remains in the lungs after a passive exhalation) is reduced in the supine position compared to the upright position, due to the relative inability of the chest wall to expand and counter increased abdominal distention [4, 5]. Upper airway structures that often contain redundant soft tissue are more prone to collapse in the supine position, which leads to an increase in upper airway resistance during sleep [4]. This is further compounded by the concurrent loss of muscle tone that occurs during rapid eye movement (REM) sleep, which will be discussed further in the next section. Additionally, minute

Table 3.1 Overview of neuromuscular and thoracic restrictive diseases at the greatest risk for sleep-disordered breathing

- Myopathies
  - Duchenne muscular dystrophy (DMD)
  - Myotonic dystrophies
  - Acid maltase deficiency (Pompe disease)
  - Limb-girdle muscular dystrophy
  - Congenital, mitochondrial, ion channel myopathies
- Anterior horn cell/motor neuron disease
  - Amyotrophic lateral sclerosis (ALS)
  - Spinal muscular atrophy
  - Post-polio syndrome
- Neuromuscular junction disorders
  - Myasthenia gravis
  - Botulism
- Peripheral nerve disorders
  - Guillain–Barre syndrome
  - Phrenic nerve diseases
- Spinal cord injury
- Thoracic cage abnormalities
  - Pectus excavatum, pectus carinatum
  - Scoliosis, kyphosis

ventilation decreases (via a tidal volume decrease) during sleep. Finally, during sleep, there is decreased chemosensitivity to hypercapnia, such that a higher CO_2 threshold is required to trigger central respiratory drive during sleep [4–6].

In patients with neuromuscular disease, night-time symptoms precede the development of daytime symptoms because the normal physiologic respiratory changes that occur during sleep are amplified. Since neuromuscular disorders represent a heterogenous group of illnesses, the underlying pathophysiology of each varies. Sleep-disordered breathing in NMD can occur due to an exaggerated reduction in lung volumes during supine sleep and profound respiratory muscle, particularly diaphragmatic, weakness [7]. Thoracic wall restriction (skeletal muscle deformities and scoliosis) can also contribute. Specific characteristics of NMD, such as pharyngeal neuropathy or weakness, macroglossia, and bulbar dysfunction, can further predispose patients to develop upper airway obstruction leading to obstructive events [7, 8]. Finally, SDB in NMD can also manifest as decreased chemosensitivity leading to decreased ventilatory response and blunted arousal thresholds despite hypercapnia [9, 10].

Night-time symptoms may manifest as sleep fragmentation, arousals, headaches, orthopnea, nocturnal sweating, vivid dreams, nightmares, or waking with a panic sensation [3, 11]. If these symptoms are not recognized early, the disease progresses and daytime symptoms ensue [12]. Nocturnal hypoventilation and sleep-disordered breathing ultimately lead to daytime hypercapnia, which causes excessive daytime sleepiness, daytime headaches, difficulty concentrating, and decreased stamina and endurance [13, 14]. Other daytime symptoms that develop are disease-specific. Manifestations of muscle weakness may include impaired cough with difficulty clearing secretions, difficulty swallowing with choking, and exhaustion with eating causing weight loss. It is important to recognize the early signs of SDB and initiate non-invasive ventilation when indicated prior to the development of debilitating daytime symptoms and overt respiratory failure [13].

REM Symptoms Precede Non-REM Symptoms

Night-time symptoms initially develop during rapid eye movement (REM) sleep, but as neuromuscular disease progresses, symptoms become evident in non-rapid eye movement (NREM) sleep as well. During REM sleep, chest wall excursion becomes dependent on preserved diaphragm function. This is due to a normal loss of muscle tone during REM sleep that profoundly affects intercostal and accessory respiratory muscles while sparing the diaphragm [7, 15]. As diaphragm weakness progresses, patients with NMD become more dependent on these respiratory muscles for ventilation. Physiologic atonia during REM occurs due to γ-aminobutyric acid and glycinergic-mediated inhibition, leading to reduced excitation of motor neurons [16]. Since this atonia occurs during REM, it is precisely during REM sleep that nocturnal hypoventilation occurs and symptoms first develop [2, 17]. Due to these mechanisms, hypoventilation in REM sleep will be noted as central apnea, in part due to failure of central drive and in part due to failure of muscle performance. As neuromuscular disease progresses and vital capacity (VC, the maximal volume of air that can be expired following maximum inspiration) further declines, hypoventilation progresses to NREM sleep.

Understanding the natural history of the progression of hypoventilation in NMD-related sleep is essential as it is by having this knowledge that providers can ensure timely recognition, diagnosis, and intervention in order to improve quality of life and potentially prolong survival for these patients.

Sleep-Disordered Breathing in Duchenne Muscular Dystrophy: REM-Related Obstructive Sleep Apnea Precedes Muscular Weakness

In Duchenne muscular dystrophy (DMD), mutations in the dystrophin gene lead to progressive cardiac and skeletal muscle degeneration that culminates in the loss of independent ambulation, which typically occurs in the teenage years. The long-term use of oral glucocorticoids, such as deflazacort, as well as cardioprotective medications, significantly prolong the lives of patients with DMD. These patients are now surviving into their 40s. Important to their long-term management is the use of NIV and cough assist devices, as well as the early recognition and treatment of malnutrition and respiratory infections [2].

Interestingly, the long-term use of oral glucocorticoids has altered the natural history of DMD and other dystrophinopathies. Chronic corticosteroid therapy has been shown to prolong ambulation by 2–5 years, preserve cardiopulmonary function, delay the need for assisted ventilation, and increase quality of life and survival [18]. This delay in the onset of significant weakness allows for paraspinal muscles to be preserved, severely reducing the risk of developing scoliosis. Scoliosis, in the past, had a significant impact on hypoventilation but is no longer as common.

Unfortunately, chronic steroid use, in conjunction with progressive physical inactivity and immobilization, leads to excessive weight gain. This weight gain then predisposes young patients with DMD to develop obstructive sleep apnea (OSA) [2, 18–21]. As a result, younger patients (8–14 years old) with DMD develop sleep-disordered breathing in the form of OSA, while older patients develop nocturnal hypoventilation due to progressive respiratory muscle, particularly diaphragmatic, weakness [19, 21, 22]. As DMD progresses, the diaphragm becomes progressively weaker until it follows a pattern of paradoxical movement, moving upward with inspiration instead of downward, thus leading to a progressively reduced tidal volume (Vt) in the supine position [21].

How to Elicit Sleep-Related History in Patients with Neuromuscular Disease

A typical sleep-related history in the general population includes questions about the presence of snoring, nocturnal choking or gasping, morning headaches, and excessive daytime sleepiness as a reflection of night-time sleep disturbance [23, 24]. The Epworth Sleepiness Scale (ESS)—a questionnaire that is routinely used to assess daytime sleepiness in patients with OSA—has respondents rate their typical chances of dozing off during a variety of activities [25]. In individuals with neuromuscular disease, this type of questionnaire does not adequately capture the symptoms they may experience. Symptoms may be non-specific, thus patients are less likely to recognize and report them to providers. Thus, a thorough tailored history is required in order to elicit evidence of sleep-disordered breathing in patients with NMD (Table 3.2).

A sleep-related history tailored for patients with NMD should focus on breathlessness since this may develop long before daytime sleepiness and fatigue. Providers should explore whether the patient experiences breathlessness in three particular situations: (1) in the supine position (orthopnea), (2) when bending forward (for instance, to tie shoelaces), and (3) when immersed in water [26]. The Sleep-Disordered Breathing in Neuromuscular Disease Questionnaire (SiNQ-5), which was designed by Steier et al., includes these three questions about breathlessness, and also asks about the following: (4) changes in position when in bed (such as sleeping more upright) and (5) changes in sleep (such as increased waking up, getting up, or poor sleep quality). These focused questions can elicit the presence of

Table 3.2 Focused sleep-related history to elicit symptoms of sleep-disordered breathing in patients with neuromuscular disease

- Breathlessness when supine, bending forward, or immersed in water
- Sleep fragmentation: Frequent night-time awakenings and arousals
- Early morning or nocturnal headaches
- Vivid dreams
- Nightmares
- Nocturnal sweating
- Waking with a panic sensation
- Daytime fatigue or decreased stamina

diaphragmatic weakness and early signs of SDB before any overt signs of respiratory failure develop. With a maximum score of ten, a cut-off of five or more points in the SINQ-5 was shown to have a sensitivity of 86.2% and a specificity of 88.5% to identify SDB in NMD patients [26, 27]. One limitation is that this questionnaire cannot be used in patients who have already developed limb and trunk paralysis [28].

In addition to symptoms of respiratory compromise and sleep-disordered breathing, it is also important to ask NMD patients about neuropathic and musculoskeletal pain, which can occur due to rigidity, spasticity, and immobility, as this can be a significant contributor to sleep disruption [3, 29]. A patient-tailored screen for possible comorbid sleep disorders should also inquire about the following symptoms: (1) dream enactment (suggestive of REM sleep behavior disorder or a non-REM parasomnia); (2) cataplexy, hypnagogic, or hypnopompic hallucinations (narcolepsy); (3) excessive worry about sleep, mind racing, hyperarousal (insomnia); (4) excessive daytime sleepiness despite adequate sleep (hypersomnia); and (5) leg discomfort with an irresistible urge to move (restless leg syndrome) [3, 24].

Use of Polysomnography in Neuromuscular Disease

Necessary Accommodations in the Sleep Lab for Patients with Disabilities

While in-lab polysomnography (PSG) remains the gold standard for diagnosing sleep-disordered breathing, there are certain difficulties that patients with disabilities may encounter in the sleep lab. Necessary accommodations for patients with difficulty ambulating include ensuring wheelchair access, the presence of a ceiling lift, a hospital bed, a bedside commode or accessible bathroom, and suction. It is also essential to have an adaptive call system to allow effective communication, specially trained staff members, and caregiver space if needed. Unfortunately, it is not standard of care for sleep laboratories to provide these accommodations, which makes it difficult for NMD patients with physical disabilities to undergo in-lab PSG.

Requirements for Assessing Sleep-Disordered Breathing in Neuromuscular Disease

In-lab PSG allows for a comprehensive assessment of sleep-disordered breathing. In-lab PSG includes video monitoring in addition to the following channels: electroencephalogram (EEG) that evaluates sleep stage, electrooculogram (EOG) that analyzes eye movements, electromyogram (EMG) that captures muscle tone and limb movements, and electrocardiogram (ECG) that detects cardiac rate and rhythm. In-lab PSG also includes an oronasal thermal airflow sensor (to detect apneas, or complete airflow obstruction) and a nasal pressure transducer (to detect hypopneas, or partial airflow limitation), in addition to thoracoabdominal belt signals (to detect respiratory effort to distinguish between central and obstructive events) and a pulse oximeter. A body position sensor and a snoring sensor are also typically included [30].

For patients with NMD, additional considerations for monitoring SDB are necessary. Since oxygen desaturation is not a reliable marker of hypoventilation in NMD, carbon dioxide measurement is essential to assess for hypoventilation and monitor efficacy of NIV [31]. The arterial partial pressure of carbon dioxide ($PaCO_2$) can be measured directly; however, capnography can be used as an acceptable alternative. The AASM recommends that acceptable surrogate markers are transcutaneous pCO_2 ($TcCO_2$) or end-tidal pCO_2 ($ETCO_2$) (for a diagnostic study) or $TcCO_2$ (for a titration study) [32]. Adequately calibrated $TcCO_2$ monitoring in patients who are hemodynamically stable has been shown to correlate well with arterial pCO_2 ($PaCO_2$) measurements [2, 13, 33, 34]. While $ETCO_2$ correlates well with $PaCO_2$ in individuals with healthy lung volumes, it is not an accurate surrogate for $PaCO_2$ in NMD patients who have small Vt and therefore inaccurate end-tidal readings.

In addition to capnography to allow for additional CO_2 monitoring, it is important to include measurement of respiratory effort and accessory muscle use to properly identify the etiology of SDB in NMD. Diaphragm electromyography, esophageal pressure monitoring, or pulse transit time can all be used as surrogate markers for inspiratory muscle effort [15, 35, 36]. See Table 3.3.

Diagnostic Standards in Polysomnography

Apneas and Hypopneas

When scoring polysomnography, an apnea is defined as a drop in the peak signal excursion of $\geq$90% from baseline that lasts at least 10 s. This signal can be measured via an oronasal thermal sensor (as in the case of a diagnostic study) or via a positive airway pressure device flow (as in the case of a titration study) [32]. The classification of an apnea as obstructive, central, or mixed is based on respiratory effort. An absence of flow despite the presence of effort indicates an obstructive event, while an absence of both flow and effort indicates a central event. A

Table 3.3 Polysomnography for patients with neuromuscular disease

Channel/monitoring device	Purpose: to monitor…
Electroencephalogram	Sleep stage, arousals, and epileptiform activity
Electrooculogram	Eye movements (assist in determining sleep stage)
Electromyogram	Muscle tone and limb movements
Electrocardiogram	Cardiac arrythmias
Oronasal thermal airflow sensor	Apnea (complete airflow obstruction)
Nasal pressure transducer	Hypopnea (partial airflow limitation)
Thoracoabdominal belt signal	Respiratory effort (to distinguish between central and obstructive events)
Pulse oximetry	Oxygen desaturation
CO_2 monitoring: • Arterial pCO_2, or • Transcutaneous CO_2, or • End-tidal CO_2	Hypercapnia
Inspiratory muscle monitoring options: • Diaphragm electromyography, or • Esophageal pressure monitoring, or • Pulse transit time	Inspiratory muscle effort
Body position sensor	Body position
Video monitoring	Movement disorders, parasomnias

hypopnea is defined as a drop in flow $\geq$30% from baseline that lasts at least 10 s and is associated with a $\geq$3% oxygen desaturation or is associated with an arousal. Of note, the Medicare-accepted definition of a hypopnea requires a $\geq$4% oxygen desaturation [32].

Evaluating Nocturnal Hypoventilation for Neuromuscular Diseases

In patients with NMD, discrete respiratory events, such as apnea and hypopneas, can be quite low [2]. Thus, it is important to evaluate nocturnal hypoventilation in NMD patients with suspected SDB.

A saw-tooth pattern on PSG—a waveform with prominent variability of oxygen desaturation in phasic REM sleep (during bursts of rapid eye movements)—may represent the earliest manifestation of respiratory muscle weakness [7, 37]. However, it is important to note that desaturation events in NMD patients are not specific and do not necessarily indicate hypoventilation. Desaturations may reflect sleep-disordered breathing, but they may also reflect low lung volumes and/or atelectasis [7]. Thoracoabdominal paradox frequently occurs in association with these low lung volumes and can be noted both during sleep and wakefulness. In PSG for NMD, it is important to consider that not all thoracoabdominal paradox is a result of upper airway obstruction.

Alternatively, normal oxygen saturation levels may be present despite nocturnal hypoventilation [7]. Since the oxyhemoglobin dissociation curve is characterized by a sigmoid shape, pulse oximetry can be relatively insensitive for detecting significant decreases in PaO_2 above 55–60 mmHg, so episodes of hypoventilation can be missed [38].

Early and moderate SDB in NMD patients is typically characterized by frequent arousals and awakenings, but as the severity of sleep hypoventilation progresses, the frequency of arousals and awakenings decreases significantly. In severe SDB, arousals occur only with prolonged desaturations, and REM (polysomnography: diagnostic standards) sleep is typically difficult to score due to the frequency of arousals and events [2].

Different Definitions of Hypoventilation

There are multiple different definitions of hypoventilation. The prevalence of hypoventilation in NMD varies widely depending on the definition used [39–41]. The American Academy of Sleep Medicine (AASM) defines nocturnal hypoventilation in adults as follows: (1) There is an increase in the $PaCO_2$, or surrogate, to a value >55 mmHg for $\geq$10 min; or (2) There is $\geq$10 mmHg increase in $PaCO_2$, or surrogate, during sleep in comparison to an awake supine state, to a value exceeding 50 mmHg for $\geq$10 min. When this first definition is used, the prevalence of nocturnal hypoventilation despite daytime normocapnia in NMD is 4%. When the second definition is used, the prevalence increases to 9% [15]. In pediatric patients, hypoventilation is scored when the $PaCO_2$ is >50 mmHg for >25% of total sleep time [11, 32]. Nocturnal hypoventilation has also been defined as a mean pCO_2 >50 mmHg [11], or a peak $TcCO_2$ $\geq$6.5 kPa, which corresponds to a $TcCO_2$ $\geq$48.8 mmHg [13]. Peak $TcCO_2$ $\geq$48.8 mmHg has been demonstrated as the best predictor of NMD patients requiring home mechanical ventilator (HMV) initiation over the next few years (Table 3.4) [42].

The Medicare Respiratory Assist Device (RAD) Guidelines define hypoventilation as the following: (1) Initial awake arterial pCO_2 $\geq$45 mmHg; (2) spirometry with FEV1/FVC $\geq$70%; and (3) $PaCO_2$ during sleep or immediately upon awakening that increases by $\geq$7 mmHg compared to the initial value, or an in-lab polysomnography or home sleep apnea test that demonstrates O_2 $\leq$ 88% for $\geq$5 min and is not caused by obstructive events [43]. While this last parameter may be validated in OSA, pulse oximetry is insufficient in identifying hypoventilation in NMD patients

Table 3.4 Different transcutaneous CO_2 cut-off values to define hypoventilation

AASM	T_cCO_2 >55 mmHg for $\geq$10 min, or increase in T_cCO_2 $\geq$10 mmHg to at least 50 mmHg for $\geq$10 min
Ward	Peak T_cCO_2 $\geq$49 mmHg[a]
Simonds	Mean pCO_2 >50 mmHg

[a] Use peak T_cCO_2 $\geq$49 mmHg as one of the criteria for initiating HMV in NMD patients

since alveolar hypoventilation is rarely accompanied by ventilation-perfusion mismatch given the absence of parenchymal lung disease [44, 45].

Scoring Polysomnography

Pseudo-Obstructive and Pseudo-Central Events

According to the AASM manual for scoring sleep-disordered breathing, events are likely obstructive when the following conditions are met: (1) flow limitation on a thermal airflow sensor or nasal pressure transducer, (2) phase opposition (i.e. paradoxical movement) in the thoracoabdominal belt signal, (3) Snoring, or (4) the event terminates in an arousal [15, 32]. Events are likely central when characterized by the following: (1) they are associated with periodic breathing, (2) arousals occur at the peak of ventilation (rather than at the resumption of ventilation), and (3) there is typically a proportional and simultaneous decrease in thoracic and abdominal belt signals without phase opposition [15].

The presence of diaphragmatic and other respiratory muscle impairment in NMD can present a significant challenge in determining the exact etiology of sleep-disordered breathing. As a result, scoring polysomnography in NMD requires special attention to the presence of possible pseudo-obstructive and pseudo-central events. Pseudo-obstructive events can be identified due to paradoxical thoracoabdominal movement (a feature that is typically used to define obstructive events) but can occur in NMD without any upper airway narrowing due to progressive diaphragm weakness [7].

Obstructive apneas may be misclassified as central apneas in NMD due to respiratory muscle (particularly diaphragmatic) weakness [7, 29, 46]. Upper airway obstruction (due to pharyngeal hypotonia, bulbar dysfunction, macroglossia, glottic closures) may be due to muscle weakness, but may also be due to factors such as overventilation, pharyngeal spasticity with lack of muscle control, and/or insufficient Vt to maintain adequate critical opening pressure. This may leave a sleep physician with a quandary—should the pressures be increased or decreased in the setting of upper airway collapse? In this case, a titration study may be necessary to find the most successful settings for any given patient. Trials of decreased expiratory pressure, increased pressure support, decreased pressure support, or change in respiratory rate could be considered. Non-ventilation-related strategies may also be beneficial, such as treatment for bulbar spasticity, reduction in aspiration, and/or addressing other irritants to the upper airway.

Although central drive may remain intact, the presence of REM atonia compounded by diaphragm dysfunction can lead to a complete loss of both chest and abdominal belt excursion on PSG, also creating the appearance of a pseudo-central event [15]. Pseudo-central events and hypoventilation are likely when events occur predominantly during phasic REM sleep and demonstrate a disproportionately greater decrease in thoracic belt excursion relative to abdominal belt excursion [7].

In patients with asymmetric or unilateral diaphragm impairment, positional variability in events and desaturations is more apparent such that SDB events are more prominent in a lateral decubitus position with the least affected side down [7]. In patients who have bilateral loss of diaphragm function, SDB events are more pronounced in the supine position.

How Scoring Polysomnography Differs in Neuromuscular Disease

The severity of obstructive sleep apnea is graded based on apnea-hypopnea indexes (AHI) and the scoring system described in section "Apneas and Hypopneas". Diagnostic standards for scoring PSG to identify SDB in NMD are not as refined, and guidelines vary. In patients with NMD, the apnea-hypopnea indexes and discrete respiratory events can be quite low compared to individuals with sleep apnea [2]. Events can also be misclassified because events reported as obstructive and central may actually be pseudo-obstructive and pseudo-central, considering the factors described above. Due to the underlying pathophysiology of NMD, scoring PSG must rely on identifying hypoventilation rather than recording apneas and hypopneas. Interpreting physicians should be aware that the presence of apnea and hypopnea events does not signify that the disease is obstructive sleep apnea or central sleep apnea—the disease is hypoventilation due to neuromuscular disease. The physician reporting a PSG should reflect this in both their diagnostic interpretation and therapeutic recommendations. A failure to provide appropriate neuromuscular-specific recommendations may generate a disastrous outcome in which insurance and/or referring services may provide an NMD patient with inappropriate treatment, such as CPAP therapy for hypoventilation.

NMD patients with nocturnal hypoventilation can present exclusively with hypercapnia, which may or may not be accompanied by hypoxemia [2]. PSG (scored by age-appropriate AASM criteria) in combination with capnography is the gold standard for assessing SDB and hypoventilation in DMD [20]. Because of the limited use and availability of sleep labs for NMD patients, no standards exist for other diagnoses [47].

Titration of Non-invasive Ventilation with Polysomnography

Location of Non-invasive Ventilation Titration

Non-invasive ventilation (NIV) has revolutionized treatment for sleep-disordered breathing and chronic respiratory failure in patients with NMD. NIV can effectively decrease symptoms related to SDB, decrease number of unplanned hospitalizations, and lead to improvement in quality of life for patients with NMD [48]. Additionally, NIV confers a survival benefit to patients such as those with ALS [49–51]. Despite its substantial benefit, practices for implementation and titration of NIV vary widely depending on multiple factors, including provider training, established protocols, and healthcare system features [52]. NIV can be initiated through polysomnography, capnography-focused hospital-based titration [53], clinic-based PAP-NAP (short daytime sleep studies) [54], or in-home titration [55].

According to the 2010 AASM guidelines, NIV titration with PSG is the recommended method to ensure adequate ventilatory support for patients with chronic alveolar hypoventilation [32]. The guidelines state that when NIV is initiated and titrated empirically in the outpatient setting, a PSG should still be done to make adjustments as necessary and to confirm that final NIV settings are optimized. Using in-lab PSG, providers can use real-time data to identify and correct patient-ventilator asynchrony (PVA), adjust mask interface and optimize leak, and understand how NIV efficacy varies throughout different stages of sleep [2]. If sleep lab titration is not feasible, an alternative monitored setting for NIV initiation and titration is in the hospital under the supervision of trained healthcare providers who can make stepwise adjustments to settings as needed [1, 53].

Despite these recommendations, in-lab PSG may be difficult for patients with NMD to attend due to mobility and positioning issues and given that most laboratories are not equipped to provide the necessary accommodations (as described in section "Requirements for Assessing Sleep-disordered Breathing in Neuromuscular Disease"). In-hospital monitoring and titration can also be logistically impractical, time consuming, and costly to the healthcare system [56]. As a result, it is common for patients with NMD to be initiated on NIV in the office without formal titration, after which close clinical follow-up is essential to ensure adequate ventilation. The development of remote monitoring and cloud applications has facilitated this practice. The advantage is that patients with complex care needs can then trial nighttime NIV at home in a more familiar and comfortable environment with caregiver support [52].

NIV devices have sophisticated built-in software that provides data regarding compliance, leak, and ventilatory support. For instance, the data download includes information about the average pressures required to generate a Vt (indicating pulmonary compliance) and the percentage of breaths spontaneously triggered and cycled (reflecting respiratory muscle weakness and progression of disease). Increases in the respiratory rate (RR) or rapid shallow breathing index (ratio of the RR divided by Vt) may also indicate insufficient ventilatory support. Providers can obtain serial downloads of data and make adjustments to settings remotely. If information from serial downloads is insufficient, it may be possible to use additional monitoring at home, such as transcutaneous capnography (that allows direct measurement of CO_2 levels), nocturnal oximetry, and pulse wave amplitude of the pulse oximetry probe (through which a drop in amplitude correlates with arousals) [57–59]. With advancements in auto-titration software and artificial intelligence, manual titration may not even be needed in the near future [60].

Several studies have evaluated the use of PSG versus in-hospital versus in-clinic and at-home NIV initiation and titration. One study randomized a group of NMD patients with nocturnal hypoventilation—defined as a transcutaneous carbon dioxide ($TcCO_2$) $\geq$49 mmHg—to initiate HMV in the inpatient setting versus the outpatient setting. After a mean inpatient stay of 3.8 days compared to a mean outpatient attendance of 1.2 sessions (out of an available three sessions), they observed a comparable peak nocturnal $TcCO_2$ reduction, oxygen saturation improvement, and compliance [61]. A PAP-NAP study demonstrated that a 4-h ambulatory stay to initiate NIV (instead of in-lab overnight PSG) led to significantly decreased wait time from diagnosis to initiation of NIV from 30 to 13.5 days, without any change in efficacy of ventilation [54].

A study randomized patients with NMD to be initiated on HMV via daytime titration alone or to receive daytime titration followed by night-time PSG titration. The results demonstrated improvement in PVA in the group that received polysomnographic titration of NIV; however, there was no difference in sleep fragmentation between the two groups after 10 weeks of treatment [62]. There were also no differences in any secondary outcomes, including gas exchange ($PaCO_2$ and O_2), sleep quality, sleepiness, and quality of life [57]. Another trial evaluated the efficacy of adaptation (the number of sessions needed) to home-based versus outpatient-based initiation of NIV in ALS patients, and found that home-based initiation was as effective with regards to $PaCO_2$ levels, NIV acceptance, and adherence [63].

Is Diagnostic Testing Needed in a Sleep Lab? Alternative Measurements of Respiratory Muscle Strength

Vital capacity (VC) directly correlates with respiratory muscle strength, thus it can be used as an early predictor for the presence of SDB, nocturnal hypoventilation, and daytime hypercapnia in patients with NMD [7, 17]. Decreased expiratory muscle strength leads to an increase in residual volume, which results in an early decline in VC as the total lung capacity remains preserved. Ragette et al. identified that a VC <60% of predicted consistently correlated with the onset of SDB. Therefore, it is these patients who should be referred for PSG. Patients with a VC <40% of predicted were found to have progressed to hypoventilation in both REM and NREM sleep [17]. For patients with scoliosis in whom true height is difficult to establish, arm span or ulnar length can be used to predict normal spirometry values [11].

Evaluation of upright and supine values is particularly valuable for assessing respiratory muscle weakness in NMD patients. A forced vital capacity (FVC) decrease from upright to supine by 8–10% is seen in healthy individuals. Diaphragmatic weakness leads to a further reduction in VC in the supine position, such that a decrease by >25% is 90% sensitive and 79% specific for diaphragm weakness [64, 65].

The maximal inspiratory pressure (MIP) is another non-invasive test in which patients are asked to perform a forceful inspiration (that follows a complete expiration to residual volume) with an open glottis against an occluded mouthpiece. MIP is a measure of global inspiratory muscle strength, correlating closely with diaphragmatic strength since the diaphragm is the major inspiratory muscle [66, 67]. In patients with ALS, MIP was found to predict diaphragm weakness prior to any significant decrease in FVC [68]. While MIP can be an excellent predictor of diaphragm dysfunction, it is important to consider that suboptimal patient effort, as well as issues with patient-device interface (bulbar or facial weakness leading to inability to form a good seal) can affect the measurement [66].

The sniff inspiratory pressure (SNIP) has also been suggested as an additional or alternative non-invasive test for measuring inspiratory respiratory muscle strength. SNIP can be particularly useful in the setting of bulbar dysfunction, facial weakness, or dental malocclusion, which may lead to MIP test inaccuracy [66]. It involves occluding one nostril and asking the patient to take short, sharp inspiratory sniffs that are measured through the contralateral nostril [69]. The SNIP was found to correlate with decline in respiratory muscle function in motor neuron disease or ALS without significant bulbar disease [11, 70]. It is important to keep in mind that SNIP has limitations, such as underestimating inspiratory muscle strength in patients with severe nasal obstructive or obstructive airway disease [66].

Based on CMS criteria, there are four criteria to guide initiation of NIV for patients with restrictive thoracic disorders (including patients with NMD): (1) Forced vital capacity (FVC) <50% of predicted (upright or supine), (2) Maximal inspiratory pressure (MIP) $\leq$60 cm H_2O (upright or supine), (3) $PaCO_2$ >45 mmHg; or (4) overnight nocturnal desaturation <88% for 5 min [43].

Because spirometry, MIP, and CO_2 testing can all be used as early markers of hypoventilation, diagnostic testing within the sleep lab may not be necessary in most adult patients if a significant deficit has already been established. This may not be the case in pediatric patients. As such, in-lab diagnostic testing in NMD is most often performed in children.

Titration Protocols for Technologists: Nuts and Bolts

Titration and adjustment of NIV settings are essential to decrease and optimize NIV efficacy. Since many NMD patients have diaphragm weakness, one of the most common forms of PVA is ineffective triggering, which is a form of trigger asynchrony [1, 71]. In addition, respiratory muscle weakness often leads to premature cycling-off of respiratory events [55].

Prior to troubleshooting and making any adjustments to settings, a proper mask fitting should take place to minimize leak. The presence of unintentional mask leak can lead to several issues: (1) increase trigger sensitivity (leading to missed trigger efforts) or decrease trigger sensitivity (leading to auto-triggering), (2) lower the effective EPAP (leading to increased upper airway resistance and ineffective ventilation), or (3) prevent device cycling by inhibiting the expected inspiratory peak flow decline [1]. In addition to providing proper education, providers should ensure careful mask fitting and a period of acclimatization to low pressure settings prior to NIV titration [32]. The following sections will provide detailed titration protocols for both fixed (bilevel spontaneous/timed) and targeted (volume-assured pressure support) modes (Table 3.5). For a more complete description of each available mode, please see 'Modes of Ventilation' in the Ventilatory Support for the Neuromuscular Patient: Noninvasive and Invasive chapter by Drs. Carmona, Graustein, and Benditt.

Bilevel Spontaneous/Timed (S/T)

In a fixed Bi-level Spontaneous/Timed (S/T) mode, the device will provide pressure support in order to augment any breath that is initiated by the patient (spontaneous), and it will also provide device-delivered breaths (timed) if the patient's RR falls below the set backup rate. The following major settings are set: back up respiratory rate (BUR), inspiratory positive airway pressure (IPAP), and expiratory positive airway pressure (EPAP). On a Respironics device, the minor settings that are set are inspiratory time (Ti) and rise. On a Resmed device, the minor settings set are the minimum inspiratory time (Ti min), maximum inspiratory time (Ti max), trigger, cycle, and rise.

Titration of S/T mode includes the following: (1) Begin with a EPAP minimum 4 cm H_2O (cwp) and a IPAP minimum 8 cwp (2). Provide incremental increases in IPAP and EPAP until obstructive respiratory events are eliminated as follows: increase EPAP by 1 cwp for obstructive apneas; increase IPAP by ≥ 2 cwp for hypopneas, respiratory effort-related arousals, hypercapnia, and hypoxia. Please be aware that increasing IPAP is most efficiently and appropriately achieved by responding to tachypnea. Tachypnea best reflects small Vt and technologists should

Table 3.5 In-lab titration protocol

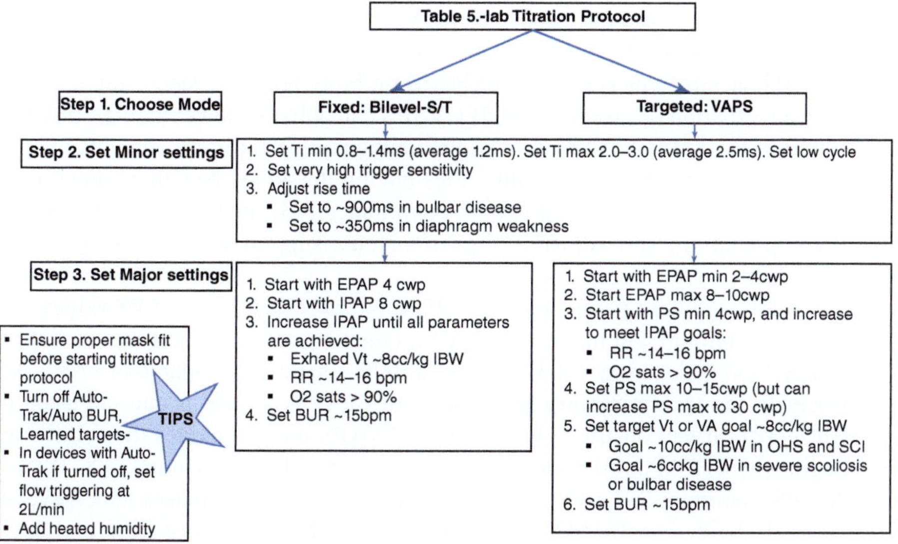

be aware that if the RR is >14–16 breaths per minute (bpm), increase in IPAP is needed. For NMD patients, low EPAP is necessary to reduce work of breathing because a higher EPAP reduces a patient's ability to trigger. In addition, technologists should be encouraged to keep the EPAP low as this will further enhance the pressure support spread, therefore augmenting delivered Vt. Too often, technologists have been trained to maintain an IPAP to EPAP difference of 4 so encouraging technologists to spread the difference may be a challenge. It is important to keep in mind that a higher EPAP may be needed for NMD patients with a history of OSA.

Increase Pressure support (PS) every 5 min to achieve target exhaled Vt, which is typically 8 cc/kg of ideal body weight (IBW) in NMD patients. PS should also be increased until the RR is approximately 14–16 bpm in adults (or 16–18 bpm in children) and SpO_2 saturations are >90%. AASM recommends a maximum IPAP 30 cwp (for adults >12 year old) or 20 cwp (for children <12 year old), and a PS minimum 4 cwp and PS maximum 20 cwp. For all patients with central hypoventilation and those who cannot reliably trigger breaths due to muscle weakness, the device must be set up with a backup rate (BUR). The starting BUR should be equal to or slightly less than the spontaneous RR during sleep, at a minimum of 10 bpm but typically 15 bpm [32, 72]. If the patient awakens and reports that the IPAP and/or EPAP feel too high, the pressure should be lowered to a more comfortable level until the patient can sleep. Incremental adjustments should then be reattempted while giving the patient time to acclimate. Heated humidification can be added to assist with nasal dryness or congestion.

Volume-Assured Pressure Support (VAPS)

Volume-assured pressure support (VAPS is an advanced mode designed to maintain a target ventilation goal or target Vt by providing variable pressure support that is automatically adjusted from breath to breath. VAPS is often preferred in NMD patients as it can achieve a more consistently reliable Vt despite changes in pressure support (PS) needs, which may occur based on body position, sleep stage, and/or disease exacerbation or progression [55]. VAPS can deliver a lower median IPAP, as compared to that set in S/T mode, while reaching equivalent improvements in nocturnal gas exchange and sleep quality, thus having the added benefit of potentially increased comfort and improved patient compliance [73]. In NMD patients, VAPS mode can potentially self-adjust settings to increase support as disease progression occurs [73].

The following major parameters in VAPS mode are set: a range of PS values that allow for a minimum and maximum IPAP, a target Vt or target alveolar ventilation [VA = RR * (Vt − dead space)], EPAP, and a BUR. On devices capable of VAPS-AE (auto-EPAP) mode, a minimum and maximum EPAP is set and is auto-adjusted to prevent upper airway obstruction. Titration of VAPS mode includes the following: (1) Begin with a EPAP minimum of 2–4 cwp, and set a EPAP maximum of 8–10 cwp (2). Set PS minimum at 4 cwp, and provide incremental PS increases to achieve an RR of 14–16 bpm, an exhaled Vt target of approximately 8 cc/kg of IBW, and SpO_2

saturation goal >90% (3). Start with a PS maximum of 10–15 cwp as this is typically the setting that is most commonly tolerated, but this can be increased to 30 cwp if needed (4). Set target Vt or alveolar ventilation goal: this is typically set to 8 cc/kg IBW, but it can be increased to 10 cc/kg IBW in obesity hypoventilation syndrome (OHS) or in spinal cord injury (SCI), or it can be decreased to 6 cc/kg IBW in severe scoliosis or bulbar disease (5). Set BUR to approximately 15 bpm, and increase BUR as needed in order to address PVA.

Whether it is in Bilevel-ST or VAPS mode, it is important to match NIV settings to the patient's underlying respiratory physiology to optimize patient comfort and patient-ventilator synchrony. Adjustments should be made to the following minor settings: (1) inspiratory time or cycle sensitivity, (2) trigger sensitivity (the inspiratory effort the patient needs to exert before the breath is augmented by the ventilator), and (3) rise time (the speed at which the inspiratory pressure increases to reach the set target pressure). For NMD patients, set Ti min between 0.8 and 1.4 ms (with an average of 1.2 ms), and Ti max from 2.0 to 3.0 ms (with an average of 2.5 ms). A long inspiratory time (or high inspiratory: expiratory ratio) and very low cycle sensitivity (late cycle) are recommended to provide a longer inhalation time in order to maximize Vt and gas exchange [1]. Set a very high trigger sensitivity so the patient with weak respiratory muscle effort needs to exert a minimal inspiratory effort before the breath is augmented by the device. Adjust rise time to enhance patient comfort. For patients with bulbar disease, set a rise time of approximately 900 ms; for patients with predominantly diaphragm weakness, set a rise time of approximately 350 ms. If the patient continues to use accessory muscles to breath—particularly if their shoulders are rising—decrease the rise time.

Importantly, NIV devices have embedded automatic software algorithms designed to adjust to changing breathing patterns and dynamic leaks in order to improve patient-ventilator synchrony. When titrating NIV for patients with NMD, it is essential to turn off these automatic settings as follows: (1) turn off Auto-Trak and auto backup rate in Respironics; (2) turn off learned targets in ResMed. This is because these automatic settings are designed to treat OSA but if used in the inappropriate context, the software will train the device to mimic the ineffective tachypnea and rapid shallow breathing pattern that prevails in neuromuscular disease.

References

1. Selim BJ, Wolfe L, Coleman JM III, Dewan NA. Initiation of noninvasive ventilation for sleep related hypoventilation disorders: advanced modes and devices. Chest. 2018;153(1):251–65. https://doi.org/10.1016/j.chest.2017.06.036. PubMed PMID: 28694199. Epub 20170708.
2. Grigg-Damberger MM, Wagner LK, Brown LK. Sleep hypoventilation in patients with neuromuscular diseases. Sleep Med Clin. 2012;7(4):667–87. https://doi.org/10.1016/j.jsmc.2012.09.001.
3. Fermin AM, Afzal U, Culebras A. Sleep in neuromuscular diseases. Sleep Med Clin. 2016;11(1):53–64. https://doi.org/10.1016/j.jsmc.2015.10.005. PubMed PMID: 26972033. Epub 20160109.

4. Newton K, Malik V, Lee-Chiong T. Sleep and breathing. Clin Chest Med. 2014;35(3):451–6. https://doi.org/10.1016/j.ccm.2014.06.001. PubMed PMID: 25156761. Epub 20140729.

5. Malik V, Smith D, Lee-Chiong T. Respiratory physiology during sleep. Sleep Med Clin. 2012;7(3):497–505. https://doi.org/10.1016/j.jsmc.2012.06.011.

6. Böing S, Randerath WJ. Chronic hypoventilation syndromes and sleep-related hypoventilation. J Thorac Dis. 2015;7(8):1273–85. https://doi.org/10.3978/j.issn.2072-1439.2015.06.10. PubMed PMID: 26380756; PubMed Central PMCID: PMC4561264.

7. Aboussouan LS. Sleep-disordered breathing in neuromuscular disease. Am J Respir Crit Care Med. 2015;191(9):979–89. https://doi.org/10.1164/rccm.201412-2224CI. PubMed PMID: 25723731.

8. Wenninger S, Jones HN. Hypoventilation syndrome in neuromuscular disorders. Curr Opin Neurol. 2021;34(5):686–96. https://doi.org/10.1097/wco.0000000000000973. PubMed PMID: 34231549.

9. Caruana-Montaldo B, Gleeson K, Zwillich CW. The control of breathing in clinical practice. Chest. 2000;117(1):205–25. https://doi.org/10.1378/chest.117.1.205. PubMed PMID: 10631221.

10. Johnson DC, Kazemi H. Central control of ventilation in neuromuscular disease. Clin Chest Med. 1994;15(4):607–17. PubMed PMID: 7867278.

11. Simonds AK. Chronic hypoventilation and its management. Eur Respir Rev. 2013;22(129):325–32. https://doi.org/10.1183/09059180.00003113. PubMed PMID: 23997060; PubMed Central PMCID: PMC9487351.

12. Pfeffer G, Povitz M. Respiratory management of patients with neuromuscular disease: current perspectives. Degener Neurol Neuromuscul Dis. 2016;6:111–8. https://doi.org/10.2147/dnnd.S87323. PubMed PMID: 30050373; PubMed Central PMCID: PMC6053085. Epub 20161118.

13. Ward S, Chatwin M, Heather S, Simonds AK. Randomised controlled trial of non-invasive ventilation (NIV) for nocturnal hypoventilation in neuromuscular and chest wall disease patients with daytime normocapnia. Thorax. 2005;60(12):1019–24. https://doi.org/10.1136/thx.2004.037424. PubMed PMID: 16299118; PubMed Central PMCID: PMC1747266.

14. Boentert M. Sleep disturbances in patients with amyotrophic lateral sclerosis: current perspectives. Nat Sci Sleep. 2019;11:97–111. https://doi.org/10.2147/nss.S183504. PubMed PMID: 31496852; PubMed Central PMCID: PMC6701267. Epub 20190809.

15. Aboussouan LS, Mireles-Cabodevila E. Sleep-disordered breathing in neuromuscular disease: diagnostic and therapeutic challenges. Chest. 2017;152(4):880–92. https://doi.org/10.1016/j.chest.2017.03.023. PubMed PMID: 28372949. Epub 20170331.

16. Brooks PL, Peever JH. Identification of the transmitter and receptor mechanisms responsible for REM sleep paralysis. J Neurosci. 2012;32(29):9785–95. https://doi.org/10.1523/jneurosci.0482-12.2012. PubMed PMID: 22815493; PubMed Central PMCID: PMC6621291.

17. Ragette R, Mellies U, Schwake C, Voit T, Teschler H. Patterns and predictors of sleep disordered breathing in primary myopathies. Thorax. 2002;57(8):724–8. https://doi.org/10.1136/thorax.57.8.724. PubMed PMID: 12149535; PubMed Central PMCID: PMC1746391.

18. Moxley RT III, Pandya S, Ciafaloni E, Fox DJ, Campbell K. Change in natural history of Duchenne muscular dystrophy with long-term corticosteroid treatment: implications for management. J Child Neurol. 2010;25(9):1116–29. https://doi.org/10.1177/0883073810371004. PubMed PMID: 20581335. Epub 20100625.

19. Sawnani H, Thampratankul L, Szczesniak RD, Fenchel MC, Simakajornboon N. Sleep disordered breathing in young boys with Duchenne muscular dystrophy. J Pediatr. 2015;166(3):640–5. e1. https://doi.org/10.1016/j.jpeds.2014.12.006. PubMed PMID: 25722267.

20. Hoque R. Sleep-disordered breathing in duchenne muscular dystrophy: an assessment of the literature. J Clin Sleep Med. 2016;12(6):905–11. https://doi.org/10.5664/jcsm.5898. PubMed PMID: 27070248; PubMed Central PMCID: PMC4877324. Epub 20160615.

21. LoMauro A, D'Angelo MG, Aliverti A. Sleep disordered breathing in Duchenne muscular dystrophy. Curr Neurol Neurosci Rep. 2017;17(5):44. https://doi.org/10.1007/s11910-017-0750-1. PubMed PMID: 28397169.
22. Polat M, Sakinci O, Ersoy B, Sezer RG, Yilmaz H. Assessment of sleep-related breathing disorders in patients with duchenne muscular dystrophy. J Clin Med Res. 2012;4(5):332–7. https://doi.org/10.4021/jocmr1075w. PubMed PMID: 23024736; PubMed Central PMCID: PMC3449431. Epub 20120912.
23. Kushida CA, Littner MR, Morgenthaler T, Alessi CA, Bailey D, Coleman J Jr, et al. Practice parameters for the indications for polysomnography and related procedures: an update for 2005. Sleep. 2005;28(4):499–521. https://doi.org/10.1093/sleep/28.4.499. PubMed PMID: 16171294.
24. Williams K, Shelgikar AV. The clinical evaluation and use of sleep studies in neurological practice. Curr Sleep Med Rep. 2015;1(2):101–7. https://doi.org/10.1007/s40675-015-0014-z.
25. Johns MW. A new method for measuring daytime sleepiness: the Epworth sleepiness scale. Sleep. 1991;14(6):540–5. https://doi.org/10.1093/sleep/14.6.540. PubMed PMID: 1798888.
26. Steier J, Jolley CJ, Seymour J, Teschler H, Luo YM, Polkey MI, et al. Screening for sleep-disordered breathing in neuromuscular disease using a questionnaire for symptoms associated with diaphragm paralysis. Eur Respir J. 2011;37(2):400–5. https://doi.org/10.1183/09031936.00036210. Epub 20100701. PubMed PMID: 20595146.
27. Zhang C, Ramsay M, Drakatos P, Steier J. The clinical usefulness of a self-administered questionnaire for sleep-disordered breathing in patients with neuromuscular disease. J Thorac Dis. 2018;10(Suppl 1):S153–9. https://doi.org/10.21037/jtd.2017.06.40. PubMed PMID: 29445539; PubMed Central PMCID: PMC5803035.
28. Lofaso F, Fauroux B, Orlikowski D, Prigent H. Daytime predictors of sleep-disordered breathing in neuromuscular patients to better schedule polysomnography. Eur Respir J. 2011;37(2):231–2. https://doi.org/10.1183/09031936.00122610. PubMed PMID: 21282806.
29. Nicolle MW. Sleep and neuromuscular disease. Semin Neurol. 2009;29(4):429–37. https://doi.org/10.1055/s-0029-1237119. Epub 20090909. PubMed PMID: 19742417.
30. Markun LC, Sampat A. Clinician-focused overview and developments in polysomnography. Curr Sleep Med Rep. 2020;6(4):309–21. https://doi.org/10.1007/s40675-020-00197-5. PubMed PMID: 33251088; PubMed Central PMCID: PMC7683038. Epub 20201123.
31. Aarrestad S, Qvarfort M, Kleiven AL, Tollefsen E, Skjønsberg OH, Janssens JP. Diagnostic accuracy of simple tools in monitoring patients with chronic hypoventilation treated with non-invasive ventilation; a prospective cross-sectional study. Respir Med. 2018;144:30–5. https://doi.org/10.1016/j.rmed.2018.09.015. Epub 20180926. PubMed PMID: 30366581.
32. Berry RB, Budhiraja R, Gottlieb DJ, Gozal D, Iber C, Kapur VK, et al. Rules for scoring respiratory events in sleep: update of the 2007 AASM manual for the scoring of sleep and associated events. Deliberations of the Sleep Apnea Definitions Task Force of the American Academy of Sleep Medicine. J Clin Sleep Med. 2012;8(5):597–619. https://doi.org/10.5664/jcsm.2172. PubMed PMID: 23066376; PubMed Central PMCID: PMC3459210. Epub 20121015.
33. Janssens JP, Perrin E, Bennani I, de Muralt B, Titelion V, Picaud C. Is continuous transcutaneous monitoring of PCO_2 ($TcPCO_2$) over 8 h reliable in adults? Respir Med. 2001;95(5):331–5. https://doi.org/10.1053/rmed.2001.1045. PubMed PMID: 11392572.
34. Duyu M, Mocan Çağlar Y, Karakaya Z, Usta Aslan M, Yılmaz S, Ören Leblebici AN, et al. Comparison of arterial CO_2 estimation by end-tidal and transcutaneous CO_2 measurements in intubated children and variability with subject related factors. J Clin Monit Comput. 2021;35(1):101–11. https://doi.org/10.1007/s10877-020-00569-w. PubMed PMID: 32720231; PubMed Central PMCID: PMC7384390. Epub 20200727.
35. Pham T, Telias I, Beitler JR. Esophageal manometry. Respir Care. 2020;65(6):772–92. https://doi.org/10.4187/respcare.07425. PubMed PMID: 32457170; PubMed Central PMCID: PMC7362579.

36. Contal O, Carnevale C, Borel JC, Sabil A, Tamisier R, Lévy P, et al. Pulse transit time as a measure of respiratory effort under noninvasive ventilation. Eur Respir J. 2013;41(2):346–53. https://doi.org/10.1183/09031936.00193911. Epub 20120420. PubMed PMID: 22523360.

37. Weinberg J, Klefbeck B, Borg J, Svanborg E. Polysomnography in chronic neuromuscular disease. Respiration. 2003;70(4):349–54. https://doi.org/10.1159/000072896. PubMed PMID: 14512668.

38. Lofaso F, Quera-Salva MA. Polysomnography for the management of progressive neuromuscular disorders. Eur Respir J. 2002;19(6):989–90. https://doi.org/10.1183/09031936.02.00752002. PubMed PMID: 12108883.

39. Pautrat J, Khirani S, Boulé M, Ramirez A, Beydon N, Fauroux B. Carbon dioxide levels during polygraphy in children with sleep-disordered breathing. Sleep Breath. 2015;19(1):149–57. https://doi.org/10.1007/s11325-014-0980-2. Epub 20140426. PubMed PMID: 24770898.

40. Wolfe LF, Benditt JO, Aboussouan L, Hess DR, Coleman JM III. Optimal NIV Medicare Access Promotion: patients with thoracic restrictive disorders: a technical expert panel report from the American College of Chest Physicians, the American Association for Respiratory Care, the American Academy of Sleep Medicine, and the American Thoracic Society. Chest. 2021;160(5):e399–408. https://doi.org/10.1016/j.chest.2021.05.075. PubMed PMID: 34339688; PubMed Central PMCID: PMC8828932. Epub 20210730.

41. Ogna A, Quera Salva MA, Prigent H, Mroue G, Vaugier I, Annane D, et al. Nocturnal hypoventilation in neuromuscular disease: prevalence according to different definitions issued from the literature. Sleep Breath. 2016;20(2):575–81. https://doi.org/10.1007/s11325-015-1247-2. Epub 20150904. PubMed PMID: 26338464.

42. Orlikowski D, Prigent H, Quera Salva MA, Heming N, Chaffaut C, Chevret S, et al. Prognostic value of nocturnal hypoventilation in neuromuscular patients. Neuromuscul Disord. 2017;27(4):326–30. https://doi.org/10.1016/j.nmd.2016.12.006. Epub 20161221. PubMed PMID: 28153460.

43. Medicare Respiratory Assist Device coverage guidelines: U.S. Centers for Medicare and Medicaid Services; 2019. [cited 15 May 2023]. https://document.resmed.com/documents/articles/1010293_RAD_Guidelines.pdf.

44. Nardi J, Prigent H, Adala A, Bohic M, Lebargy F, Quera-Salva MA, et al. Nocturnal oximetry and transcutaneous carbon dioxide in home-ventilated neuromuscular patients. Respir Care. 2012;57(9):1425–30. https://doi.org/10.4187/respcare.01658. Epub 20120217. PubMed PMID: 22348449.

45. Trucco F, Pedemonte M, Fiorillo C, Tan HL, Carlucci A, Brisca G, et al. Detection of early nocturnal hypoventilation in neuromuscular disorders. J Int Med Res. 2018;46(3):1153–61. https://doi.org/10.1177/0300060517728857. PubMed PMID: 29210305; PubMed Central PMCID: PMC5972237. Epub 20171206.

46. Ferguson KA, Strong MJ, Ahmad D, George CF. Sleep-disordered breathing in amyotrophic lateral sclerosis. Chest. 1996;110(3):664–9. https://doi.org/10.1378/chest.110.3.664. PubMed PMID: 8797409.

47. Zhang Y, Ren R, Yang L, Nie Y, Zhang H, Shi Y, et al. Sleep in amyotrophic lateral sclerosis: a systematic review and meta-analysis of polysomnographic findings. Sleep Med. 2023;107:116–25. https://doi.org/10.1016/j.sleep.2023.04.014. Epub 20230424. PubMed PMID: 37163838.

48. Annane D, Orlikowski D, Chevret S. Nocturnal mechanical ventilation for chronic hypoventilation in patients with neuromuscular and chest wall disorders. Cochrane Database Syst Rev. 2014;2014(12):Cd001941. https://doi.org/10.1002/14651858.CD001941.pub3. PubMed PMID: 25503955; PubMed Central PMCID: PMC7068159. Epub 20141213.

49. Bourke SC, Tomlinson M, Williams TL, Bullock RE, Shaw PJ, Gibson GJ. Effects of noninvasive ventilation on survival and quality of life in patients with amyotrophic lateral sclerosis: a randomised controlled trial. Lancet Neurol. 2006;5(2):140–7. https://doi.org/10.1016/s1474-4422(05)70326-4. PubMed PMID: 16426990.

50. Berlowitz DJ, Sheers N. Not only about the drugs: improved survival with noninvasive ventilation in amyotrophic lateral sclerosis. Ann Am Thorac Soc. 2021;18(3):419–20. https://doi.org/10.1513/AnnalsATS.202011-1404ED. PubMed PMID: 33646079; PubMed Central PMCID: PMC7919150.
51. Lechtzin N, Scott Y, Busse AM, Clawson LL, Kimball R, Wiener CM. Early use of non-invasive ventilation prolongs survival in subjects with ALS. Amyotroph Lateral Scler. 2007;8(3):185–8. https://doi.org/10.1080/17482960701262392. PubMed PMID: 17538782.
52. Kampelmacher MJ. Moving from inpatient to outpatient or home initiation of non-invasive home mechanical ventilation. J Clin Med. 2023;12(8):2981. https://doi.org/10.3390/jcm12082981. PubMed PMID: 37109317; PubMed Central PMCID: PMC10144297. Epub 20230419.
53. Patout M, Arbane G, Cuvelier A, Muir JF, Hart N, Murphy PB. Polysomnography versus limited respiratory monitoring and nurse-led titration to optimise non-invasive ventilation set-up: a pilot randomised clinical trial. Thorax. 2019;74(1):83–6. https://doi.org/10.1136/thoraxjnl-2017-211067. Epub 20180330. PubMed PMID: 29602814.
54. Sheers N, Berlowitz DJ, Rautela L, Batchelder I, Hopkinson K, Howard ME. Improved survival with an ambulatory model of non-invasive ventilation implementation in motor neuron disease. Amyotroph Lateral Scler Frontotemporal Degener. 2014;15(3–4):180–4. https://doi.org/10.3109/21678421.2014.881376. Epub 20140220. PubMed PMID: 24555916.
55. Nicholson TT, Smith SB, Siddique T, Sufit R, Ajroud-Driss S, Coleman JM III, et al. Respiratory pattern and tidal volumes differ for pressure support and volume-assured pressure support in amyotrophic lateral sclerosis. Ann Am Thorac Soc. 2017;14(7):1139–46. https://doi.org/10.1513/AnnalsATS.201605-346OC. PubMed PMID: 28410001.
56. Janssens JP, Cantero C, Pasquina P, Georges M, Rabec C. Monitoring long term noninvasive ventilation: benefits, caveats and perspectives. Front Med (Lausanne). 2022;9:874523. https://doi.org/10.3389/fmed.2022.874523. PubMed PMID: 35665357; PubMed Central PMCID: PMC9160571. Epub 20220519.
57. Borel JC, Gonzalez-Bermejo J. Is it still relevant to consider polysomnography as essential for noninvasive ventilation titration? Eur Respir J. 2019;53(5):1900619. https://doi.org/10.1183/13993003.00619-2019. PubMed PMID: 31123024. Epub 20190523.
58. Janssens JP, Borel JC, Pépin JL. Nocturnal monitoring of home non-invasive ventilation: the contribution of simple tools such as pulse oximetry, capnography, built-in ventilator software and autonomic markers of sleep fragmentation. Thorax. 2011;66(5):438–45. https://doi.org/10.1136/thx.2010.139782. PubMed PMID: 20971980. Epub 20101022.
59. Delessert A, Espa F, Rossetti A, Lavigne G, Tafti M, Heinzer R. Pulse wave amplitude drops during sleep are reliable surrogate markers of changes in cortical activity. Sleep. 2010;33(12):1687–92. https://doi.org/10.1093/sleep/33.12.1687. PubMed PMID: 21120131; PubMed Central PMCID: PMC2982739.
60. Sahni AS, Wolfe L. Respiratory care in neuromuscular diseases. Respir Care. 2018;63(5):601–8. https://doi.org/10.4187/respcare.06210. PubMed PMID: 29692352. Epub 20180424.
61. Chatwin M, Nickol AH, Morrell MJ, Polkey MI, Simonds AK. Randomised trial of inpatient versus outpatient initiation of home mechanical ventilation in patients with nocturnal hypoventilation. Respir Med. 2008;102(11):1528–35. https://doi.org/10.1016/j.rmed.2008.07.019. PubMed PMID: 18774702. Epub 20080907.
62. Hannan LM, Rautela L, Berlowitz DJ, McDonald CF, Cori JM, Sheers N, et al. Randomised controlled trial of polysomnographic titration of noninvasive ventilation. Eur Respir J. 2019;53(5):1802118. https://doi.org/10.1183/13993003.02118-2018. PubMed PMID: 30880286. Epub 20190523.
63. Volpato E, Vitacca M, Ptacinsky L, Lax A, D'Ascenzo S, Bertella E, et al. Home-based adaptation to night-time non-invasive ventilation in patients with amyotrophic lateral sclerosis: a randomized controlled trial. J Clin Med. 2022;11(11):3178. https://doi.org/10.3390/jcm11113178. PubMed PMID: 35683562; PubMed Central PMCID: PMC9181816. Epub 20220602.

64. Fromageot C, Lofaso F, Annane D, Falaize L, Lejaille M, Clair B, et al. Supine fall in lung volumes in the assessment of diaphragmatic weakness in neuromuscular disorders. Arch Phys Med Rehabil. 2001;82(1):123–8. https://doi.org/10.1053/apmr.2001.18053. PubMed PMID: 11239298.

65. Allen SM, Hunt B, Green M. Fall in vital capacity with posture. Br J Dis Chest. 1985;79(3):267–71. PubMed PMID: 4015957.

66. Schoser B, Fong E, Geberhiwot T, Hughes D, Kissel JT, Madathil SC, et al. Maximum inspiratory pressure as a clinically meaningful trial endpoint for neuromuscular diseases: a comprehensive review of the literature. Orphanet J Rare Dis. 2017;12(1):52. https://doi.org/10.1186/s13023-017-0598-0. PubMed PMID: 28302142; PubMed Central PMCID: PMC5353799. Epub 20170316.

67. ATS/ERS statement on respiratory muscle testing. Am J Respir Crit Care Med. 2002;166(4):518–624. https://doi.org/10.1164/rccm.166.4.518. PubMed PMID: 12186831.

68. Mendoza M, Gelinas DF, Moore DH, Miller RG. A comparison of maximal inspiratory pressure and forced vital capacity as potential criteria for initiating non-invasive ventilation in amyotrophic lateral sclerosis. Amyotroph Lateral Scler. 2007;8(2):106–11. https://doi.org/10.1080/17482960601030188. PubMed PMID: 17453639.

69. Lofaso F, Nicot F, Lejaille M, Falaize L, Louis A, Clement A, et al. Sniff nasal inspiratory pressure: what is the optimal number of sniffs? Eur Respir J. 2006;27(5):980–2. https://doi.org/10.1183/09031936.06.00121305. Epub 20060202. PubMed PMID: 16455823.

70. Lyall RA, Donaldson N, Polkey MI, Leigh PN, Moxham J. Respiratory muscle strength and ventilatory failure in amyotrophic lateral sclerosis. Brain. 2001;124(Pt 10):2000–13. https://doi.org/10.1093/brain/124.10.2000. PubMed PMID: 11571218.

71. Ramsay M, Mandal S, Suh ES, Steier J, Douiri A, Murphy PB, et al. Parasternal electromyography to determine the relationship between patient-ventilator asynchrony and nocturnal gas exchange during home mechanical ventilation set-up. Thorax. 2015;70(10):946–52. https://doi.org/10.1136/thoraxjnl-2015-206944. PubMed PMID: 26197816. Epub 20150721.

72. Kushida CA, Chediak A, Berry RB, Brown LK, Gozal D, Iber C, et al. Clinical guidelines for the manual titration of positive airway pressure in patients with obstructive sleep apnea. J Clin Sleep Med. 2008;4(2):157–71. PubMed PMID: 18468315; PubMed Central PMCID: PMC2335396

73. Selim B, Ramar K. Sleep-related breathing disorders: when cpap is not enough. Neurotherapeutics. 2021;18(1):81–90. https://doi.org/10.1007/s13311-020-00955-x. PubMed PMID: 33150546; PubMed Central PMCID: PMC8116389. Epub 20201104.

Chapter 4
Ventilatory Support for the Neuromuscular Patient: Noninvasive and Invasive Ventilation

Hugo Carmona, Andrew Graustein, and Joshua Benditt

Introduction

Many patients with neuromuscular disease will require respiratory assistance to aid in ventilation, cough, and symptom management. In this chapter, we will review the role of noninvasive (NIV) and invasive mechanical ventilation to support patients. In general, there is both provider and patient preference for noninvasive ventilation whenever possible, as it is better tolerated, reduces care requirements compared to invasive mechanical ventilation, and has more flexibility with regards to options. In this chapter, we will discuss the indications and contraindications for choosing noninvasive ventilation, the interface types and modes of ventilation, along with suggested monitoring for safe use of NIV. We will then discuss the need for transitioning to invasive mechanical ventilation when NIV is no longer safe or is contraindicated, along with a discussion around tracheostomy selection, modes of ventilation, and monitoring as well. Finally, we will review when hospice care should be considered and the ethical considerations around the care of patients with neuromuscular disease.

H. Carmona (✉) · J. Benditt
Division of Pulmonary, Critical Care and Sleep Medicine, Department of Medicine,
University of Washington, Seattle, WA, USA
e-mail: hcarmona@uw.edu; benditt@uw.edu

A. Graustein
Division of Pulmonary, Critical Care and Sleep Medicine, Department of Medicine,
University of Washington, Seattle, WA, USA

Division of Pulmonary, Critical Care and Sleep Medicine, Department of Medicine,
Veterans Affairs Puget Sound Health Care System, Seattle, WA, USA
e-mail: adg2001@uw.edu

N. Lechtzin (ed.), *Pulmonary Complications of Neuromuscular Disease*,
Respiratory Medicine, https://doi.org/10.1007/978-3-031-65335-3_4

Indications and Considerations for Eligibility

Noninvasive ventilation (NIV) is the use of ventilatory support devices that avoid the use of invasive tracheostomy or endotracheal tubes. The goal of NIV is to improve sleep disturbances, improve hypoventilation that occurs during sleep as well as during the day, and possibly improve mortality. For many neuromuscular diseases, initiation of NIV is usually based on the presence of symptoms of sleep disturbance or dyspnea, the presence of hypoventilation with hypercapnia, as well as objective testing such as a reduced vital capacity or reduced respiratory muscle pressure generation [1]. However, the optimal timing for initiating NIV is unknown. A variety of consensus statements exist that recommend the initiation of NIV with criteria that vary by disease state (see Table 4.1). For patients with evidence of hypoventilation based on direct or indirect measurement of $PaCO_2$ levels via blood gas, end-tidal, or transcutaneous testing, NIV support is recommended. However, if hypoventilation is not yet present, a combination of the trajectory of the disease along with pulmonary function testing can be used to establish timing for NIV. As an example, in ALS, a decreasing vital capacity is the most common measure used by specialists in the United States to initiate NIV [2]. Due to Medicare reimbursement criteria in the United States, often NIV is initiated only after the VC has decreased below 50%, though one retrospective analysis found that early initiation of NIV in ALS while the VC was still preserved had a mortality advantage [3].

For most patients who have chronic hypoventilation, noninvasive ventilation is the standard of care if they are able to tolerate the interface. That being said, there are few randomized trials of NIV in the NMD population. Many of the diseases are rare and the question of withholding ventilation from those with evidence of respiratory failure to serve as a control group in an RCT had been a controversial question in the past, and is unlikely to be acceptable today, though there remain insurance coverage barriers. Two diseases where more data are available are Duchenne muscular dystrophy (DMD) and amyotrophic lateral sclerosis (ALS). In a single-center retrospective review covering 35 years and 197 patients, there was an additional mean survival benefit of 6 years with the use of NIV in Duchenne muscular dystrophy [4]. Likewise, in a Japanese cohort, there was shown to be a survival benefit with use of NIV. The mean survival was 20.1 years without NIV and 30.4 years with nasal NIV [5]. The advent of mouthpiece ventilation for diurnal support has also likely improved survival in patients with DMD [6]. The use of NIV to prolong ALS survival is more evident, even with only using NIV for a few hours a day [7, 8]. In a trial that used orthopnea or symptomatic hypercapnia as initiation points for NIV, the use of NIV vs standard of care prolonged survival in patients with ALS [9]. A subsequent Cochrane Review also supported the suggestion that NIV provides a survival benefit in ALS [10]. Consensus statements have been established based on these and other studies, endorsing the commencement of noninvasive ventilation (NIV) for both symptomatic patients and those at risk of hypoventilation, as well as for patients with ALS and DMD [11, 12] who are experiencing hypoventilation. Other expert opinion-based consensus statements support using NIV for patients

Table 4.1 Guidelines for initiation of noninvasive positive-pressure ventilation in neuromuscular and chest wall disorders [1] (adapted from Box 6)

NAMDRC national consensus conference[a], 1999, restrictive thoracic disorders
- Symptoms of hypoventilation (fatigue, dyspnea, and morning headache)

and
- One of the following:
  - $PaCO_2$ ≥45 mmHg
  - Nocturnal oximetry with SpO_2 ≤88% for 5 consecutive minutes
  - For NMD only: MIP less than 60 cm H_2O or FVC <50%

American Thoracic Society, 2004, DMD
- Sleep-related upper airway obstruction or
- Chronic respiratory insufficiency

American Academy of Neurology, 2009, ALS
- One of
  - Orthopnea
  - SNP <40 cm H_2O or MIP less than 60 cm H_2O
  - Abnormal nocturnal oximetry
  - FVC <50%

International Standard of Care Committee for Congenital Muscular Dystrophy, 2010, MD
- Symptomatic daytime hypercapnia
- Symptomatic nocturnal hypoventilation
- Nonsymptomatic nocturnal hypercapnia and hypopneas
- Failure to thrive
- Recurrent chest infections (>3/year)
- Fatigue
- Respiratory muscle weakness as documented by pulmonary function tests

Germany Society for Pneumonology, 2010, neuromuscular diseases
- Clinical signs of chronic respiratory failure and at least one of
  - Chronic daytime hypercapnia $PaCO_2$ ≥45 mmHg
  - Nocturnal hypercapnia with rise in $PtcCO_2$ of ≥10 mmHg during the night
  - Rapid significant reduction in vital capacity

Canadian Thoracic Society, 2011, ALS
- Any one of
  - Orthopnea
  - Daytime hypercapnia
  - Symptomatic sleep-disordered breathing
  - FVC <50%
  - SNP <40 cm H_2O or MIP <40 cm H_2O

Canadian Thoracic Society, 2011, kyphoscoliosis
- Chronic hypercapnic respiratory failure

Canadian Thoracic Society, 2011, DMD
- Diurnal hypercapnia ($PaCO_2$ >45 mmHg) or
- Nocturnal hypercapnia and symptoms consistent with hypoventilation

Canadian Thoracic Society, 2011, MD
- Daytime hypercapnia or
- Symptomatic nocturnal hypoventilation

Canadian Thoracic Society, 2011, postpolio syndrome
- Chronic hypoventilation

British Thoracic Society, 2012, children with neuromuscular weakness
- Symptomatic nocturnal hypoventilation or
- Daytime hypercapnia

(continued)

Table 4.1 (continued)

European Federation of Neurological Societies, 2012, ALS
- Symptoms/signs related to respiratory muscle weakness. At least one of
  - Dyspnea
  - Tachypnea
  - Orthopnea
  - Disturbed sleep due to nocturnal desaturation/arousals
  - Morning headache
  - Use of accessory muscles at rest
  - Paradoxic respiration
  - Daytime fatigue
  - Excessive daytime sleepiness (ESS >9)
- Abnormal respiratory function tests. At least one of
  - FVC <80%
  - SNP <40 cm H_2O
  - MIP <60 cm H_2O
  - Significant nocturnal desaturation on overnight oximetry
  - Morning blood gas $PaCO_2$ >45 mmHg

DMD Duchenne muscular dystrophy, *ESS* Epworth Sleepiness Scale, *FiO₂* fraction of inspired oxygen, *FVC* forced vital capacity, *MD* myotonic dystrophy, *MIP* maximal inspiratory pressure, *NMD* neuromuscular disease, *SNP* sniff nasal pressure

[a] Note: The NAMDRC National Consensus Conference (1999) was convened and organized by the National Association for the Medical Direction of Respiratory Care (NAMDRC) and included representatives from American Academy of Home Care physicians, American Association for Respiratory Care, American College of Chest Physicians, American College of Physicians, American Sleep Disorders Association, Mayo Clinic, and National Association for Medical Direction of Respiratory Care. Reproduced from Hilbert [1]

with restrictive thoracic disease and nocturnal hypoventilation [13]. When considering whether a patient with neuromuscular disease should be started on noninvasive ventilation outside of these guidelines, the clinician should also consider the patient's stage in their disease, their expected trajectory, their ability to manage secretions, and their level of caregiver support.

In the United States, initiation of NIV is often guided by reimbursement guidelines from the Centers for Medicare and Medicaid Services (CMS), which stipulate that reimbursement requires certain criteria for patients with neuromuscular disease or thoracic cage abnormalities as noted below [14]:

1. Documentation of restrictive thoracic disorder with respiratory symptoms
2. One of the following:

    (a) $PaCO_2$ on awake arterial blood gas $\geq$45 mmHg while breathing the prescribed fraction of oxygen
    (b) Sleep oximetry with SpO_2 of 88% or lower for 5 min or more while breathing the prescribed fraction of oxygen
    (c) Either a maximal inspiratory pressure <60 cm H_2O or forced vital capacity <50% predicted

3. COPD is not a significant contributor to the pulmonary limitation

Contraindications

There are few contraindications to the initiation of NIV in the setting of neuromuscular disease. An important aspect of NIV use with face masks is that patients may not be able to don and doff the masks themselves, requiring caregiver assistance. Without the ability to remove their mask, patients using full-face masks are at risk of aspiration in the setting of emesis. Therefore, patients using a full-face mask should have immediate caregiver support or be able to remove the masks easily themselves. In most settings, a nasal mask or pillow interface is usually preferred as they are found to be more comfortable by most patients, as they also allow speech and oral intake. Facial anatomy that does not favorably allow for a seal with an oral, nasal, or full-face mask may also limit the efficacy of NIV, though often adjustments can be made and leak can be tolerated except in the most severe cases. In some patients with advanced bulbar disease, both insufflation and exsufflation have been shown to cause airway adduction [15]. Therefore, advanced bulbar disease may prevent the successful use of NIV at desired levels of pressure support due to airway closure from supraglottic and glottic collapse with inspiratory pressures from bilevel support or inability to use the mouthpiece with mouthpiece ventilation. Attention to airway collapse with titration of inspiratory pressures will be important and trials with individual patients to see if they tolerate NIV is helpful [16].

Interface Type

Interfaces for NIV provide air pressure for ventilation via a full-face mask, oral, nasal, or combination oral-nasal mask, or via a mouthpiece [17, 18]. Proper sizing and fit are very important to the success of NIV [17, 19, 20]. Poor fitting interfaces will cause discomfort, pressure points [21], and allow for leak around the mask seal, providing ineffective and inefficient ventilatory support [22] and, thus, poor sleep [19]. Individual facial architecture will dictate that some masks may fit and seal better than others [20, 23]. Custom mask fabrication, which used to be common, is generally no longer needed due to the abundance of commercially available mask types.

Nasal Masks

Given the soft silicone features of modern masks, a common comfortable option is a nasal-only mask, both as nasal pillows or nasal-covering masks. These masks route air pressure only through the nasal passages and leave the mouth clear, allowing for speech and eating while still providing ventilation. They can be utilized both diurnally and nocturnally. A wide variety of nasal masks exist [20]. Due to the pressure utilized as well as patient factors such as muscle tone and control, some patients may not be able to keep their mouths closed and oral leaks can occur, limiting the efficacy of the pressure settings from NIV [19, 22]. A chin strap can be considered to gently close the mouth and reduce leak, prior to switching to a different interface, though their efficacy is limited and variable [24, 25].

Oral and Full-Face Masks

If a nasal mask is not comfortable, significant pressure is required, or there is excessive leak through the mouth that is not abated by a chin strap, then either a combined nasal/oral hybrid mask or a full-face mask can be employed. These masks provide full seals around the chin and cheeks, routing air pressure through both nasal and oral passages and can be more comfortable with higher pressures [26]. As they cover the mouth, there is no oral air leaks. Patients with beards or no dentition may have a harder time fitting a full-face mask without air leak. The major drawback to these masks is that they do not allow for easy speech or eating, as they cover the mouth, and they increase the surface area where skin breakdown can occur [20]. For patients who progress from needing just nocturnal NIV support to diurnal support as well, even if they were using a full-face mask during sleep, they can often utilize a nasal-only mask or mouthpiece when they are awake, have more muscle tone, and are less prone to obstruction.

Mouthpiece Ventilation

Mouthpiece ventilation (MPV) allows for "on-demand" breaths with the use of an angled mouthpiece or straight tube or straw connected to a ventilator that is adapted for mouthpiece ventilation. The mouthpiece is mounted on a custom or commercially available articulating arm that can be clamped to a patient's wheelchair, side table, or other nearby structure and positioned to be within a few degrees' turn of their head. Some patients will maintain the mouthpiece in their mouth entirely, while many will move their mouth to and from the mouthpiece. The patient activates ventilation by placing their mouth over the mouthpiece to initiate a breath. The breath is delivered until the patient is satisfied, at which point they remove their mouth or open their lips to allow leak and exhalation. This movement also allows speech in between breaths and can augment the quality of speech. As such, it is an excellent option for patients who can tolerate the interface [27, 28]. When considering a patient for MPV, clinicians should assure that the patient can form a seal around the mouthpiece in order to be able to initiate and receive breaths; thus, patients with significant bulbar symptoms such as in bulbar-onset or advanced ALS may not be appropriate candidates. Likewise, patients with significant secretions and hypersalivation are at increased risk of aspiration and caution should be taken

[29]. As it is an active mode, generally patients will be on mouthpiece ventilation during the daytime but switch to a mask interface during sleep to utilize a mode that can provide a mandated backup respiratory rate [6, 29, 30]. Similar to how patients with face masks may require assistance donning and doffing their mask, if the patient who uses MPV is moved or repositioned by a caregiver, or likewise their device is, care should be taken to reposition it to where they can reach. An expert consensus panel suggested that patients should have at least 5° of turning motion with their heads to safely be able to use MPV [26].

Modes of Ventilation

The choice of mode is dependent on the patient's needs and comfort along with the experience of the provider, with the understanding that multiple modes can all accomplish the goal of providing an adequate minute ventilation. Additionally, it may be necessary for patients to alternate mode of NIV depending on their activity level—that is, they may use a daytime mode of NIV and a different nocturnal mode to accomplish different goals. For the vast majority of patients with neuromuscular respiratory disease, the continuous positive airway pressure (CPAP) mode does not provide enough ventilatory support and, as such, is infrequently used unless they only have obstructive sleep apnea. Therefore, we will focus on NIV modes that provide separate inspiratory support, mainly various forms of bilevel positive airway pressure.

Spontaneous, Spontaneous/Timed, and Pressure-Control Modes

Standard bilevel therapy consists of an inspiratory positive airway pressure (IPAP) settings and an expiratory positive airway pressure (EPAP) setting. The addition of IPAP allows for ventilatory assistance by increasing the volumes during tidal breathing, thus improving overall minute ventilation. In this mode, if no back-up respiratory rate (BUR) is set, then it is referred to as spontaneous bilevel, and the patient is unprotected against low minute ventilation due to a low respiratory rate during sleep. Therefore, this mode is usually not recommended for patients with neuromuscular disease. A more commonly used modality is spontaneous/timed (S/T) bilevel, where a BUR is set. Thus, if the patient's intrinsic respiratory rate falls below the BUR threshold, they are assured at least a minimum respiratory rate. The calculation for the intrinsic respiratory rate and the decision point to initiate a backup breath is managed by proprietary algorithms that differ between manufacturers but all work in essentially the same way. The algorithmic differences are attempts to provide a more comfortable transition between backup and intrinsic breaths. In bilevel S/T, spontaneous breaths are flow-cycled and the mandatory ("timed") breaths from the BUR are time-cycled. Bilevel S/T is a common mode that is easily titrated as a result. One pitfall of this mode is that because tidal volume is still dependent on patient effort and compliance (in addition to the setting IPAP), a specific minute ventilation is not assured if there is a change in respiratory system compliance or patient effort, such as with acute respiratory illness or progressive disease. However, the mode is well tolerated by many patients.

To initiate bilevel S/T therapy, we typically target a tidal volume of 8 mL/kg of ideal body weight for most patients. Most patients require some acclimation to using PAP therapy, and thus often are started on lower pressures than might be ultimately adequate to achieve the targeted tidal volume. IPAP of approximately 10 cm H_2O and EPAP of approximately 5 cm H_2O along with a backup rate of 12 are comfortable settings for most patients to start. They will require a reevaluation of their bilevel use after a few weeks (see the section on monitoring), generally increasing the IPAP to achieve the targeted tidal volume and increasing the EPAP to obliterate any residual apnea. As well, we target a backup rate of just 2–3 breaths under their natural respiratory rate.

For patients with severe weakness as well as occasionally for comfort as well as to maintain a uniform inspiratory time (Ti), it may be better to utilize a pressure-control mode. In pressure-control, the same inspiratory and expiratory pressure settings are set as in S/T mode, but all breaths are time-cycled. This allows for sustained and consistent breath lengths, even in the setting of severe weakness.

VAPS

Volume-assured pressure support (VAPS) is a ventilatory mode that attempts to target an alveolar ventilation or total minute ventilation by dynamically altering the amount of inspiratory pressure in response to patient effort and respiratory mechanics [31]. VAPS is usually set in either of the above S/T or pressure-control modes, depending on the manufacturer device and provider preference. While the algorithms are proprietary to each manufacturer, they calculate the average minute or alveolar ventilation based on exhaled breaths and then adjust IPAP within a specified range to maintain consistent ventilation. We typically target a goal tidal volume of 8 mL/kg of the patient's ideal body weight. Whereas in bilevel S and bilevel S/T, the IPAP-EPAP difference must be changed manually by the provider to achieve that targeted goal based on the patient's respiratory system compliance, in VAPS mode, the machine will continuously adjust the IPAP-EPAP difference to achieve this. The purported benefit of VAPS is that it aims to maintain consistent minute or alveolar ventilation over time in spite of changes in the patient's respiratory system compliance, such as with progressive disease. This could be beneficial for a patient with variable respiratory effort, such as throughout a sleep night where the movement between non-REM and REM sleep causes shallower breathing, or during an acute respiratory infection. VAPS theoretically allows for improved support with dynamic disease processes, such as in ALS where there will be a decline in respiratory strength, mechanics, or dead space over time, all of which might impact the ultimate tidal volume for any given pressure settings [32]. However, patient tolerance may be limited by the higher tidal volumes that the manufacturers recommend for VAPS [33]. Studies on the use of VAPS have included heterogenous neuromuscular patient populations with ultimately conflicting outcomes or equivalence to bilevel S/T [3, 33–36]. There are also auto-adjusting EPAP algorithms that work along VAPS on several advanced respiratory assist devices that similarly adjust not only the inspiratory pressure but also the EPAP itself in response to obstructive apneas, known as VAPS-AE [37].

Mouthpiece Ventilation

Mouthpiece ventilation (MPV) is an essential diurnal mode that allows for freedom from facial masks but has unique characteristics that place unusual demands on the ventilators that support it. While the first ventilator that was specifically designed to allow MPV was developed in 2012 [18], other ventilators have been adapted for this use since the 1950s [38]. The fundamental difference between NIV with MPV and other modes of ventilation, other than interface, is that in MPV, air leak is a fundamental characteristic that is expected and needed as part of its use. In essence, from one breath to another, patients may have varying levels of a lip seal or choose to not connect to the mouthpiece at all, and this variation necessitates dynamic air leak. Patients actively choose how large a tidal volume they can receive (up to 100% of the set tidal volume) by shortening or extending the time on the mouthpiece and adjusting the amount of lip seal they allow with each breath. This will also vary by their speech cadence, their breathlessness, and their activity level, all of which are dynamic throughout the day. In addition, patients are able to provide their own cough augmentation through breath stacking [29], which requires repetitive triggers punctuated by breaks from the circuit in quick succession.

In order to manage all of the above demands, most MPV modes of ventilation will be accomplished in a volume-cycled mode rather than a pressure-cycled mode [18, 29]. The main advantage is that volume-cycled modes will have consistent set tidal volumes and will not engage in leak compensation, allowing for the purposeful leak described above. As a result, the tidal volume is also often set higher (500–1500 mL) to allow the patient a broader range of volumes to receive [39]. Pressure-cycled modes will engage in leak compensation, leading to possible safety issues related to high volumes, more aerophagia, and patient discomfort. Additionally, dedicated MPV modes provide for very easy breath triggering. As with most ventilators, a ventilator with MPV capability can have a breath triggered by the patient generating an inspiratory effort (with a flow or pressure trigger) via their mouthpiece. However, modern MPV ventilators allow patients with neuromuscular disease and an inability to generate any inspiratory effort to trigger a breath by forming a seal around their mouthpiece and interrupting a continuous flow through the ventilator circuit, thus providing a very sensitive trigger [39]. This greatly extends the accessibility of MPV for many patients with neuromuscular disease.

In addition to the above settings, ventilators with a specific MPV mode also have a variety of other settings, including alarm settings, that are consistent with the needs of someone using MPV. Usually PEEP is set to zero, though with pressure-cycled modes, this is usually set to a low nonzero value. A backup rate is only included if the patient cannot have more than a small amount of time off NIV. Non-MPV-specific ventilators should have their alarms changed to facilitate MPV. Disconnection alarms may need to be turned off unless a backup rate is used [40]. Generally, the apnea alarm should also be turned off, especially if the patient can tolerate several hours off of ventilation. Low-pressure alarms should likewise be lowered or turned off.

Monitoring Non-Invasive Ventilation

Effective monitoring of NIV is crucial to assure correct settings and support for patients who are initiated on NIV. The most important aspect to be monitored is improvement in patient's symptoms, followed by diurnal and nocturnal arterial CO_2 levels. Patient symptoms of dyspnea, fatigue, morning headache, and daytime somnolence should all improve with improved nocturnal (and diurnal, if needed) ventilatory support, if the primary dysfunction is hypoventilation. Additionally, frequent checks with the patient regarding their sense of synchrony with the device, discomfort with breathing and the amount of pressure, mask fit, and sleep disruption due to noise can also assist in assessing the quality of support given. The use of a survey tool can help standardize this assessment for efficacy of NIV [41, 42].

Additionally, most respiratory assist devices have capabilities for either downloading respiratory data onto a memory card or uploaded to a website for easy access by clinicians. The use of cellular signaling technology in these devices means that essentially real-time data can be accessed from these devices for monitoring. The data can be sorted by minute, hourly, or daily use and provides information such as overall time used in hours and days, average and 95th percentile respiratory rates, inspiratory and expiratory pressures, tidal volumes (and thus minute ventilation), leak, I:E time, trigger and cycling data, among other information. Combined with patient reported symptoms, settings can then be titrated for patient comfort.

Carbon-dioxide tension ($PaCO_2$) monitoring for hypercapnia and reduction in hypercapnia should be monitored. The use of arterial blood gases is often impractical in the outpatient setting and so surrogates are often employed. Intermittent diurnal end-tidal CO_2 testing in the absence of parenchymal lung disease is a common, noninvasive modality that may be utilized to monitor the efficacy of nocturnal ventilatory support in the outpatient setting such as in clinic or a PFT laboratory. However, it cannot reliably be used by patients on continuous NIV and may have limited accuracy if dead space is elevated due to weak expiratory muscles. Transcutaneous CO_2 has been developed as an alternative that may track more reliably with $PaCO_2$, though both measures suffer from accuracy, especially in the non-invasively ventilated patient [43–46]. While the regular use of polysomnography is not necessary, transcutaneous CO_2 monitoring is frequently used in a sleep lab for PAP titration. Home use of either modality is not covered currently by healthcare insurance in the United States.

Indications for Tracheostomy with Mechanical Ventilation

The question of whether or not to choose tracheostomy in a patient with respiratory failure has been described as a "threshold moment" that requires thoughtful consideration prior to proceeding [47, 48]. In patients with NMD, the decision to transition from NIV to tracheostomy with mechanical ventilation (TMV) is based both on clinical parameters such as the inability to adequately ventilate with NIV as well as other factors such as local standards of care and the experience of the patient's clinicians. The use of TMV for patients with NMD is controversial and some experts argue that most patients with NMD can be maintained indefinitely on NIV [49, 50], the exception being those with bulbar weakness who are unable to prevent aspiration and cannot tolerate mechanically assisted cough [51]. The American College of Chest Physicians recommends that, in patients with NMD, both TMV and full-time NIV should be considered acceptable options based on patient preferences, tolerability, ability to maintain mouthpiece ventilation, and availability of resources [52].

The use of TMV can prolong survival and improve sleep quality relative to no ventilatory support in people with NMD and may be needed if a patient wishes to prolong survival but cannot tolerate NIV. It is also important to note that, while TMV may prolong survival, it does not slow disease progression due to the NMD. In a recent ACCP Clinical Practice Guideline, the authors suggest invasive home mechanical ventilation via tracheostomy as an alternative to NIV under the following circumstances in patients with NMD: failure of NIV or inability to tolerate NIV, worsening bulbar function, frequent aspiration, insufficient cough, recurrent chest infection despite secretion management, or declining lung function [52]. However, the authors also note that full-time NIV may be an acceptable alternative.

In patients with ALS, elective tracheostomy with mechanical ventilation is considered either when adequate oxygenation or ventilation cannot be achieved with noninvasive ventilation or when secretions cannot be sufficiently managed [12]. The American Academy of Neurology specifically recommends consideration for TMV with pO_2 <90% or pCO_2 >50 mmHg despite adequate NIV therapy [12]. Insufficient oxygenation or ventilation may occur due to bulbar dysfunction precluding use of an effective mask interface or the inability of NIV to provide sufficient support as respiratory muscle weakness progresses. In some cases, patients simply cannot tolerate NIV despite education, desensitization, clinical evaluation, and ongoing NIV mode and setting titration. Nevertheless, use of TMV in people with ALS is very uncommon in the U.S. Bach and colleagues have argued that among patients with NMD who eventually become dependent on continuous ventilatory support, the only indication for tracheostomy is oxygen desaturation to SpO_2 <95% in the setting of saliva aspiration due to bulbar dysfunction [53]. While such bulbar dysfunction is common in ALS, it is uncommon in most other types of NMD.

A recent DMD Care Considerations Working Group [11] recognizes that the question of whether to manage patients with late, nonambulatory DMD with tracheostomy or noninvasively is controversial. Some centers use time on a ventilator (EG over 16 h/day) as a tracheostomy indication. The working group supports noninvasive ventilation for most circumstances. Indications for tracheostomy suggested by the working group are:

1. Patient preference
2. Inability to use noninvasive ventilation
3. Three failed extubation attempts during critical illness despite optimal cough assistance
4. Failure of noninvasive cough assistance to prevent aspiration due to bulbar weakness

The authors note that the decision is also influenced by other factors such as the usual practices and skill of the patient's clinicians, local standards of care, and the availability of home resources [11].

Rates of TMV in NMD vary by country and are best studied in patients with ALS, and range from 2% to 38% [54–56]. In the United States, rates of TMV are roughly 5–8% of ALS patients [57]. In Korea rates are higher at approximately 13% [58]. In the United Kingdom less than 1% of patients with ALS undergo TMV, which is usually undertaken in response to a crisis rather than electively [59]. In Japan, where rates of TMV are relatively high at a recent estimate of 33%, it has been suggested that physician behavior is shaped by concerns over legal action with regards to end-of-life care. However, an additional factor is that in Japan, the full cost of TMV is covered by the government and medical insurance, whereas in other countries such as the United States and the United Kingdom this is not the case [56]. A majority of physicians would not pursue tracheostomy when faced with a hypothetical ALS diagnosis [60]. In the United States, patients with ALS who elect for TMV are younger, have young children, have higher education and socioeconomic status, and display optimism and positive reflections of their daily lives [55, 57].

Invasive Versus Noninvasive Ventilation for Acute Respiratory Failure

Acute respiratory failure can occur in acute onset NMDs such as myasthenia gravis as well as in exacerbations of chronic NMDs such as ALS. While evidence supports trialing NIV rather than endotracheal intubation in acute respiratory failure with COPD and cardiogenic pulmonary edema [61], less is known about the benefits of NIV for patients with NMD in acute respiratory failure relative to endotracheal intubation. A 2017 Cochrane Review attempted to understand this question, with the primary objective to compare efficacy of NIV with invasive ventilation in improving short-term survival in acute respiratory failure with NMD [62]. The authors found no randomized control trials with which to generate evidence-based recommendations, concluding there is a need for further research in this important area.

Desirable Versus Undesirable Effects of Tracheostomy with Mechanical Ventilation

Survival

Multiple retrospective, observational studies suggest a survival benefit in patients with ALS with the use of TMV relative to either no ventilatory support or NIV, though the level of certainty is low because of lack of randomized trials [52]. Spataro et al. followed 87 ALS patients receiving TMV and 192 ALS patients either receiving NIV or no ventilatory support at a single ALS center in Italy [63]. The patients with TMV lived significantly longer, with a median survival from disease onset to death of 47 months compared to 31 months for non-tracheostomized patients, with a stronger effect on younger patients less than 60 years old at disease onset. The authors did not specifically compare survival between patients with TMV and those using NIV. In a single-center retrospective cohort study from Germany [64], 2702 ALS patients were examined for utilization of NIV (358 patients) and TMV (164 patients). Relative to the non-NIV cohort, median survival was longer in the NIV cohort (33.6 months versus 40.8 months) and in the TMV cohort (33.6 months versus 82.1 months) with a median survival after TMV of 25 months. In ALS patients with tracheostomy in Italy the most common causes of death were respiratory tract infection (48%), nonrespiratory medical conditions (30%), and acute complications of tracheostomy (15%) [65].

While most survival analyses comparing TMV to its alternatives have been in patients with ALS, some data exists for DMD as well. Soudon et al. conducted an observational cohort study of 42 patients with end-stage DMD who were being ventilated for a minimum of 15 h/day at a single center in Belgium [66]. Sixteen patients were ventilated via tracheostomy and 26 via noninvasive techniques. Patients with both TMV and NIV had similar ages and causes of death. The use of TMV resulted in some morbidity that was avoided with NIV including higher rates of tracheal injuries, mucus hypersecretion, and lung infection in the TMV group. The authors did not measure quality of life but did observe that, when living at home was no longer possible, most TMV patients required hospitalization while patients with NIV were able to find placement more easily in nursing homes.

Quality of Life and Caregiver burden

TMV can place a burden not only on the patient but also on their caregivers. It is important to understand this dynamic when discussing tracheostomy decisions in patients with NMD. A cross-sectional survey conducted by the German Association for Neuromuscular Disease studied quality of life in patients with ALS and their caregivers specifically in patients receiving ventilatory support [67]. There were no significant differences between the scales used to assess QoL with either ventilatory strategy; 94% of NIV patients and 81% of TMV patients would choose ventilation again and similar numbers would advise others to do the same. However, important differences were seen in surveys provided by the patients' caregivers. Ninety-seven percent of NIV caregivers would advise choosing ventilation again; this number was only 75% for TMV. In addition, 94% of caregivers would choose NIV if facing the same decision, whereas 50% would choose TMV. Surprisingly, 30% of TMV caregivers reported that their own quality of life was worse than that of the patient. The authors conclude that while TMV provides an adequate QoL for patients with ALS, it creates a very high burden for their caregivers.

A recent cross-sectional study of adults with slowly progressive neuromuscular disease throughout France assessed health-related quality of life (HRQoL) in patients using mechanical ventilation [68]. Individuals were eligible if they were wheelchair-bound or bedridden, dependent on either NIV or TMV for 16 h or more daily, and did not carry a diagnosis of ALS, myasthenia, polyradiculoneuritis, or metabolic neuropathy. DMD was the most common diagnosis, followed by limb–girdle muscular dystrophy. Of the 119 participants, 33% used NIV while 72% used TMV. Perhaps surprisingly, tracheostomy was not associated with poorer HRQoL. More than 80% of patients who initiated TMV did not need to move to a medical institution and two of five lived alone, compared to one of five patients using NIV. Patients with TMV had fewer respiratory complaints and anxiety. It is important to recognize that these outcomes were specific to patients primarily with muscular dystrophy and did not include more rapidly progressive NMDs.

Tracheostomy Impact on Speech and Swallowing

The introduction of a tracheostomy tube impacts both speech and swallow function. In some patients, this will not be important, for example, in an ALS patient with bulbar dysfunction who has already lost the ability to speak and receives nutrition via a feeding tube. However, patients who have maintained the ability to speak and/or eat should be aware of potential changes to both following tracheostomy. Speech is possible following tracheostomy tube placement and can be supported through the use of a one-way valve, attached in-line with the ventilator, that blocks air from flowing back into the ventilator circuit and thus redirects it past the tracheostomy tube and through the vocal cords. Extreme caution must be taken using a one-way valve in patients with a cuffed tracheostomy tube: if the cuff is not deflated prior to one-way valve insertion then exhalation will not be possible, leading quickly to increased intrathoracic pressure and potentially death. While oral feeding is still possible with TMV, the presence of the tracheostomy tube adjacent to the esophagus impacts swallowing sensation [55]. Often, patients with a progressive neuromuscular disease who are at a point of requiring invasive ventilation already receive nutritional support via a feeding tube.

Cost

In general, the cost of long-term NIV management is less than that of TMV, primarily due to the need for more highly trained caregivers at home or admission to a healthcare facility for TMV. Bach et al. performed a retrospective cost assessment for all DMD patients presenting to a single center in the United States who became continuously ventilator dependent either with NIV or TMV [69]. Costs for physician RVU, equipment, and intercurrent hospitalization were far less important than personal care and facility costs. In 2015, the annual cost of TMV averaged $269,000 at home with 16 h/day of licensed practical nurse/registered nurse care and $237,000 annually in an institution. Cost of NIV was generally much lower, but was dependent on the type of caregiver hired for support. Annual cost of NIV was $9800 without caregiver support, $45,000 with nurse's aide support, $81,400/year for unskilled personal assistance services, and $240,000/year for licensed practical nurse/registered nurse support.

In an earlier study from 1992, Moss et al. compared costs associated with care for patients with ALS having undergone TMV receiving long-term care either at home or in an institution in two regions of the United States [70]. The annual cost of home management was 37% that of management in an institution. Similar results have been found in other countries. A recent cost analysis of ALS patients in the Czech Republic with TMV managed either at home or in a healthcare facility found that the annual cost of home management was approximately ¼ that of the cost at a healthcare facility [71]. To summarize the available data, the cost of long-term management of NIV is substantially less than TMV, while the cost of TMV management at home is lower than management in a healthcare facility. The annual cost for the management of a patient requiring TMV can easily range in the hundreds of thousands of dollars [72].

Tracheostomy Selection with NMD

A few different surgical options exist for patients with NMD who are interested in pursuing long-term invasive mechanical ventilation. Tracheotomy with tracheostomy tube placement is by far the most common. Tracheotomy is a procedure that creates an opening in the trachea and a tract through the skin of the neck through which a tracheostomy tube is usually placed. The tracheostomy tube can be either cuffed or non-cuffed. The presence of the cuff may reduce aspiration risk though does not entirely eliminate it [73]. In the United Kingdom, the majority (~80%) of patients with ALS receive a cuffed tracheostomy tube [56]; this number may be lower in patients with other forms of NMD where bulbar dysfunction is not common and secretion management is less of a concern.

Total laryngectomy (TL) is an alternative to tracheotomy in patients with bulbar dysfunction. During total laryngectomy, the larynx is removed and the pharyngeal mucosa is closed to create a single digestive tube from the mouth to the stomach. The trachea is mobilized and sewn to the skin of the neck, completely separating the airway from the digestive tract. Total laryngectomy eliminates the chance of oral aspiration since the esophagus and trachea no longer share a common origin. Garvey et al. describe the findings of a retrospective chart review of a single ALS center over a 9-year period during which 15 patients were considered candidates for TL and 5 underwent the procedure [73]. Criteria for consideration included dysphagia, evidence of aspiration, and the inability to phonate intelligibly since for these patients the larynx serves no purpose. There is also a subset of ALS patients who may choose TL despite preserved speech in order to eliminate aspiration risk.

Laryngotracheal separation (LTS) is a third surgical technique that is an option for patients with bulbar dysfunction [74]. Rather than resection of the larynx, the procedure involves the transection of the trachea at the level of the second or third tracheal ring and the anastomosis of the upper trachea to the esophagus. The lower trachea is connected to the skin of the neck in a similar manner as the TL. As with the TL, this procedure eliminates the possibility of aspiration of oral contents into the lungs. It also offers the potential of reversibility, though this is usually less relevant for patients with progressive neuromuscular weakness. To our knowledge, there have not been comparisons in outcomes in patients with NMD receiving TL versus LTS and, if one of the procedures is to be considered, it may be at the discretion of the surgical team performing the procedure.

Modes of Invasive Mechanical Ventilation and Monitoring

There is no specific mode of mechanical ventilation that is known to be superior in patients with NMD requiring invasive mechanical ventilation. Generally, a mode with a set respiratory rate, such as volume or pressure limited assist control ventilation, is preferred. A pressure-control mode may be more comfortable due to its decelerating flow waveform. In our practice, we target a tidal volume of 8 mL/kg of ideal body weight and then adjust ventilator settings to achieve normocarbia and comfort. For patients with tracheostomy who are able to communicate, multiple modes including assist-control volume, assist-control pressure, as well as a volume or pressure limited mode incorporating synchronized intermittent mandatory ventilation (SIMV), can be trialed to optimize patient comfort. Often, patients with NMD on invasive ventilation do not require supplemental oxygen since the source of their respiratory failure does not involve the lung parenchyma. A pulse oximetry reading less than 95% may indicate a problem such as mucus plugging and that more aggressive cough assistance is needed [51].

Depending on post-tracheostomy disposition, comprehensive patient and caregiver training may be necessary prior to discharge from the hospital. For patients who are planning to go home following elective tracheostomy, this training often starts well before the surgical date is even set and can include a home remodel, providing a backup ventilator and ensuring an adequate backup power supply is available, and identifying caregivers among family members and paid care providers.

In our practice, postoperative tracheostomy patients are managed in an intensive care unit until they are ready either for discharge to home or to a healthcare facility that manages ventilators. Patients who are planning to go home with tracheostomy and mechanical ventilation require caregiver support 24 h a day. Caregivers receive the majority of their training, while the patient is postoperative in the intensive care unit. Some institutions have comprehensive protocols and training checklists in place to ensure that caregivers have not only been taught, but also are comfortable with, all necessary aspects of ventilator and tracheostomy management. A thorough discussion of home ventilator and tracheostomy management is beyond the scope of this chapter. However, a basic checklist for home caregiver training, individualized as much as possible to the patient's circumstances, is shown in Table 4.2 [75].

In our practice, the more time that home caregivers can spend post-tracheostomy in the hospital assisting with management, the better prior to patient discharge. We try to steadily increase the home caregiver responsibility for the patient in the presence of nursing and respiratory therapy backup support, to the point where the primary caregiver is able to manage all aspects of ventilator and tracheostomy management for the 24 h preceding hospital discharge to home.

Table 4.2 Basic checklist for tracheostomy care (adapted from Lewarski [75])

Basic airway anatomy
Tracheostomy tube description and operation
Clinical signs of respiratory distress
Clinical signs of aspiration
Suction techniques
Tracheostomy tube cleaning and maintenance
Stoma-site assessment and cleaning
Cardiopulmonary resuscitation and bag mask ventilation
Emergency decannulation and reinsertion
Tracheostomy tube exchange
Ventilator high- and low-pressure alarm troubleshooting

Decannulation of "Unweanable" Patients

Some NMD experts advocate for decannulation of most patients with NMD even if they are considered "unweanable." Bach et al. argue that any patient whose bulbar muscle strength is sufficient to prevent aspiration and who has a peak cough flow >120 L/min is a candidate for decannulation [76]. A recent multicenter review recorded rates of progression to continuous noninvasive ventilatory support in 1623 patients with ALS, DMD, or SMA1 who were initially requiring <23 h/day of noninvasive ventilatory support [77]. At the time of data collection, 494 patients were dependent on continuous noninvasive ventilatory support, while 110 patients had undergone tracheotomies, the majority of whom had bulbar ALS. The authors note that many intubated patients with neuromuscular disease who are considered "unweanable" can actually be extubated to continuous noninvasive ventilatory support and MI-E, noting an exception with upper motor neuron ALS patients.

In the above review, the authors note a 99% success rate at extubating so-called unweanable patients with NMD to continuous noninvasive ventilatory support and MI-E. Again, this was applicable to patients without bulbar dysfunction [77]. Bach et al. provide data from 157 consecutive "unweanable" patients who were either transferred from other facilities for help with decannulation or had refused tracheostomy [51]. Patients met a number of criteria including a vital capacity <20% predicted and failure of recent spontaneous breathing trial (see Table 4.3). Patients were extubated to noninvasive ventilation with either assist/control volume of 800–1500 mL or pressure control of at least 18 cm H_2O if abdominal distension developed. A variety of mouthpiece interfaces were provided. Manually assisted cough were provided with breath stacking and abdominal thrusts. Extubation was considered successful if the patient was discharged without reintubation. Using this approach, 95% of patients were successfully extubated on the first attempt,

Table 4.3 Extubation criteria for unweanable ventilator-dependent patients (from Bach et al. [51])

Afebrile and normal WBC count
Aged 4 years and older
No ventilator-free breathing tolerance with 7-cm pressure support in ambient air on the basis of NMD or CCM
VC <20% of normal
$PaCO_2$ ≤40 mmHg at peak inspiratory pressures <35 cm H_2O on full-setting assist/control mode at a rate of 10–13/min
SpO_2 ≥95% for 12 h or more in ambient air
All oxyhemoglobin desaturations <95% reversed by MAC and suctioning via translaryngeal tube
Fully alert and cooperative, receiving no sedative medications
Chest radiograph abnormalities cleared or clearing
Air leakage via upper airway sufficient for vocalization upon cuff deflation

CCM critical care myopathy, *MAC* mechanically assisted coughing, *NMD* neuromuscular disease, *SpO₂* pulse oxyhemoglobin saturation, *VC* vital capacity including all patients with assisted peak cough flow $\geq$160 L/min. The authors conclude that the use of continuous noninvasive ventilation and manually assisted cough can permit safe extubation of "unweanable"' patients with NMD.

Transition to Hospice Care

For many diseases that are progressive, NIV may fail at some point to provide adequate ventilatory or symptomatic support. As discussed in a prior section, some patients may choose to "progress" to TMV, while others would rather choose hospice care. For patients on TMV, at some point their quality of life may fall below an acceptable level and this may not be related to their physical function, but rather to their social or cognitive function [78, 79]. If patients decide they no longer have an acceptable quality of life, they will require support to make informed decisions as to when and how to withdraw care [80, 81]. A well-formed clinician-patient relationship and adequate palliative care services are necessary for a smooth transition, along with a clear plan for symptomatic control during and after withdrawal of mechanical respiratory assistance [82]. Withdrawal of ventilatory support and symptom management is beyond the scope of this chapter.

Ethical Considerations in Noninvasive Ventilation

NIV offers the possibility of extending life expectancy, as has been demonstrated in certain diseases such as ALS and DMD. This level of data, however, does not exist for all neuromuscular and restrictive thoracic cage diseases. However, the authors of this chapter would argue there is not equipoise about the use of NIV in those diseases for patients showing evidence of hypoventilation or symptomatic hypercapnia. As such, though it adds significant resource utilization, NIV should be offered to patients who have a neuromuscular condition, the symptoms stated above in the "indications" section of this chapter, and no contraindications.

Many of the other ethical considerations around the use of NIV center around the decision to initiate and discontinue NIV, particularly in the setting of prognostic uncertainty or with patients who cannot fully consent to therapy such as with children or those with cognitive impairment. When counseling patients and caregivers on whether to initiate NIV, transition to invasive mechanical ventilation, or to withdraw care, clinicians should be aware of their own biases and aim to provide honest information to allow patients and their families to make the best treatment decisions [83–85]. It is clear that clinicians should not assume that they can accurately assess patients' quality of life and, thus, extreme caution should be taken to imply or assume how a patient may feel about a specific choice [86]. In fact, even caregivers may underestimate patients' own perceived quality of life. Clinicians should lay out, as best known, the expected respiratory function trajectory and how NIV or TMV might impact that trajectory, as well as describing realistic respiratory care needs. Multidisciplinary input from physical and occupational therapists, respiratory therapists, general and subspecialty medical providers, and social workers (or case managers) is recommended to provide the most holistic approach. It is notable that patients may often rate their quality of life more highly than caregivers and may choose to undergo TMV again at a higher rate than caregivers would choose for those patients [87, 88]. While ultimately the decision to pursue or withdraw care is the patient's (or their legal decision-maker), that care choice will certainly have positive and possibly negative impact on their caretakers and/or family [67, 89]. The care burden placed on caregivers can lead to isolation and loneliness. If patients choose continuation of care initially, some may decide at a later point to then withdraw care, particularly those with progressive disease like ALS. Prior to initiation of invasive mechanical ventilation, patients should be informed of their ability to make this choice and clinicians should assist them in considering when that may be the case [85].

Patients on NIV or TMV require a relatively high amount of caregiving and utilize high amounts of health care [90, 91], with there being a higher cost burden for those with invasive mechanical ventilation when compared to NIV [69]. It is likely that the variability in cultural norms and expectations, legal and medical frameworks, and cost burden in different healthcare systems also impacts how patients make choices around respiratory support [92]. Limited access to qualified healthcare professionals trained to support NIV and other disabilities propagates poor outcomes and health inequity [93]. Other social determinants of health including health insurance coverage and availability of well-staffed durable medical equipment suppliers may also contribute to health inequity in these patients, especially in healthcare systems that do not provide state-coverage or single-payer coverage for the necessary resources [85].

Summary

Noninvasive ventilation is the standard of care for most patients with neuromuscular respiratory disease. Recommendations for the timing and modality of NIV are based on expert opinion, consensus statements, and small clinical or observational trials. For some patients, NIV is not appropriate due to specific features of their disease, comorbidities, or due to disease progression and, as such, invasive mechanical ventilation can be considered. Caregiver burden is high for the entire population, but particularly high for those using invasive mechanical ventilation, so appropriate education and counseling prior to proceeding with tracheostomy is necessary. Finally, there are ethical challenges that should be considered when considering individual and system-level care for these patients to improve decision-making and communication around their care.

References

1. Hilbert J. Sleep-disordered breathing in neuromuscular and chest wall diseases. Clin Chest Med. 2018;39(2):309–24. https://doi.org/10.1016/j.ccm.2018.01.009.
2. Parsons EC, Carter JC, Wrede JE, Donovan LM, Palen BN. Practical implementation of noninvasive ventilation in amyotrophic lateral sclerosis: lessons learned from a clinical case series. Can J Respir Ther. 2019;55:13–5. https://doi.org/10.29390/CJRT-2018-020.
3. Nicholson TT, Smith SB, Siddique T, et al. Respiratory pattern and tidal volumes differ for pressure support and volume-assured pressure support in amyotrophic lateral sclerosis. Ann Am Thorac Soc. 2017;14(7):1139–46. https://doi.org/10.1513/AnnalsATS.201605-346OC.
4. Eagle M, Baudouin SV, Chandler C, Giddings DR, Bullock R, Bushby K. Survival in Duchenne muscular dystrophy: improvements in life expectancy since 1967 and the impact of home nocturnal ventilation. Neuromuscul Disord. 2002;12(10):926–9. https://doi.org/10.1016/S0960-8966(02)00140-2.
5. Yasuma F, Sakai M, Matsuoke Y. Effects of noninvasive ventilation on survival in patients with Duchenne's muscular dystrophy. Chest. 1996;109(2):590. https://doi.org/10.1378/CHEST.109.2.590.
6. Toussaint M, Steens M, Wasteels G, Soudon P. Diurnal ventilation via mouthpiece: survival in end-stage Duchenne patients. Eur Respir J. 2006;28(3):549–55. https://doi.org/10.118 3/09031936.06.00004906.
7. Kleopa KA, Sherman M, Neal B, Romano GJ, Heiman-Patterson T. Bipap improves survival and rate of pulmonary function decline in patients with ALS. J Neurol Sci. 1999;164(1):82–8. https://doi.org/10.1016/S0022-510X(99)00045-3.
8. Khamankar N, Coan G, Weaver B, Mitchell CS. Associative increases in amyotrophic lateral sclerosis survival duration with non-invasive ventilation initiation and usage protocols. Front Neurol. 2018;9:578. https://doi.org/10.3389/FNEUR.2018.00578.
9. Bourke SC, Tomlinson M, Williams TL, Bullock RE, Shaw PJ, Gibson GJ. Effects of noninvasive ventilation on survival and quality of life in patients with amyotrophic lateral sclerosis: a randomised controlled trial. Lancet Neurol. 2006;5(2):140–7. https://doi.org/10.1016/S1474-4422(05)70326-4.
10. Radunovic A, Annane D, Rafiq MK, Brassington R, Mustfa N. Mechanical ventilation for amyotrophic lateral sclerosis/motor neuron disease. Cochrane Database Syst Rev. 2017;10(10):CD004427. https://doi.org/10.1002/14651858.CD004427.PUB4.
11. Birnkrant DJ, Bushby K, Bann CM, et al. Diagnosis and management of Duchenne muscular dystrophy, part 2: respiratory, cardiac, bone health, and orthopaedic management. Lancet Neurol. 2018;17(4):347. https://doi.org/10.1016/S1474-4422(18)30025-5.
12. Miller RG, Jackson CE, Kasarskis EJ, et al. Practice parameter update: the care of the patient with amyotrophic lateral sclerosis: multidisciplinary care, symptom management, and cognitive/behavioral impairment (an evidence-based review): report of the Quality Standards Subcommittee of the American. Neurology. 2009;73(15):1227–33. https://doi.org/10.1212/WNL.0B013E3181BC01A4.
13. Clinical indications for noninvasive positive pressure ventilation in chronic respiratory failure due to restrictive lung disease, COPD, and nocturnal hypoventilation—a consensus conference report. Chest. 1999;116(2):521–34. https://doi.org/10.1378/CHEST.116.2.521.
14. Sunwoo BY, Mulholland M, Rosen IM, Wolfe LF. The changing landscape of adult home noninvasive ventilation technology, use, and reimbursement in the United States. Chest. 2014;145(5):1134–40. https://doi.org/10.1378/CHEST.13-0802.
15. Andersen T, Sandnes A, Brekka AK, et al. Laryngeal response patterns influence the efficacy of mechanical assisted cough in amyotrophic lateral sclerosis. Thorax. 2017;72(3):221–9. https://doi.org/10.1136/thoraxjnl-2015-207555.
16. Simonds AK. Progress in respiratory management of bulbar complications of motor neuron disease/amyotrophic lateral sclerosis? Thorax. 2017;72(3):199–201. https://doi.org/10.1136/thoraxjnl-2016-208919.

17. Hess DR. Noninvasive ventilation for neuromuscular disease. Clin Chest Med. 2018;39(2):437–47. https://doi.org/10.1016/j.ccm.2018.01.014.

18. Toussaint M, Chatwin M, Gonçalves MR, et al. Mouthpiece ventilation in neuromuscular disorders: narrative review of technical issues important for clinical success. Respir Med. 2021;180:106373. https://doi.org/10.1016/j.rmed.2021.106373.

19. Hess DR. Noninvasive ventilation in neuromuscular disease: equipment and application. Respir Care. 2006;51(8):896–912.

20. Nava S, Navalesi P, Gregoretti C. Interfaces and humidification for noninvasive mechanical ventilation. Respir Care. 2009;54(1):71–84.

21. Worsley P, Prudden G, Gower G, Bader D. Investigating the effects of strap tension during noninvasive ventilation mask application: a combined biomechanical and biomarker approach. MDER. 2016;9:409–17. https://doi.org/10.2147/MDER.S121712.

22. Teschler H, Stampa J, Ragette R, Konietzko N, Berthon-Jones M. Effect of mouth leak on effectiveness of nasal bilevel ventilatory assistance and sleep architecture. Eur Respir J. 1999;14(6):1251–7. https://doi.org/10.1183/09031936.99.14612519.

23. Visscher MO, White CC, Jones JM, Cahill T, Jones DC, Pan BS. Face masks for noninvasive ventilation: fit, excess skin hydration, and pressure ulcers. Respir Care. 2015;60(11):1536–47. https://doi.org/10.4187/respcare.04036.

24. Gonzalez J, Sharshar T, Hart N, Chadda K, Raphaël JC, Lofaso F. Air leaks during mechanical ventilation as a cause of persistent hypercapnia in neuromuscular disorders. Intensive Care Med. 2003;29(4):596–602. https://doi.org/10.1007/S00134-003-1659-5.

25. Wilson GN, Piper AJ, Norman M, et al. Nasal versus full face mask for noninvasive ventilation in chronic respiratory failure. Eur Respir J. 2004;23(4):605–9. https://doi.org/10.1183/09031936.04.00051604.

26. Navalesi P, Fanfulla F, Frigerio P, Gregoretti C, Nava S. Physiologic evaluation of noninvasive mechanical ventilation delivered with three types of masks in patients with chronic hypercapnic respiratory failure. Crit Care Med. 2000;28(6):1785–90. https://doi.org/10.1097/00003246-200006000-00015.

27. Bach JR, Alba AS, Saporito LR. Intermittent positive pressure ventilation via the mouth as an alternative to tracheostomy for 257 ventilator users. Chest. 1993;103(1):174–82. https://doi.org/10.1378/CHEST.103.1.174.

28. Garuti G, Nicolini A, Grecchi B, Lusuardi M, Winck JC, Bach JR. Open circuit mouthpiece ventilation: concise clinical review. Rev Port Pneumol. 2014;20(4):211–8. https://doi.org/10.1016/j.rppneu.2014.03.004.

29. Chatwin M, Gonçalves M, Gonzalez-Bermejo J, Toussaint M, ENMC Respiratory Therapy Consortium. 252nd ENMC international workshop: developing best practice guidelines for management of mouthpiece ventilation in neuromuscular disorders. March 6th to 8th 2020, Amsterdam, The Netherlands. Neuromuscul Disord. 2020;30(9):772–81. https://doi.org/10.1016/J.NMD.2020.07.008.

30. Finder JD, Birnkrant D, Carl J, et al. Respiratory care of the patient with Duchenne muscular dystrophy: ATS consensus statement. Am J Respir Crit Care Med. 2004;170(4):456–65. https://doi.org/10.1164/RCCM.200307-885ST.

31. Pluym M, Kabir AW, Gohar A. The use of volume-assured pressure support noninvasive ventilation in acute and chronic respiratory failure: a practical guide and literature review. Hosp Pract. 2015;43(5):299–307. https://doi.org/10.1080/21548331.2015.1110475.

32. Patel SI, Gay P, Morgenthaler TI, et al. Practical implementation of a single-night split-titration protocol with BPAP-ST and AVAPS in patients with neuromuscular disease. J Clin Sleep Med. 2018;14(12):2031–5. https://doi.org/10.5664/jcsm.7530.

33. Crescimanno G, Marrone O, Vianello A. Efficacy and comfort of volume-guaranteed pressure support in patients with chronic ventilatory failure of neuromuscular origin. Respirology. 2011;16(4):672–9. https://doi.org/10.1111/j.1440-1843.2011.01962.x.

34. Jaye J, Chatwin M, Dayer M, Morrell MJ, Simonds AK. Autotitrating versus standard noninvasive ventilation: a randomised crossover trial. Eur Respir J. 2009;33(3):566–71. https://doi.org/10.1183/09031936.00065008.
35. Annane D, Orlikowski D, Chevret S. Nocturnal mechanical ventilation for chronic hypoventilation in patients with neuromuscular and chest wall disorders. Cochrane Database Syst Rev. 2014;2014(12):CD001941. https://doi.org/10.1002/14651858.CD001941.pub3.
36. Kelly JL, Jaye J, Pickersgill RE, Chatwin M, Morrell MJ, Simonds AK. Randomized trial of "intelligent" autotitrating ventilation versus standard pressure support non-invasive ventilation: impact on adherence and physiological outcomes. Respirology. 2014;19(4):596–603. https://doi.org/10.1111/resp.12269.
37. Patout M, Gagnadoux F, Rabec C, et al. AVAPS-AE versus ST mode: a randomized controlled trial in patients with obesity hypoventilation syndrome. Respirology. 2020;25(10):1073–81. https://doi.org/10.1111/resp.13784.
38. Affeldt JE. Roundtable conference on poliomyelitis equipment. National Foundation for Infantile Paralysis-March of Dimes; 1953.
39. Toussaint M, Chatwin M, Verhulst S, Reychler G. Preference of neuromuscular patients regarding equipment for daytime mouthpiece ventilation: a randomized crossover study. Clin Respir J. 2020;14(3):214–21. https://doi.org/10.1111/crj.13118.
40. Boitano LJ, Benditt JO. An evaluation of home volume ventilators that support open-circuit mouthpiece ventilation. Respir Care. 2005;50(11):1457–61.
41. Steier J, Jolley CJ, Seymour J, et al. Screening for sleep-disordered breathing in neuromuscular disease using a questionnaire for symptoms associated with diaphragm paralysis. Eur Respir J. 2011;37(2):400–5. https://doi.org/10.1183/09031936.00036210.
42. Dupuis-Lozeron E, Gex G, Pasquina P, et al. Development and validation of a simple tool for the assessment of home noninvasive ventilation: the S^3-NIV questionnaire. Eur Respir J. 2018;52(5):1801182. https://doi.org/10.1183/13993003.011822018.
43. Sanders MH, Kern NB, Costantino JP, et al. Accuracy of end-tidal and transcutaneous PCO_2 monitoring during sleep. Chest. 1994;106(2):472–83. https://doi.org/10.1378/chest.106.2.472.
44. Lermuzeaux M, Meric H, Sauneuf B, et al. Superiority of transcutaneous CO_2 over end-tidal CO_2 measurement for monitoring respiratory failure in nonintubated patients: a pilot study. J Crit Care. 2016;31(1):150–6. https://doi.org/10.1016/j.jcrc.2015.09.014.
45. Won YH, Choi WA, Lee JW, Bach JR, Park J, Kang SW. Sleep transcutaneous vs. end-tidal CO_2 monitoring for patients with neuromuscular disease. Am J Phys Med Rehabil. 2016;95(2):91–5. https://doi.org/10.1097/PHM.0000000000000345.
46. Orlikowski D, Prigent H, Ambrosi X, et al. Comparison of ventilator-integrated end-tidal CO_2 and transcutaneous CO_2 monitoring in home-ventilated neuromuscular patients. Respir Med. 2016;117:7–13. https://doi.org/10.1016/j.rmed.2016.05.022.
47. Venkat A. The threshold moment: ethical tensions surrounding decision making on tracheostomy for patients in the intensive care unit. J Clin Ethics. 2013;24(2):135–43.
48. Macauley R. To trach or not to trach, that is the question. Paediatr Respir Rev. 2019;29:9–13. https://doi.org/10.1016/j.prrv.2018.05.004.
49. Cheng G, Bach JR. Avoidance of tracheostomy in patients with neuromuscular disease. Chron Respir Dis. 2008;5(4):243; author reply 245. https://doi.org/10.1177/1479972308097464.
50. McKim DA, Griller N, LeBlanc C, Woolnough A, King J. Twenty-four hour noninvasive ventilation in Duchenne muscular dystrophy: a safe alternative to tracheostomy. Can Respir J. 2013;20(1):e5–9. https://doi.org/10.1155/2013/406163.
51. Bach JR, Gonçalves MR, Hamdani I, Winck JC. Extubation of patients with neuromuscular weakness: a new management paradigm. Chest. 2010;137(5):1033–9. https://doi.org/10.1378/chest.09-2144.
52. Khan A, Frazer-Green L, Amin R, et al. Respiratory management of patients with neuromuscular weakness: an American College of Chest Physicians clinical practice guideline and expert panel report. Chest. 2023;164(2):394–413. https://doi.org/10.1016/j.chest.2023.03.011.

53. Bach JR. Tracheostomy for advanced neuromuscular disease. Con. Chron Respir Dis. 2007;4(4):239–41. https://doi.org/10.1177/1479972307084081.

54. Takei K, Tsuda K, Takahashi F, Hirai M, Palumbo J. An assessment of treatment guidelines, clinical practices, demographics, and progression of disease among patients with amyotrophic lateral sclerosis in Japan, the United States, and Europe. Amyotroph Lateral Scler Frontotemporal Degener. 2017;18(sup1):88–97. https://doi.org/10.1080/21678421.2017.1361445.

55. Niedermeyer S, Murn M, Choi PJ. Respiratory failure in amyotrophic lateral sclerosis. Chest. 2019;155(2):401–8. https://doi.org/10.1016/j.chest.2018.06.035.

56. Turner MR, Faull C, McDermott CJ, Nickol AH, Palmer J, Talbot K. Tracheostomy in motor neurone disease. Pract Neurol. 2019;19(6):467–75. https://doi.org/10.1136/practneurol-2018-002109.

57. Rabkin JG, Albert SM, Tider T, et al. Predictors and course of elective long-term mechanical ventilation: a prospective study of ALS patients. Amyotroph Lateral Scler. 2006;7(2):86–95. https://doi.org/10.1080/14660820500515021.

58. Bae JS, Hong YH, Baek W, et al. Current status of the diagnosis and management of amyotrophic lateral sclerosis in Korea: a multi-center cross-sectional study. J Clin Neurol. 2012;8(4):293–300. https://doi.org/10.3988/jcn.2012.8.4.293.

59. Wilson E, Turner N, Faull C, Palmer J, Turner MR, Davidson S. Understanding living with tracheostomy ventilation for motor neuron disease and the implications for quality of life: a qualitative study protocol. BMJ Open. 2023;13(3):e071624. https://doi.org/10.1136/bmjopen-2023-071624.

60. Rabkin J, Ogino M, Goetz R, et al. Tracheostomy with invasive ventilation for ALS patients: neurologists' roles in the US and Japan. Amyotroph Lateral Scler Frontotemporal Degener. 2013;14(2):116–23. https://doi.org/10.3109/17482968.2012.726226.

61. Rochwerg B, Brochard L, Elliott MW, et al. Official ERS/ATS clinical practice guidelines: noninvasive ventilation for acute respiratory failure. Eur Respir J. 2017;50(2):1602426. https://doi.org/10.1183/13993003.02426-2016.

62. Luo F, Annane D, Orlikowski D, et al. Invasive versus non-invasive ventilation for acute respiratory failure in neuromuscular disease and chest wall disorders. Cochrane Database Syst Rev. 2017;12(12):CD008380. https://doi.org/10.1002/14651858.CD008380.pub2.

63. Spataro R, Bono V, Marchese S, La Bella V. Tracheostomy mechanical ventilation in patients with amyotrophic lateral sclerosis: clinical features and survival analysis. J Neurol Sci. 2012;323(1–2):66–70. https://doi.org/10.1016/j.jns.2012.08.011.

64. Spittel S, Maier A, Kettemann D, et al. Non-invasive and tracheostomy invasive ventilation in amyotrophic lateral sclerosis: utilization and survival rates in a cohort study over 12 years in Germany. Eur J Neurol. 2021;28(4):1160–71. https://doi.org/10.1111/ene.14647.

65. Chiò A, Calvo A, Ghiglione P, et al. Tracheostomy in amyotrophic lateral sclerosis: a 10-year population-based study in Italy. J Neurol Neurosurg Psychiatry. 2010;81(10):1141–3. https://doi.org/10.1136/jnnp.2009.175984.

66. Soudon P, Steens M, Toussaint M. A comparison of invasive versus noninvasive full-time mechanical ventilation in Duchenne muscular dystrophy. Chron Respir Dis. 2008;5(2):87–93. https://doi.org/10.1177/1479972308088715.

67. Kaub-Wittemer D, Von Steinbüchel N, Wasner M, Laier-Groeneveld G, Borasio GD. Quality of life and psychosocial issues in ventilated patients with amyotrophic lateral sclerosis and their caregivers. J Pain Symptom Manag. 2003;26(4):890–6. https://doi.org/10.1016/S0885-3924(03)00323-3.

68. Delorme M, Reveillere C, Devaux C, Segovia-Kueny S, Lofaso F, Boussaid G. Quality of life in patients with slowly progressive neuromuscular disorders dependent on mechanical ventilation. Thorax. 2023;78(1):92–6. https://doi.org/10.1136/thorax-2022-219211.

69. Bach JR, Tran J, Durante S. Cost and physician effort analysis of invasive vs. noninvasive respiratory management of Duchenne muscular dystrophy. Am J Phys Med Rehabil. 2015;94(6):474–82. https://doi.org/10.1097/PHM.0000000000000228.

70. Moss AH, Oppenheimer EA, Casey P, et al. Patients with amyotrophic lateral sclerosis receiving long-term mechanical ventilation. Advance care planning and outcomes. Chest. 1996;110(1):249–55. https://doi.org/10.1378/chest.110.1.249.
71. Gajdoš O, Rožánek M, Donin G, Kamenský V. Cost–utility analysis of home mechanical ventilation in patients with amyotrophic lateral sclerosis. Healthcare (Basel). 2021;9(2):142. https://doi.org/10.3390/healthcare9020142.
72. MacIntyre EJ, Asadi L, Mckim DA, Bagshaw SM. Clinical outcomes associated with home mechanical ventilation: a systematic review. Can Respir J. 2016;2016:6547180. https://doi.org/10.1155/2016/6547180.
73. Garvey CM, Boylan KB, Salassa JR, Kennelly KD. Total laryngectomy in patients with advanced bulbar symptoms of amyotrophic lateral sclerosis. Amyotroph Lateral Scler. 2009;10(5–6):470–5. https://doi.org/10.3109/17482960802578373.
74. Snyderman CH, Johnson JT. Laryngotracheal separation for intractable aspiration. Ann Otol Rhinol Laryngol. 1988;97(5 Pt 1):466–70. https://doi.org/10.1177/000348948809700506.
75. Lewarski JS. Long-term care of the patient with a tracheostomy. Respir Care. 2005;50(4):534–7.
76. Bach JR. Noninvasive respiratory management of patients with neuromuscular disease. Ann Rehabil Med. 2017;41(4):519–38. https://doi.org/10.5535/arm.2017.41.4.519.
77. Gonçalves MR, Bach JR, Ishikawa Y, Saporito L, Winck JC, International Study Group on Continuous Noninvasive Ventilatory Support in Neuromuscular Disease (CNVSND). Continuous noninvasive ventilatory support outcomes for patients with neuromuscular disease: a multicenter data collaboration. Pulmonology. 2021;27(6):509–17. https://doi.org/10.1016/j.pulmoe.2021.06.007.
78. Simmons Z, Bremer BA, Robbins RA, Walsh SM, Fischer S. Quality of life in ALS depends on factors other than strength and physical function. Neurology. 2000;55(3):388–92. https://doi.org/10.1212/WNL.55.3.388.
79. Chiò A, Gauthier A, Montuschi A, et al. A cross sectional study on determinants of quality of life in ALS. J Neurol Neurosurg Psychiatry. 2004;75(11):1597–601. https://doi.org/10.1136/jnnp.2003.033100.
80. Mitsumoto H, Bromberg M, Johnston W, et al. Promoting excellence in end-of-life care in ALS. Amyotroph Lateral Scler Other Motor Neuron Disord. 2005;6(3):145–54. https://doi.org/10.1080/14660820510028647.
81. Connolly S, Galvin M, Hardiman O. End-of-life management in patients with amyotrophic lateral sclerosis. Lancet Neurol. 2015;14(4):435–42. https://doi.org/10.1016/S1474-4422(14)70221-2.
82. Danel-Brunaud V, Touzet L, Chevalier L, et al. Ethical considerations and palliative care in patients with amyotrophic lateral sclerosis: a review. Rev Neurol (Paris). 2017;173(5):300–7. https://doi.org/10.1016/j.neurol.2017.03.032.
83. Simonds AK. Respiratory support for the severely handicapped child with neuromuscular disease: ethics and practicality. Semin Respir Crit Care Med. 2007;28(3):342–54. https://doi.org/10.1055/s-2007-981655.
84. Ray S, Brierley J, Bush A, et al. Towards developing an ethical framework for decision making in long-term ventilation in children. Arch Dis Child. 2018;103(11):1080–4. https://doi.org/10.1136/archdischild-2018-314997.
85. Magelssen M, Holmøy T, Horn MA, Fondenæs OA, Dybwik K, Førde R. Ethical challenges in tracheostomy-assisted ventilation in amyotrophic lateral sclerosis. J Neurol. 2018;265(11):2730–6. https://doi.org/10.1007/s00415-018-9054-x.
86. Slevin ML, Plant H, Lynch D, Drinkwater J, Gregory WM. Who should measure quality of life, the doctor or the patient? Br J Cancer. 1988;57(1):109–12.
87. Moss AH, Casey P, Stocking CB, Roos RP, Brooks BR, Siegler M. Home ventilation for amyotrophic lateral sclerosis patients: outcomes, costs, and patient, family, and physician attitudes. Neurology. 1993;43(2):438–43. https://doi.org/10.1212/WNL.43.2.438.

88. Marchese S, Lo Coco D, Lo Coco A. Outcome and attitudes toward home tracheostomy ventilation of consecutive patients: a 10-year experience. Respir Med. 2008;102(3):430–6. https://doi.org/10.1016/j.rmed.2007.10.006.
89. Rossi Ferrario S, Zotti AM, Zaccaria S, Donner CF. Caregiver strain associated with tracheostomy in chronic respiratory failure. Chest. 2001;119(5):1498–502. https://doi.org/10.1378/chest.119.5.1498.
90. Sevick MA, Bradham DD. Economic value of caregiver effort in maintaining long-term ventilator-assisted individuals at home. Heart Lung. 1997;26(2):148–57. https://doi.org/10.1016/S0147-9563(97)90075-3.
91. Nonoyama ML, McKim DA, Road J, et al. Healthcare utilisation and costs of home mechanical ventilation. Thorax. 2018;73(7):644–51. https://doi.org/10.1136/thoraxjnl-2017-211138.
92. Dybwik K, Tollåli T, Nielsen EW, Brinchmann BS. Why does the provision of home mechanical ventilation vary so widely? Chron Respir Dis. 2010;7(2):67–73. https://doi.org/10.1177/1479972309357497.
93. Sabatello M, Burke TB, McDonald KE, Appelbaum PS. Disability, ethics, and health care in the COVID-19 pandemic. Am J Public Health. 2020;110(10):1523–7. https://doi.org/10.2105/AJPH.2020.305837.

Chapter 5
Non-invasive Approaches to Secretion Clearance in Neuromuscular Disease

Douglas McKim and Mirna Attalla

Introduction

Respiratory muscle weakness due to neuromuscular disease (NMD) can lead to impaired airway clearance. Healthy subjects produce 10–100 mL of airway mucus per day. A build-up of secretions and reduced mucociliary clearance can increase risk for respiratory tract infection and lead to acute or chronic respiratory failure. Impaired airway clearance and retained secretions can increase the risk for infection and may reduce lung function and respiratory system compliance. Impaired airway clearance during chest infections is a leading cause of morbidity and mortality for individuals with neuromuscular diseases. Most episodes of respiratory failure in patients with ventilatory compromise are related to ineffective airway clearance [1]. Airway clearance becomes impaired as a result of abnormal lung mechanics, change in mucus quality, and reduced mucociliary clearance [2]. Interventions and therapies, focused on airway clearance, can augment cough effectiveness, improve respiratory system compliance, improve alveolar ventilation and gas exchange with the goal of preventing acute or chronic respiratory failure in individuals with NMD.

D. McKim (✉)
Department of Medicine, University of Ottawa, Ottawa, ON, Canada

CANVent Respiratory Rehabilitation Services, Ottawa, ON, Canada
e-mail: dmckim@toh.ca

M. Attalla
Division of Respirology, University of Ottawa, Ottawa, ON, Canada
e-mail: attalla.m@queensu.ca

N. Lechtzin (ed.), *Pulmonary Complications of Neuromuscular Disease*,
Respiratory Medicine, https://doi.org/10.1007/978-3-031-65335-3_5

Respiratory Parameters in Patients with Neuromuscular Diseases

Pulmonary function testing can help predict the risk of respiratory failure during acute illness, assess cough effectiveness, monitor progression of respiratory failure, and guide the timing of initiation of airway clearance measures [3]. Pulmonary function, including vital capacity, inspiratory and expiratory flow rates, and SaO_2, can be affected by the retention of secretions. Reduced vital capacity and cough effectiveness are associated with severe respiratory distress when secretions accumulate [4]. Spirometry can be used to monitor vital capacity and the maximal insufflation capacity (MIC). For patients with a vital capacity less than 50% of the predicted normal values or when peak cough flow falls below 270 L/min, lung volume recruitment techniques should be promptly initiated [5, 6].

Cough is an important defence mechanism to prevent foreign material from entering the lower airways, and for clearance of secretions and retained material. An effective cough relies on both inspiratory and expiratory muscle forces and can be measured by peak cough flow (PCF, L/min). It can also be estimated from the peak expired flow (PEF) from the forced vital capacity flow volume loop (L/s). Maximum expiratory pressure (MEP) is a function of lung and chest wall recoil and expiratory muscle strength at full inspiration. Cough flows depend on chest wall and lung recoil, expiratory muscle force, vital capacity, airway calibre, and glottic function. While chest wall compliance may be expected to be low in neuromuscular disease, resulting in increased recoil, this is usually offset by reduced VC, weak expiratory muscles, at unfavourable length-tension relation, and reduced airway calibre at low lung volumes.

The PCF should be routinely measured in patients with neuromuscular disease and spinal cord injuries [6–8]. PCF is a useful measurement for monitoring pulmonary function and management of airway clearance related to muscle weakness. PCF can be measured by instructing a patient to cough as forcefully as possible through a peak flow meter, wearing a nose clip, after maximal inspiration. Alternatively, a face mask can be attached to a peak flow meter for patients who cannot form a seal around a mouthpiece. Assisted peak cough flow can also be measured following lung volume augmentation to one's MIC with or without an abdominal thrust timed with glottic opening [4]. An inability to generate a PCF greater than 270 L/s, even if MIC after volume recruitment improves, is associated with upper airway obstruction, significant bulbar dysfunction, or hypopharyngeal collapse during the manoeuvre [9–11].

Insufflation capacity

Maximum Insufflation Capacity (MIC) and Maximum Insufflation Capacity–Vital Capacity Difference (MIC–VC Difference)

The MIC, which is measured on exhalation, is a measurement of the lung volume, following volume augmentation or volume 'recruitment' by a breath-stacking manoeuvre. The lower limit of the MIC is the residual volume (RV) [12]. The effectiveness of airway clearance techniques can be assessed by measuring the difference between maximum insufflation capacity and vital capacity (MIC-VC difference) before and after airway clearance measures. The MIC-VC difference measures how much additional volume has been recruited with the intervention (see Fig. 5.1). A larger MIC-VC difference is associated with more effective airway clearance and lower risk of developing respiratory complications. Monitoring the MIC-VC difference can also be useful for assessing the effectiveness of a volume recruitment strategy over time. Although a lower vital capacity may be associated with a lower MIC, a lower vital capacity with preserved lung compliance will be associated with a greater MIC-VC difference.

Peak Cough Flow (PCF)

Cough becomes ineffective when respiratory muscles are too weak or when mucus develops an altered quality and adheres to the airway wall. Peak cough flow (PCF), a measure of the maximum airflow generated during cough, correlates with effective airway clearance. It is determined by the linear velocity of airflow, the diameter of the airway, and dynamic airway compression [13]. Effective PCF requires inspiration to 85–90% of vital capacity and generation of high intrathoracic pressure, to allow exhalation of at least 2.3–2.5 L at a PCF of 6–20 L/s. The broadly accepted normal range for PCF is 360–849 L/min [14]. Bach et al. have suggested that a PCF of 160 L/min is required for successful extubation in the context of neuromuscular weakness.

In a Canadian/UK cross-sectional survey of clinicians who care for patients with spinal cord injuries that included 155 participants, peak cough flow was the most

Fig. 5.1 Forced vital capacity flow volume loop, spontaneous (red), following lung volume recruitment (blue, MIC). MIC-VC difference is 1 L

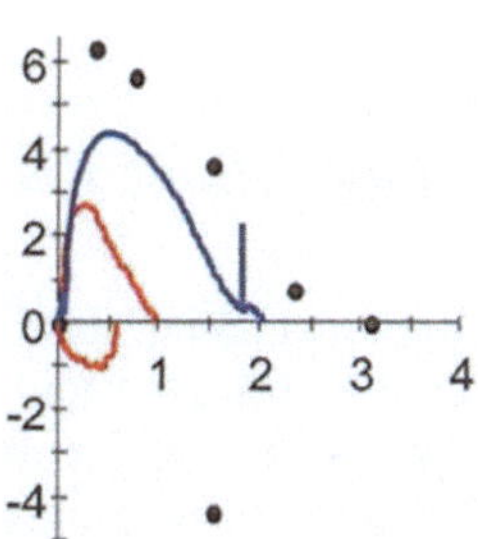

common method of monitoring cough effectiveness in both countries. Peak cough flow was used less often in Canada before initiation of airway clearance (81% versus 97%). Both groups similarly used PCF to ensure adequate airway clearance technique, the most common interventions being mechanical insufflation-exsufflation, lung volume recruitment and manually assisted cough when PCF was less than 270 L/min [15].

Smina et al. demonstrated in 95 patients undergoing 115 extubations, that successful extubation was associated with a cough flow, measured through the ETT, of over 60 L/min [16]. Monlagh et al. conducted a similar study demonstrating improved ETT secretion clearance and mean airway pressure after using a secretion-clearance device at a flow rate of 60 L/min [17].

It has also been observed that patients with a PCF >270 L/min are at lower risk of developing respiratory failure during respiratory tract infections. Those with a PCF <270 L/min are more likely to experience a PCF <160 L/min during acute respiratory illnesses, which is suggestive of cough ineffectiveness during acute respiratory illnesses [18]. A retrospective study by Donha-Schwake et al. demonstrated that a PCF <160 L/min was sensitive (75.2) and specific (79.2) for increased risk of severe respiratory infections requiring hospitalization [19].

Maximum expiratory pressure (MEP), measured from total lung capacity (TLC), correlates well with cough effectiveness. A MEP >60 cm H_2O is correlated with an effective cough, and a MEP <45 cm H_2O is associated with ineffective cough [3].

Coughing from MIC has been demonstrated to lead to a higher PCF. The increased lung volume at MIC results in a larger airway diameter and increased elastic recoil. However, the measurement should only be noted as a trend to monitor for progression of respiratory failure [12]. When mucociliary clearance is impaired, secretion clearance depends on flow generated during the expulsive phase of cough [19].

Cough Augmentation

Effective coughing requires adequate inspiration followed by adequate contraction of expiratory muscles [20] and active closure and release of glottic structures. Cough impairment is one of the leading causes of hospitalization in patients with ALS [21].

Lung Volume Recruitment (Breath Stacking)

Breath stacking has been recommended as the first-line intervention for lung volume recruitment and cough augmentation for ALS patients. Breath stacking is a manoeuvre that involves inflating the lungs by 'stacking' one inhaled breath on top of another, without exhaling, over a short period of time. Breath stacking is done to recruit volume and increase cough effectiveness. It may recruit volume in more dependent areas of the lung to improve ventilation and gas exchange. This can be achieved with several methods, the most common being the use of a manual resuscitation bag with a one-way valve. Other techniques include glossopharyngeal breathing, breath stacking with mouthpiece ventilation, or a more prolonged inspiratory breath-hold with a cough assist device [4, 5].

Kang and Bach described performing breath stacking using a manual resuscitation bag or portable volume ventilator to increase maximum insufflation capacity [5]. Breath stacking with a manual resuscitation bag can be achieved by attaching extension tubing and one-way valve to the bag. A patient can achieve maximal insufflation capacity using this equipment. It is important to emphasize that this is not an emergency resuscitation device, as it is a closed circuit and will not allow the patient to exhale. Caution should be used in patients at risk for pneumothorax.

Breath stacking can also be achieved with glossopharyngeal breathing (GPB). Glossopharyngeal breathing, often referred to as 'frog breathing', involves the use of oropharyngeal muscles to force air into the lungs. Patients can be instructed to sit in an upright position, breathe in deeply and hold, and say the word 'gup' back to back at a rate of 100 times per min 6–9 times to allow maximal inhalation and/or cough. GBP can increase inspiratory capacity, initiate a stronger cough, prevent atelectasis, improve phonation, and improve chest compliance [22].

Breath stacking or air stacking usually requires adequate glottic closure and bulbar function to be effective in increasing MIC to a volume greater than vital capacity. However, Bach has referred to the achievement of lung insufflation capacity (LIC) performed with an in-line one-way valve and mask, in the absence of voluntary activity or adequate glottic function [23].

Reduced chest wall and lung compliance can also limit the volume recruitment that can be achieved by breath stacking. Regular breath stacking can maintain lung and chest wall compliance while increasing cough effectiveness [8]. Breath stacking can also significantly improve peak cough flow and allow for more effective cough for secretion clearance [1].

Sheers et al. conducted a randomized controlled trial evaluating the effect of regular lung volume recruitment using a manual resuscitation bag on the maintenance of chest wall flexibility and decline in lung function in a sample of 76 participants and demonstrated that regular LVR did increase MIC and MIC-VC difference without clear evidence of modification of lung mechanics or slowing the rate of lung volume decline or rate of respiratory tract infections. The study also demonstrated that increasing the frequency or duration of LVR manoeuvres did not have a greater effect on increasing MIC. Those patients, did, however, have a higher tolerability to increased insufflation capacity, which may or may not lead to increased treatment adherence and tolerance over time [24].

For patients with Duchenne muscular dystrophy, LVR can maintain MIC-VC difference over time, even if vital capacity declines, which suggests stability of pulmonary compliance over time [25].

Manually Assisted Cough

Coughing without adequate abdominal muscle contraction can often lead to impaired cough effectiveness. The 2023 American College of Chest Physicians (ACCP) guidelines on respiratory management of patients with neuromuscular weakness recommends manually assisted cough for patients with neuromuscular disease and reduced cough effectiveness, with or without the addition of other cough augmentation modalities [26].

Manually assisted cough involves the patient spontaneously inspiring to TLC, closing the glottis and generating a cough by contracting any functional expiratory muscles while an assistant applies an inward and upward thrust to their epigastric abdomen or anterior chest well, also known as an abdominal thrust or 'Heimlich-type assisted cough' [27]. Manually assisted cough can be performed by encouraging the patient to inhale until maximal inspiratory capacity, to maximize elastic recoil during exhalation, followed by augmentation of exhalation using abdominal thrust or thoracic squeeze technique. Combining deep inspiration with LVR to MIC with manually assisted cough via abdominal thrust can significantly increase PCF. Manually assisted cough can also achieve a faster expiratory flow rate and greater volume exhaled by reducing residual volume, as illustrated by Fig. 5.2 [9, 27]. An increase in PCF can also be achieved by abdominal thrust alone, although it is more effective when it follows insufflation to MIC, following breath stacking. Inhaling to MIC has been shown to have a greater effect on PCF than MAC [30, 31].

Some patients have demonstrated independent discovery and performance of manually assisted cough by, for example, advancing their power chair into the edge of a table or counter, and compressing their abdomen during a breath hold at TLC, then performing their own assisted cough manoeuvre. Individuals with paraplegia can be taught a similar autonomous method of manually assisted cough, inspiring to TLC (or better MIC, with GPB or assistance with LVR), folding their arms over their abdomen and rolling forward over their arms. The mass of the arms

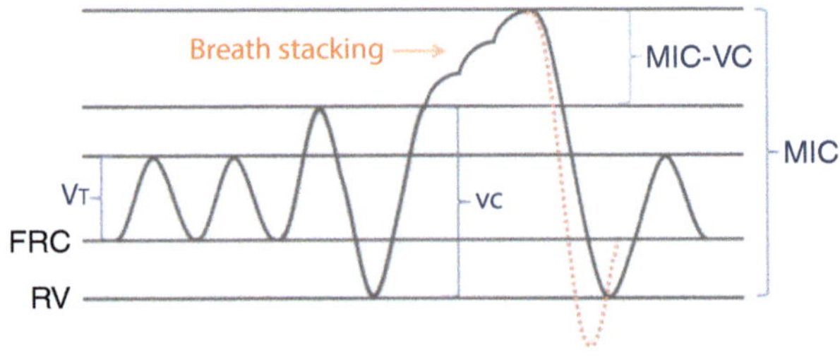

Fig. 5.2 Lung volume recruitment (LVR) with breath stacking and effect of manually assisted cough. (*Adapted from ACI Respiratory Network, Domiciliary Non-Invasive Ventilation in Adult Patients* (www.aci.health.nsw.gov.au) [28, 29])

compresses and pressurizes the abdomen and thorax, increasing expiratory cough flows.

There are limitations to the effectiveness of manually assisted cough. It requires the patient to be able to cooperate with the manoeuvre and to coordinate with the caregiver assisting. Another limitation is that glottic closure must be intact for manually assisted cough to be effective. Reduced chest wall compliance can also reduce the effectiveness of manually assisted cough, as it reduces the achievable maximum insufflation capacity. Obesity and spinal deformities significantly limit chest wall compliance and often lead to ineffectiveness of manually assisted cough [28].

As manually assisted cough can increase the risk of vomiting and aspiration, it should only be performed before or at least 1–1.5 h after a meal. Thoracic thrust techniques should be performed with caution in patients with osteoporosis due to risk of rib fractures [29]. Manually assisted cough should also be avoided in pregnancy.

Mechanical Insufflation/Exsufflation

Mechanical insufflation/exsufflation devices are frequently applied to enhance cough efficiency for patients with neuromuscular disorders. Cough augmentation can be achieved by delivering positive pressure to assist with deep inspiration, followed by a rapid switch to negative pressure to augment forced expiration [32–34]. Mechanical insufflation/exsufflation (MI-E) can provide similar exsufflation flows to suctioning without the associated discomfort or airway trauma and can be more effective than conventional suctioning. When mucous plugs are present, MI-E can increase vital capacity by 300% and normalize oxygen levels [35]. When routine airway suctioning is used, secretions in the left mainstem bronchus are missed about 90% of the time [33, 34].

Mechanical insufflation/exsufflation devices can be used to apply forces to the chest or intermittent pressure changes to the airway to support expiratory muscle function and secretion clearance. The MI-E can deliver deep insufflation, for example, at pressures of +30 to +50 cm H_2O, followed immediately by deep exsufflation at negative pressures of −30 to −50 cm H_2O. The timing of these pressures can be adjusted. Using a lung model, it has been suggested that an inspiratory time of 2 s and expiratory time of 3 s is optimal for generating the goal pressures and flow [36]. MI-E can be provided via a mouthpiece, oronasal mask, endotracheal tube, or tracheostomy tube. If MI-E is to be used via tracheostomy, the cuff should be inflated to eliminate leak for adequate delivery of pressures [37]. MI-E can still be performed with a cuffless tracheostomy tube, but upper airway closure must be ensured for effectiveness and to avoid movement of oropharyngeal secretions into the airway during negative pressure application. MI-E should be strongly considered, when appropriate, via the endotracheal tube, particularly prior to extubation in the context of neuromuscular weakness [38]. Considerably more negative exsufflation pressures may be required to overcome ETT resistance and achieve clinically effective expiratory flows.

When MI-E is applied through an oronasal mask, PCFs greater than 270 L/s can be generated in motor neurone disease, although this can be compromised by bulbar dysfunction and upper airway instability [11, 39]. The MI-E can be used in automatic, manual, or combined mode. Manually cycled MI-E allows caregiver and patient timing and coordination of inspiration and expiration [40].

Figure 5.3 demonstrates flow, volume, and pressure tracings from three cycles of mechanical cough assistance. The inspiratory flow is brief, despite continuous inspiratory pressure delivery. Higher inspiratory pressures might generate higher inspiratory flow if there is reasonable chest wall compliance. The expiratory flow rises and falls with higher frequency following the peak expiratory flow; this indicates transient airway closure resulting in high local expiratory flow rates and possibly enhanced airway secretion clearance. A mask interface, rather than a tracheostomy or endotracheal tube, will sometimes lead to overestimated expiratory flow, as it includes unintentional leaks around the mask. Because flow and pressure tracing data are now readily available from device data downloads, parameters, such as pressures and timing, can be optimized to achieve maximal comfort and effective expiratory flows for individual patients.

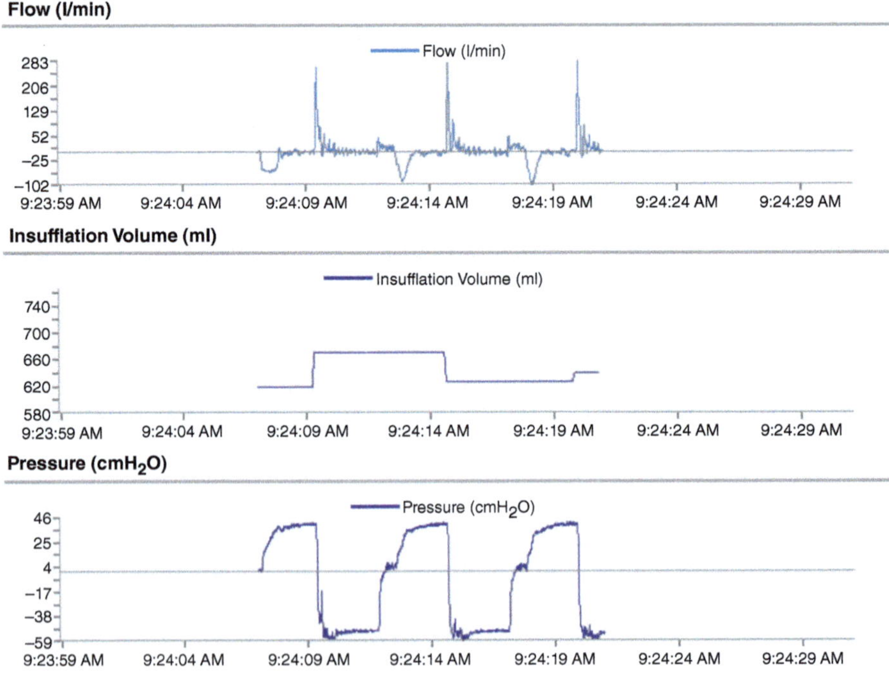

Fig. 5.3 Flow, volume, and pressure tracings from three cycles of mechanical cough assistance. Peak expired flows approximate 270 L/min

A Cochrane review of 11 studies with 287 participants assessed cough augmentation techniques, their safety, and effectiveness, but did not identify reliable evidence regarding the safety of these techniques. It also did not identify superiority of one technique over another or the impact on important clinically relevant outcomes, such as unscheduled hospitalizations due to chest infections, survival, functional status, or quality of life [41]. However, according to the authors, the inadequately reported results and limited information 'severely restricted the number of analyses that could be performed'. Cochrane reviews are useful in the analysis of multiple RCTs, which is rare in this population. The review also excluded several studies that demonstrated safety of cough augmentation, on the basis of perceived bias and concerns about the methodology.

Although there is limited robust data on the effectiveness of MI-E on outcomes in neuromuscular disorders, they are commonly used in practice, possibly due to the lack of available alternatives, particularly those that could be used at home. The British Thoracic Society has recommended considering MI-E for patients with neuromuscular disease and bulbar involvement who are unable to do breath stacking or other effective methods of airway clearance. They also recommended combining MI-E with manually assisted cough when possible, if MI-E is insufficient [42]. The 2023 American College of Chest Physicians (ACCP) guidelines on respiratory management of patients with neuromuscular weakness recommends the use of MI-E in patients with reduced cough effectiveness not improved with alternative techniques, such as glossopharyngeal breathing, breath stacking with a manual resuscitation bag or manually assisted cough [11, 26, 39].

MI-E can simulate a cough in a triphasic manoeuvre: (1) high-pressure insufflation followed by (2) high negative pressure exsufflation phase, and then (3) pause between the exsufflation and insufflation [12]. A single MI-E treatment generally consists of about five cycles of MI-E, followed by short periods of normal breathing or ventilator use to avoid hyperventilation. Additional treatments can be used during acute illness or need for coughing. Insufflation and exsufflation pressures typically range from +35 to 60 cm H_2O and −35 to −60 cm H_2O. Most patients are managed with 35–45 cm H_2O pressures for insufflation and exsufflation. Faroux et al. conducted a prospective cohort study investigating the effects of MI-E on PCF, and demonstrated a significant improvement with MI-E, particularly at higher settings, up to 45 cm H_2O for insufflation and exsufflation pressure, and demonstrated an improvement in PCF and symptoms, but no effect on vital capacity [43]. Higher settings can be used, up to +60 and −60 cm H_2O. Settings may need to be adjusted to adapt during acute illness, as lung mechanics can change.

Chatwin et al. measured spontaneous PCF before and after insufflation-exsufflation assisted cough and demonstrated a significant improvement in PCF, at a greater increase than other cough manoeuvres including manually assisted cough, physiotherapy-assisted cough, non-invasive ventilator-assisted cough, or exsufflation assisted cough [12]. They also demonstrated that the use of MI-E reduced treatment times and improved symptoms. Chatwin et al. [44] also conducted a randomised controlled trial in a respiratory physiotherapy practice comparing airway clearance with and without the use of MI-E [29] and compared SpO_2, PEF, $PtCO_2$, and heart rate between two groups, and observed no difference between the two groups, with and without MI-E. These findings are likely a reflection of the lack of robust data on the use of MI-E for airway clearance. The impact on SpO_2, $PtCO_2$, heart rate, and PEF are valuable measurements, but patient-relevant outcomes such as hospitalization rates, mortality, or quality of life are lacking.

Bach et al. also investigated the difference in PCF before and after airway clearance measures and found that the increase in PCF was greater after MI-E compared to manually assisted cough alone. There was, however, no significant difference in PCF before and after MI-E during periods of secretion production [27]. Sivasothy et al. compared the effect of MI-E alone to MI-E combined with manually assisted cough on PCF in patients with neuromuscular respiratory disease without scoliosis and found that there was a significant increase from baseline PCF when manually assisted cough and MI-E were used in combination. Manually assisted cough alone did increase PCF, but MI-E alone did not [27]. Another study performed by Mustafa et al. comparing manually assisted cough alone to manually assisted cough combined with MI-E found an 11% increase in PCF in bulbar patients and 13% in non-bulbar patients with manually assisted cough alone, and a 26% increase in bulbar and 28% increase in non-bulbar patients when manually assisted cough and MI-E were used in combination [45].

Lacombe et al. [46] conducted a study comparing the effects of different coughing techniques in 18 patients with neuromuscular respiratory failure, including MI-E alone, MI-E with manually assisted cough, and intermittent positive pressure supported breaths with manually assisted cough. They found that intermittent positive pressure supported breathing combined with manually assisted cough resulted in higher PCF than MI-E alone or MI-E combined with manually assisted cough. Interestingly, the authors suggested that adding MI-E to manually assisted cough may not improve PCF and may lead to less-effective cough in patients with neuromuscular disease who can generate high PCF with intermittent positive pressure supported breathing combined with manually assisted cough.

Andersen et al. conducted a cross sectional study in 20 patients with ALS and conducted video-recorded flexible transnasal fibre-optic laryngoscopy during MI-E, applying pressure of ±20 to ±50 cm H_2O to assess laryngeal movements on the effect on upper and lower motor neurone symptoms. All patients with ALS and bulbar symptoms ($n = 14$) adducted the supraglottic laryngeal structures during insufflation and abducted at the glottic level during insufflation and exsufflation [47]. Healthy subjects and patients with ALS and no bulbar symptoms, by contrast, demonstrated normal cough coordination while using MI-E [48]. These findings suggest that there may be limited effectiveness of MI-E in patients with bulbar symptoms. They suggested that ALS patients with significant bulbar impairment likely experience adduction of supraglottic structures during insufflation leading to a reduction in airflow.

The use of MI-E has not demonstrated any change in outcomes in terms of mortality, hospitalization, length of stay, or quality of life in comparison to breath stacking [49]. Vianello et al. evaluated 11 adults with neuromuscular disease during episodes of respiratory tract infections and found that MI-E did not have an impact on length of hospital stay [50]. However, studies have generally been small without sufficient follow-up time to adequately power these clinical outcomes. MI-E was, however, associated with a lower rate of endotracheal intubation and tracheostomy related to treatment failure, compared to conventional chest physiotherapy.

In patients who are weaning from mechanical ventilation, MI-E can be an effective tool to facilitate extubation. MI-E can also be used to avoid intubation by clearing airway secretions during acute respiratory infections [50, 51]. The combined use of MI-E, manually assisted cough, oximetry monitoring, and home non-invasive intermittent positive pressure ventilation has been shown to decrease rates of hospitalization, respiratory complications, and mortality in patients with neuromuscular disease [52, 53].

Contraindications to the use of MI-E include barotrauma after previous use, bullae, emphysema, and bronchial reactivity. Avoiding its use in these circumstances is important to avoid the risk of pneumothorax, aspiration, or haemoptysis [35]. In patients with spinal shock, it can also provoke bradycardia, and should be used with caution in this population with gradual increases in pressures. Progressive increase in pressures is also recommended for patients with low vital capacities to avoid thoracic discomfort. There are no data on complications such as barotrauma in patients with associated primary lung disease (e.g. COPD), but inspiratory pressures may be reduced and exsufflation pressures made more negative to minimize risk for pneumothorax. Interventions that increase cough should be avoided in patients with raised intracranial pressure or severe head injury [54].

It has been documented that MI-E can be safely applied, following abdominal or thoracic surgery without interrupting the surgical wounds [55, 56]. The increase in expiratory flows immediately following exsufflation using the MI-E also does not provoke airflow obstruction [57].

The impact of MI-E on healthcare utilization, costs, and survival trajectory in 106 patients with neuromuscular disease determined that fewer hospital days and physician specialist visits occurred following MI-E approval. On the other hand, home care nursing and personal support service visits increased. As a result, costs associated with physician billing and access to secondary care decreased, but costs associated with community support services increased. Risk of death was determined to be higher in patients using more medical devices at home (hazard ratio 1.12), although this may be related to the severity of illness associated with need for home airway clearance device use [58].

Expiratory Muscle Training (EMT)

EMT is a technique that increases subglottic pressure for airway clearance [59]. A study by Reyes et al. demonstrated that EMT in combination with breath stacking improved voluntary and reflex coughing for patients with Parkinson's disease [60]. Another study by Plowman et al. sought to determine whether there could be improvements in respiratory and bulbar function when EMT is combined with breath stacking compared to breath stacking alone, but only demonstrated an improvement in mean expiratory pressure. It is unclear whether this effect is sustainable [59].

Andersen et al. conducted a review of the use of respiratory muscle exercise training for patients with Duchenne muscular dystrophy and found that there was no significant improvement in lung function, and limited certainty about its effect on health-related quality of life [61].

Assisted Insufflation

Non-invasive Ventilation

Ventilatory support can reliably provide volume and pressure only if airway is clear of mucus and debris [5, 12, 23].

Intermittent Positive Pressure Ventilation (i.e. Mouthpiece Ventilation)

A ventilator can be used for breath stacking in a similar way to a manual resuscitation bag. Although a ventilator with a nasal or oronasal mask can also be used, a mouthpiece interface is often the most comfortable interface. In a study performed by Dohna-Schwake et al., intermittent positive pressure breathing using a mouthpiece interface was used for 29 patients with neuromuscular disease with a PCF <160 L/min or a history of chest infections, and demonstrated an improvement in PCF, particularly patients with a lower vital capacity [62].

Glossopharyngeal Breathing

Glossopharyngeal breathing (GPB) can be performed by using the glossopharyngeal muscles to repeatedly inhale through the glottis, which closes between breaths to stack air. The patient does not exhale between breaths. Once breath stacking has been achieved using glossopharyngeal breathing, spontaneous or cough augmentation manoeuvres can be introduced to clear secretions.

An important benefit of GPB is that patients can perform the manoeuvre independently without assistance. If caregiver assistance is available, breath stacking with a manual resuscitation bag can be combined with GPB to significantly increase PCF.

One of the limitations of GPB is that it is limited by bulbar function and coordination of glottic closure between breaths. It also cannot be used with patients with a tracheostomy.

Manual Airway Clearance Techniques

Manual airway clearance techniques can be effective in removing pulmonary secretions, facilitating inspiration, and increasing alveolar ventilation.

Percussion

Manual chest compression is a common technique used for airway clearance. It consists of manual rhythmic clapping with cupped hands to the back, chest, and dorsal sides of the thorax at a frequency of approximately 3–6 Hz. Percussion is often applied during postural drainage for 10–20-min treatment sessions to increase its effectiveness. There have been some concerns that chest percussion can worsen obstruction or hypoxemia, possibly related to mobilization of secretions to well-ventilated areas [63]. However, when chest percussion is combined with chest expansion exercises or active airway clearance techniques, oxygen saturation does not fall [64]. Research regarding the use of chest percussion with the assistance of physiotherapists or respiratory therapists demonstrated no effect on airway clearance [65].

Vibration

Vibration is another manual chest therapy technique that can be used for secretion clearance. Vibration is a technique that applies oscillation that is transmitted to the lower airways to move mucous. The aim is to improve mucociliary clearance in the peripheral airways. Vibration is often used in combination with postural drainage and is likely not effective in isolation [4, 66–68].

Secretion Clearance Devices

Intrapulmonary Percussive Ventilation

Intrapulmonary percussive ventilation (IPV), such as the percussionaire, is a device used for airway clearance that can deliver aerosolized solution and intrathoracic percussion. IPV can be delivered through a face mask, mouthpiece, an endotracheal tube, or tracheostomy. IPV can deliver intermittent positive pressure breathing with high-frequency small bursts of air (at 50–550 cycles/min) from the patient's respiration, which can help clear secretions from the peripheral airways. Percussions are delivered continuously through air-entrainment equipment. The high-frequency pulsations can also expand the lungs and large airways and deliver air into the distal airways [66, 69, 70]. Pressures delivered through IPV can be adjusted to clinical effect and patients' individual comfort. After the patient initiates airflow, pulsations are delivered by internal percussion, and then interrupted to allow passive expiration. The main goal of treatment with IPV is to reduce the viscosity of secretions, promote volume recruitment, improve ventilation and perfusion matching, improve gas exchange, and protect against barotrauma.

Contraindications to IPV include diffuse alveolar haemorrhage and hemodynamic instability. Relative contraindications include recent pneumothorax, oesophageal surgery, spinal injury, uncontrolled hypertension, bronchospasm, acute pulmonary oedema, or large pleural effusions.

High-Frequency Chest Wall Oscillations or Compression

High-frequency chest wall oscillations (HFCWO) are rapidly alternating negative and positive pressure under an outer chest shell by applying external oscillation at 5–25 Hz and vibration applied throughout the breathing cycle or during expiration only. The inspiration to expiration ratio can be adjusted, and different pressures can be applied during inspiration or expiration. Higher exsufflation pressures are required to mobilize secretions, particularly in the peripheral airways [4]. The pressure settings can be adapted to patient comfort. Treatment sessions can vary in length based on patient tolerance, the effectiveness of therapy, and the amount of secretions. Inhaled therapies are recommended for use during therapy sessions to make secretions less viscous. Air can also be humidified to increase mobilization of secretions. Lechtzin et al. conducted a cohort study that determined that HFCWO reduces medical costs, hospitalizations, and pneumonia for patients with a variety of neuromuscular diseases [71]. Recommendations from the 2023 American College of Chest Physicians (ACCP) guidelines suggest that HFCWO should be used in conjunction with other airway clearance therapies, such as LVR or MI-E [26].

Contraindications to HFCWO are similar to IPV, with the addition of burns, head and neck injuries, rib fractures, pulmonary contusions, chest wall pain, osteoporosis, coagulopathy, or abdominal dysfunction. Perhaps the greatest concern with HFCWO or IPV is performing these techniques in a patient who is unable to cough and clear the secretions mobilized. These strategies must be combined with effective airway clearance to prevent mobilized secretions from worsening gas exchange by affecting lung units with better V/Q ratios. The high cost associated with a HFCWO device, along with caregiver assistance and training, should also be taken into consideration before implementation [71].

Inhaled Therapies

Inhaled therapies may be considered for improvement of ciliary function and reducing viscosity of secretions. However, there is a lack of clinical research on these therapies in the neuromuscular population.

Inhaled hypertonic saline (3–7% solution) triggers the cough reflex and has mucolytic properties, reducing the mucus viscosity by breaking down protein and molecular bonds. It also increases the volume of airway mucus, at a lower viscosity, through osmosis [72]. It has not been studied in patients with neuromuscular disorders, but may be considered for patients with tenacious secretions where other measures have provided limited benefit. Inhaled hypertonic saline should be used with caution, however, as it can increase the risk of bronchospasm, particularly in patients with obstructive airways disease or airway hyperreactivity.

Dornase-alpha (recombinant human DNAse) has been regularly used as a mucolytic medication to reduce the viscosity of secretions for patients with cystic fibrosis. In this cystic fibrosis population, it has shown improvement in lung function and a reduction in the frequency of exacerbations [73]. In a randomized-controlled trial of patients with non-cystic fibrosis bronchiectasis, it has been associated with an increased risk of exacerbations and decline in lung function [74]. The use of dornase-alpha in patients with neuromuscular disease has not been studied and cannot be routinely recommended. However, in patients with tenacious secretions in whom other therapies have been unsuccessful, a trial may be considered on an individual basis [72].

N-acetylcysteine is another mucolytic, available in oral and inhaled formulations, that has demonstrated inconsistent benefit in most respiratory diseases, and has not been studied in patients with neuromuscular disorders. It may be considered for patients with copious secretions in whom other measures have not been sufficiently effective. Inhaled n-acetylcysteine has been associated with bronchospasm and should be used with caution, particularly with patients with obstructive airways disease [75].

It is important to note that inhaled therapies, including n-acetylcysteine, hypertonic saline, and dornase-alpha should be used in conjunction with well-established airway clearance measures discussed above but should not replace them.

Conclusion

Effective airway clearance is an important part of management of respiratory failure in patients with neuromuscular disease. Respiratory muscle weakness can lead to impaired lung mechanics and weakened cough, increasing the risk of infection and respiratory failure. Airway clearance interventions, including breath stacking, mechanical insufflation exsufflation, and positive pressure ventilation may mitigate these risks. Further robust research is required to determine the impact of interventions for airway clearance on patient important outcomes including morbidity, mortality, hospitalization days, and quality of life.

References

1. Gauld L. Airway clearance in neuromuscular weakness. Dev Med Child Neurol. 2009;51:350–5.
2. Sheers NL, et al. A randomised controlled trial of lung volume recruitment in adults with neuromuscular disease. ATS. 2023;20:1445.
3. Szeinberg A. Cough capacity in patients with muscular dystrophy. Chest. 1998;94:1232–5.
4. Adir Y. Ventilatory support for chronic respiratory failure. Nicolino Ambrosino RSG, editor. vol. 225. Haifa: European Respiratory Review; 2009.
5. Kang SBJ. Maximum insufflation capacity: vital capacity and cough flows in neuromuscular disease. Am J Phys Med Rehabil. 2000;70:222–7.
6. Bach JR, Ishikawa Y, Kim H. Prevention of pulmonary morbidity for patients with Duchenne muscular dystrophy. Chest. 1997;112(4):1024.
7. Bach JR, Alba AS. Noninvasive options for ventilatory support of traumatic high level quadriplegic. Chest. 1990;98(3):613–9.
8. Bach JR. New approaches in the rehabilitation of the traumatic high level quadriplegic patient. Am J Phys Med Rehabil. 2000;79(3):222–7.
9. Bach JR, et al. Expiratory flow manoeuvres in patients with neuromuscular diseases. Am J Phys Med Rehabil. 2006;85(2):105–11.
10. Sancho J, et al. Effect of lung mechanics on mechanically assisted flows and volumes. Am J Phys Med Rehabil. 2004;83(9):698–703.
11. Sancho J, et al. Efficacy of mechanical insufflation-exsufflation in medically stable patients with amyotrophic lateral sclerosis. Chest. 2004;125(4):1400–5.
12. Chatwin M, et al. Airway clearance techniques in neuromuscular disorders: a state of the art review. vol. 136. Respiratory medicine. W.B. Saunders Ltd; 2018. p. 98–110.
13. Quanjer PH, et al. Lung volumes and forced ventilatory flows. Eur Respir J. 1993;6(5):5–40.
14. Leiner GC, et al. Expiratory peak flow rate. Standard values for normal subjects. Use as a clinical test of ventilatory function. Am Rev Respir Dis. 1963;88:644–51.
15. Rose L, et al. Monitoring cough effectiveness and use of airway clearance strategies: a Canadian and UK survey. Respir Care. 2018;63(12):1506–13.
16. Smina M, et al. Cough peak flows and extubation outcomes. Chest. 2003;124(1):262–8.
17. Waters C, et al. Ex vivo evaluation of secretion-clearing device in reducing airway resistance within endotracheal tubes. Crit Care Res Pract. 2018;2018:3258396.
18. Tzeng AC, et al. Prevention of pulmonary morbidity for patients with neuromuscular disease. Chest. 2000;118(5):1390.
19. Donha-Schwake C, et al. Predictors of severe chest infections in pediatric neuromuscular disorders. Neuromuscul Disord. 2006;16:325–8.

20. King M, et al. Clearance of mucus by simulated cough. J Appl Physiol. 1985;58(6):1776.
21. Farrero E, et al. Normativa sobre el manejo de las complicaciones respiratorias de los pacientes con enfermedad neuromuscular. Arch Bronconeumol. 2013;49(7):306–13.
22. Bach JR, et al. Lung insufflation capacity in neuromuscular disease. Am J Phys Med Rehabil. 2008;87(9):720–5.
23. Sheers NL, Howard ME, Rochford PD, Rautela L, Chao C, McKim D, Berlowitz DJ. A randomised controlled clinical trial of lung volume recruitment in adults with neuromuscular disease. Ann Am Thorac Soc. 2023;20(10):1445–55.
24. Katz S, et al. Long-term effects of lung volume recruitment on maximal inspiratory capacity and vital capacity in Duchenne muscular dystrophy. ATS. 2015;13(2):217–22.
25. Akram K, et al. Respiratory management of patients with neuromuscular weakness: an American College of Chest Physicians clinical practice guideline and expert panel report. CHEST J. 2023;164(2):394–413.
26. Sivasothy P, et al. Effect of manually assisted cough and mechanical insufflation on cough flow of normal subjects, patients with chronic obstructive pulmonary disease (COPD), and patients with respiratory muscle weakness. Thorax. 2001;56:438–44.
27. Bach JR. Mechanical insufflation-exsufflation: comparison of peak expiratory flows with manually assisted and unassisted coughing techniques. Chest. 1993;104(5):1553–62.
28. Bach JR, et al. Standards of care in MDA clinics. Muscular dystrophy association. Am J Phys Med Rehabil. 2000;79(2):193–6.
29. Chatwin M, et al. Mechanical insufflation-exsufflation: considerations for improving clinical practice. J Clin Med. 2023;12(7):2626.
30. Bach JR. Don't forget the abdominal thrust. Chest. 2004;126(4):1389–90.
31. Finder JD. Airway clearance modalities in neuromuscular disease. Paediatr Respir Rev. 2010;11:31–4.
32. Garstang SV, et al. Patient preference for in-exsufflation for secretion management with spinal cord injury. J Spinal Cord Med. 2000;23(2):80–5.
33. Sancho J, et al. Mechanical insufflation-exsufflation vs. tracheal suctioning via tracheostomy tubes for patients with amyotrophic lateral sclerosis: a pilot study. Am J Phys Med Rehabil. 2003;82(10):750–3.
34. Servara E, et al. Non-invasive management of an acute chest infection for a patient with ALS. J Neurol Sci. 2003;209(1–2):111–3.
35. Gomez-Merino E, et al. Mechanical insufflation-exsufflation: pressure, volume and flow relationships and the adequacy of the manufacturer's guidelines. Am J Phys Med Rehabil. 2002;81(8):579–83.
36. Bach JR, et al. Airway secretion clearance by mechanical exsufflation for post-poliomyelitis ventilator-assisted individuals. Arch Phys Med Rehabil. 1993;74(2):170–7.
37. Guérin C, et al. Performance of the coughassist insufflation-exsufflation device in the presence of an endotracheal tube or tracheostomy tube: a bench study. Respir Care. 2011;56(8):1108–14.
38. Farrero E, et al. Survival in amyotrophic lateral sclerosis with home mechanical ventilation: the impact of systematic respiratory assessment and bulbar involvement. Chest. 2005;127(6):2132–8.
39. Servara E, et al. Cough and neuromuscular diseases. Noninvasive airway secretion management. Arch Bronconeumol. 2003;39(9):418–27.
40. Catherine Auger VH, et al. Use of mechanical insufflation-exsufflation devices for airway clearance in subjects with neuromuscular disease. Respir Care. 2017;62(2):236.
41. Morrow B, et al. Cough augmentation techniques for people with chronic neuromuscular disorders (review). Cochrane Database Syst Rev. 2021;4(4):CD013170.
42. Hull J, et al. British Thoracic Society guideline for respiratory management of children with neuromuscular weakness. BTS guidelines. Thorax. 2012;67(1):i1–40.
43. Fauroux B, et al. Physiologic benefits of mechanical insufflation-exsufflation in children with neuromuscular diseases. Chest. 2008;133:161–8.

44. Chatwin M, et al. Cough augmentation with mechanical insufflation/exsufflation in patients with neuromuscular weakness. Eur Respir J. 2003;21:503.
45. Mustfa N, et al. Cough augmentation in amyotrophic lateral sclerosis. Neurology. 2003;61(9):1285–7.
46. Lacombe M, et al. Comparison of three cough-augmentation techniques in neuromuscular patients: mechanical insufflation combined with manually assisted cough, insufflation-exsufflation alone and insufflation-exsufflation combined with manually assisted cough. Respiration. 2014;88(3):215–22.
47. Andersen T, et al. Laryngeal response patterns influence the efficacy of mechanical assisted cough in amyotrophic lateral sclerosis. Thorax. 2017;72(3):221–9.
48. Rafiq MK, et al. A preliminary randomized trial of the mechanical insufflator-exsufflator versus breath-stacking technique in patients with amyotrophic lateral sclerosis. Amyotroph Lateral Scler Frontotemporal Degener. 2015;16(7–8):448–55. https://doi.org/10.310 9/21678421.2015.1051992.
49. Vianello A, et al. Mechanical insufflation-exsufflation improves outcomes for neuromuscular disease patients with respiratory tract infections. Am J Phys Med Rehabil. 2005;84(2):83–8.
50. Servara E, et al. Alternatives to endotracheal intubation for patients with neuromuscular diseases. Am J Phys Med Rehabil. 2005;84(11):851–7.
51. Bach JR. Prevention of morbidity and mortality with the use of physical medicine aids: the obstructive and paralytic conditions. In: Bach J, editor. Pulmonary rehabilitation. Philadelphia: Hanley & Belfus Inc.; 1996. p. 303–29.
52. Bach J, et al. Ventilatory weaning by lung expansion and decanulation. Am J Phys Med Rehabil. 2004;83:560–8.
53. Dunn LT. Raised intracranial pressure. J Neurol Neurosurg Psychiatry. 2002;73(1):i23.
54. Williams EK, et al. The use of exsufflation with negative pressure in postoperative patients. Am J Surg. 1955;90(4):637–40.
55. Marchant WA, et al. Postoperative use of cough assist device in avoiding prolonged patients. Br J Anaesth. 2002;89(4):644–7.
56. Bach JR. Cough in SCI patients. Arch Phys Med Rehabil. 1994;75(5):610.
57. Rose L, et al. Health care use, costs, and survival trajectory of home mechanical insufflation-exsufflation. Respir Care. 2022;67(2):191.
58. Plowman EK, et al. Impact of expiratory strength training in amyotrophic lateral sclerosis: results of a randomized, sham-controlled trial. Muscle Nerve. 2018;59(1):40.
59. Reyes A, et al. Effects of expiratory muscle training and air stacking on peak cough flow in individuals with Parkinson's disease. Lung. 2020;198:207–2011.
60. Stian H, et al. Exercise training in Duchenne muscular dystrophy: a systematic review and meta-analysis. J Rehabil Med. 2021;53.
61. Dohna-Schwake C, et al. IPPB-assisted coughing in neuromuscular disorders. Pediatr Pulmonol. 2006;41:551–7.
62. Wolmer P, et al. Inefficiency of chest percussion in the physical therapy of chronic bronchitis. Eur J Respir Dis. 1985;66(4):233–9.
63. Bach PB, et al. Management of acute exacerbation of chronic obstructive pulmonary disease: a summary and appraised of published evidence. Ann Intern Med. 2001;134(7):600–20.
64. Pryor JA, et al. Effect of chest physiotherapy on oxygen saturation in patients with cystic fibrosis. Thorax. 1990;45(1):77.
65. Langenderfer B. Alternatives to percussion and postural drainage. A review of mucus clearance therapies: percussion and postural drainage, autogenic drainage, positive expiratory pressure, flutter valve, intrapulmonary percussive ventilation and high frequency chest compressions with the ThAIRapy Vest. J Cardpulm Rehabil. 1998;18(4):283–9.
66. Oldenburg FA, et al. Effects of postural drainage, exercise and cough on mucus clearance in chronic bronchitis. Respir Care. 2001;46(11):1276–93.
67. Pryor JA. Physiotherapy for airway mucus clearance in adults. Eur Respir J. 1999;14(6):1418–24.

68. Lechtzin N, et al. The impact of high-frequency chest wall oscillation on healthcare use in patients with neuromuscular diseases. Ann Am Thorac Soc. 2016;13(6):904.
69. Toussant M, et al. Effect of intrapulmonary percussive ventilation on mucus clearance in Duchenne muscular dystrophy patients: a preliminary report. Respir Care. 2003;48(10):940–7.
70. Gosman AJ, et al. Airway clearance in patients with neuromuscular disease. Paediatr Respir Rev. 2023;47:33–40.
71. Hess JR. The evidence for secretion clearance techniques. Respir Care. 2001;46(11):1276–93.
72. Yang C, Montgomery M. Dornase alfa for cystic fibrosis. Cochrane Database Syst Rev. 2021;3:CD001127.
73. O'Donnell AE, et al. Treatment of idiopathic bronchiectasis with aerosolized recombinant human DNase I. rhDNase Study Group. Chest. 1998;113(5):1329–34.
74. Rubin BK. The pharmacologic approach to airway clearance: mucoactive agents. Paediatr Respir Rev. 2006;7:S215–9.
75. Calverley P, et al. Safety of N-acetylcysteine at high doses in chronic respiratory diseases: a review. Drug Saf. 2021;44:273–90. https://doi.org/10.1007/s40264-020-01026-y.

Chapter 6
Monitoring Patients on Long-Term Noninvasive Ventilation

Jason Ackrivo

Introduction

Home ventilation technology has progressed significantly since the 1950s when the iron lung promoted domiciliary respiratory care [1, 2]. The original piston-driven devices were replaced by turbine flow generators around the turn of the twenty-first century, enabling more compact ventilators [3]. Further refinements in machine capability have enabled multiple programs, a variety of mode options, portability with internal batteries, and the ability to collect device usage and performance data.

Originally, data were stored locally on the device, but advent of telemonitoring enables data transmission wirelessly to cloud-based web servers. The availability of such data has encouraged clinicians to employ a granular analysis of ventilation efficacy and thereby has streamlined troubleshooting. Despite the intuitive benefits, there is a paucity of literature supporting the dissemination of telemonitoring as standard of care for home ventilation. Caveats include prolonged care time as well as vague responsibilities from legal and ethical perspectives.

Pioneers in home ventilation in Europe have previously described an expert consensus on ideal approaches to home monitoring [2, 4–7]. The following chapter incorporates prior literature and focuses on an approach to home ventilation for adults with neuromuscular disease that is specific to the United States health system [8]. However, many of the concepts are broadly applicable for home ventilation strategies regardless of age, geographic location, or payer system.

J. Ackrivo (✉)
Pulmonary, Allergy, and Critical Care Division, Department of Medicine and Neurology,
Perelman School of Medicine at the Hospital of the University of Pennsylvania, Philadelphia,
PA, USA
e-mail: jason.ackrivo@pennmedicine.upenn.edu

N. Lechtzin (ed.), *Pulmonary Complications of Neuromuscular Disease*,
Respiratory Medicine, https://doi.org/10.1007/978-3-031-65335-3_6

Ventilation Devices

In the United States, Centers for Medicare & Medicaid Services (CMS) recognizes three categories of home ventilation devices: (1) respiratory assist devices (RADs), (2) mechanical ventilators, and (3) multifunctional respiratory devices.

Complex sleep apnea gave rise to RADs, as a secondary, higher inspiratory pressure setting was necessary to improve ventilation. RADs can be identified by the Healthcare Common Procedural Coding System (HCPCS) codes E0470 and E0471 by the absence or presence of a backup respiratory rate, respectfully. Most RADs provide bilevel positive airway pressure (bilevel PAP) in fixed inspiratory and expiratory pressure settings via single-limb passive circuits. A select few RADs can deliver more advanced settings, such as volume-assured pressure support (VAPS). Some notable advantages for RADs over ventilators include built-in humidification, ability to adjust settings remotely via online data monitoring software, and lower cost. An example of a commonly available RAD in the United States today is the ResMed AirCurve (Fig. 6.1).

Adaptations to inpatient acute care ventilators permitted home use of portable ventilators since at least the 1970s [9]. CMS considers home mechanical ventilators for the purpose of "life support" and are designated by HCPCS codes E0465 (invasive interface) and E0466 (noninvasive interface). Some of the most commonly used home ventilators in the United States are shown in Fig. 6.2. Most home ventilators support the use of multiple circuit types, including single limb passive, single limb active, and dual limb active. Compared to RADs, home ventilators offer internal battery power for portability, customizable alarms, a wider variety of modes with unique settings for VAPS (such as auto-titrating EPAP and IPAP adjustment speed), and mouthpiece ventilation. Mouthpiece ventilation will be discussed in further detail in Chap. 4. A humidifier is usually incorporated by inserting it in-line with the circuit tubing.

More recently, the multifunction ventilator has emerged as a third category of home respiratory assistance, designated by HCPCS code E0467. As of this writing, the only multifunction device used in the United States is the React Health VOCSN (Fig. 6.3), named after its capability of providing ventilation, supplemental oxygen, cough assistance, suctioning, and nebulizer delivery. To qualify for a

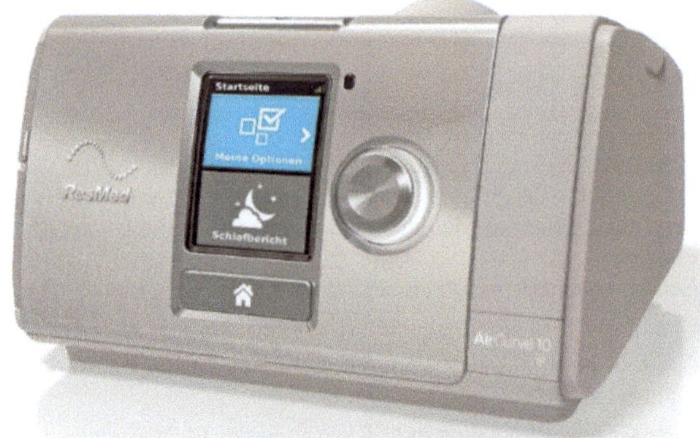

Fig. 6.1 ResMed AirCurve 10 ST, an example of a respiratory assist device available in the United States

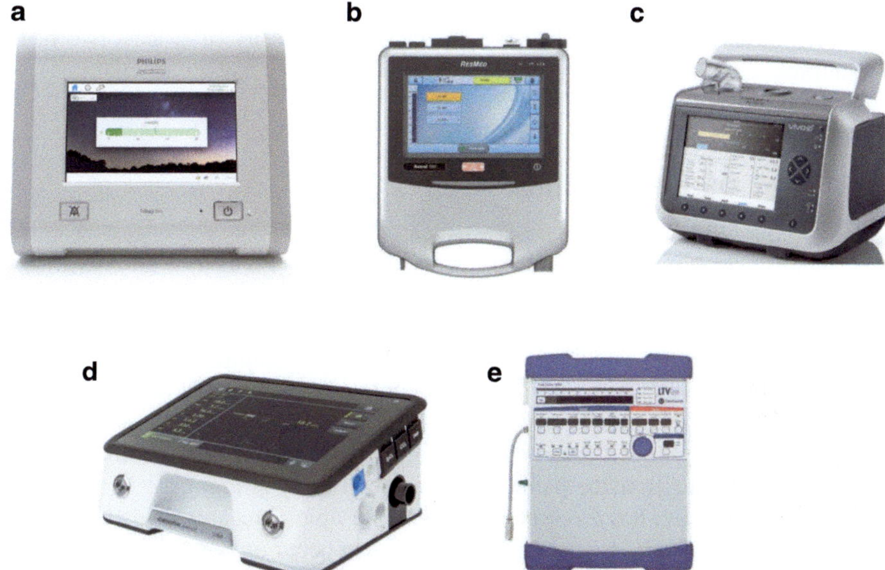

Fig. 6.2 Most common home mechanical ventilators available for use in the United States, (**a**) Trilogy Evo, (**b**) ResMed Astral, (**c**) Breas Vivo 45 LS, (**d**) Löwenstein Luisa, (**e**) CareFusion LTV

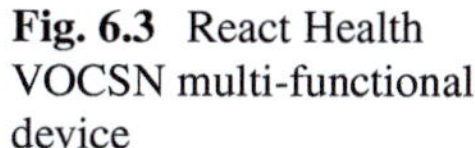

Fig. 6.3 React Health VOCSN multi-functional device

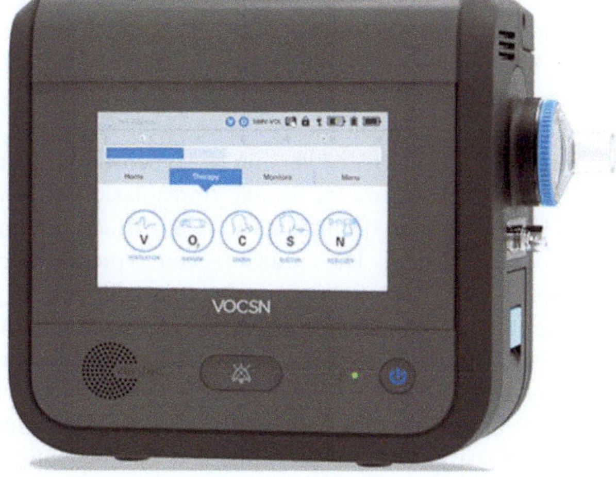

multifunctional device, a patient must meet several criteria, including (a) have no prior use of a ventilator and (b) have documented necessity of at least two of the modalities.

Ventilator Data Acquisition

The majority of noninvasive ventilation in the home is delivered via single-limb passive circuits. Under this setup, a respiratory device can directly measure airway pressure, flow rates, triggering events, cycling times, and duration of device use. Several parameters are calculated, including leak, tidal volume, and minute ventilation (as discussed later in section "Data Components, Reliability, and Accuracy"). Depending on the manufacturer, an apnea-hypopnea index may also be calculated. All of the aforementioned parameters are recorded by RADs and ventilators to an internal memory anytime the patient uses the device day or night.

Each manufacturer has proprietary software for uploading and reviewing ventilation usage and performance data. Data transfer can occur on a synchronous (instantaneous) or asynchronous (deferred) basis [5, 6]. Outpatient home ventilation device data transfer occurs on an asynchronous basis, as determined by The US Federal Drug Administration.

The original method for asynchronous data acquisition involved downloading the data via universal serial bus (USB) storage device or Secure Digital (SD card). This process required a clinician to access the device or have the patient mail an SD card. A durable medical equipment (DME) representative could also access the device at home and send a report by Health Insurance Portability and Accountability Act (HIPAA)-compliant secure fax or electronic mail.

Recently, a modernized version of asynchronous data acquisition has arisen from online-based platforms for remote transmission of device usage and performance data. Uploading can occur via a wireless Bluetooth connection to a transmitter or via a wired modem. Data transmission typically occurs on a daily basis in an encrypted HIPAA-compliant fashion via cellphone signal transmission, and thus requires the patient to have adequate local cellular service. Each manufacturer has a proprietary online data portal for clinician access with a personalized account and password.

There are several advantages to this telemonitoring capability. Given the frequency of daily data transfer, clinicians can instantly access device data up to the previous 24 h, thus bypassing delays inherent to the aforementioned USB and SD card method. Clinicians can customize data views on a variety of scales from monthly averages down to minute-by-minute changes within a single night (Fig. 6.4). Each account enables customizable reports, layouts, document and note uploading, message transmission with the DME, and creation of alerts to specific data thresholds. These features create an environment for rapid troubleshooting of ventilation issues. Several disadvantages include data overload, liability, and security concerns as discussed later in section, "Legal and Ethical Issues with Telemonitoring."

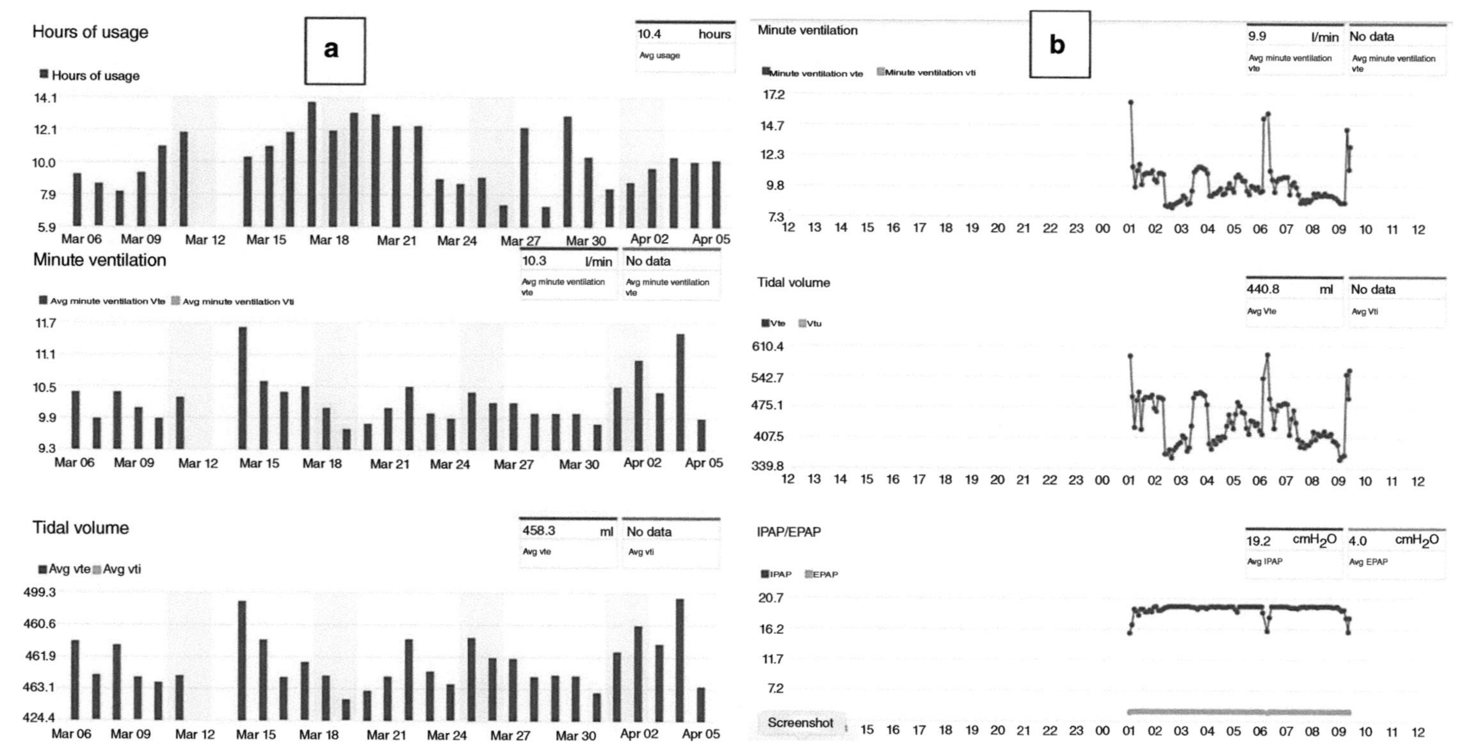

Fig. 6.4 Philips Respironics Care Orchestrator data displayed over different intervals. (**a**) Daily data for 1 month, (**b**) Hourly data for one night

Ventilator Manufacturer-Specific Platforms

Each manufacturer has developed proprietary software for reviewing ventilation data. Clinicians wishing to care for patients across a variety of manufacturers must familiarize themselves with the various programs. Each program is password-protected and requires a unique user or clinician group account.

ResMed

ResMed AirView is a cloud-based platform compatible with many of the ResMed devices, such as the ResMed AirSense, AirMini, AirCurve, Stellar, and Astral. The Stellar and Astral require wired connection to a physical modem (Fig. 6.5), while the AirCurve and AirSense have internal modems.

The ResMed AirView platform permits viewing data on multiple scales. Clinicians can view data over customized time periods, which can range from a broad overview of several months to granular minute-by-minute data. When viewing time intervals beyond a single day, parameters are summarized as medians with 5–95% ranges. Selecting a single day enables adjusting the analysis period from the entire 24-h period down to a single hour. Within a single hour, the data are displayed in minute-by-minute intervals.

In addition to the typical parameters (e.g., tidal volume, minute ventilation, respiratory rate, and leak), AirView displays apneas with apnea index and hypopnea index, percentage of both spontaneous triggers *and* spontaneous cycles, inspiratory time, and rapid-shallow breathing index. For patients on machines with multiple preset ventilator settings (e.g., ResMed Astral), AirView clearly indicates within a

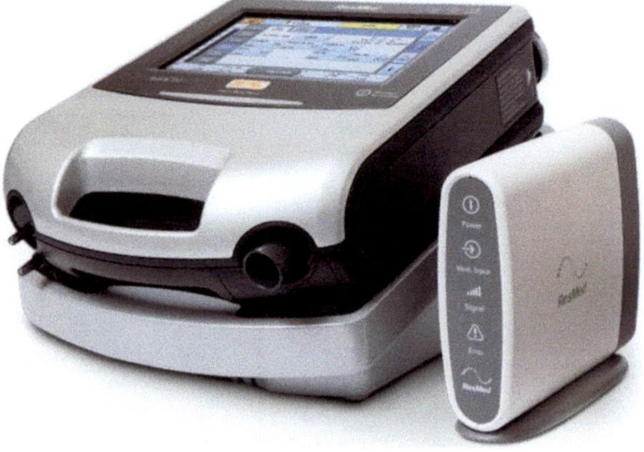

Fig. 6.5 ResMed Astral ventilator shown with modem

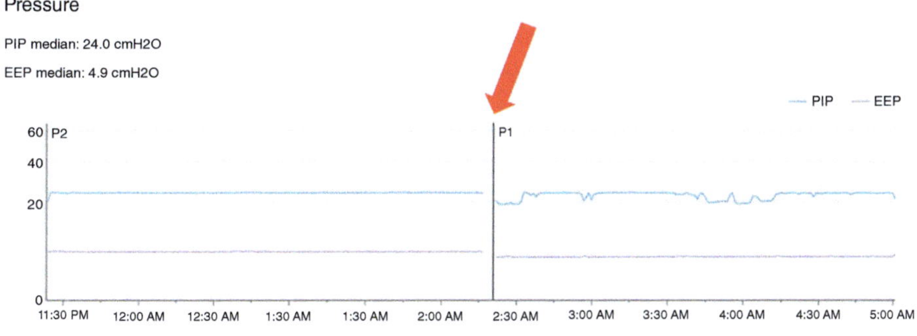

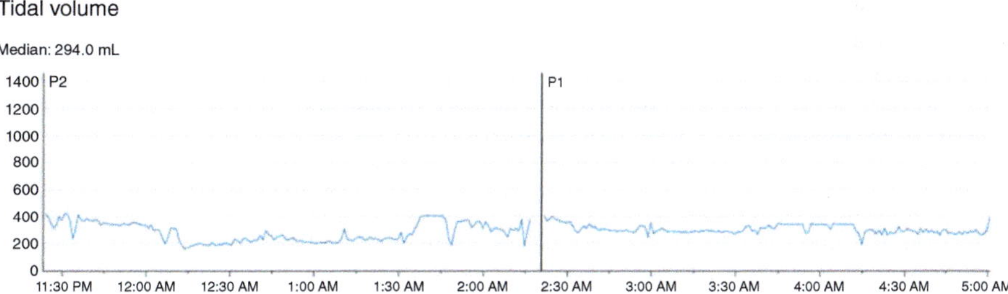

Fig. 6.6 ResMed AirView for a ResMed Astral ventilator, shown over a 5.5 h interval. Notice the vertical bar indicating a switch from use of Program 2 (P2) to Program 1 (P1) marked by the red arrow

specific day when the patient switches from one preset to another (Fig. 6.6). Clinicians can categorize patients by disease process, device adherence, mode of ventilation, and within specific alarm types.

Philips Respironics

Philips Respironics previously used Encore Anywhere as their mainstream software for data analysis. Encore Anywhere required proprietary software loaded onto a specific computer and typically accepted data downloads from device SD cards. Compared to more modern data monitoring platforms, Encore Anywhere has limited flexibility for customizing data reports.

Philips Respironics now uses a cloud-based data platform known as Care Orchestrator, which can be accessed via the Internet. Philips Respironics Trilogy Legacy and Trilogy Evo series ventilators can communicate wirelessly with Bluetooth hubs plugged into a nearby electrical outlet. As long as the hub and the ventilator come within range of one another, uploads to Care Orchestrator will occur every 8 h. Similar to ResMed AirView (above) data can be reviewed on a spectrum of timelines from months down to 5-min intervals. Users of Care

Orchestrator can build personalized reports, rules, and can leave messages for other clinicians (such as respiratory therapists from the DME company). Some unique features of Care Orchestrator include (1) viewing waveform data (requires direct USB download from device) and (2) integrating transcutaneous carbon dioxide (CO_2) reading via wired connection between a Sentec transcutaneous digital monitor and Trilogy Evo (Fig. 6.7).

Ventec Life Systems

Ventec Life Systems (Ventec), the original manufacturer of the VOCSN, offers an online telemonitoring platform known as Multi-View. As of this writing, data transmission can occur wirelessly via modem or using a USB stick with FAT32 formatting. Unique to Multi-View includes the ability to display usage data across all five functions by calendar day or within a specific day (Fig. 6.8).

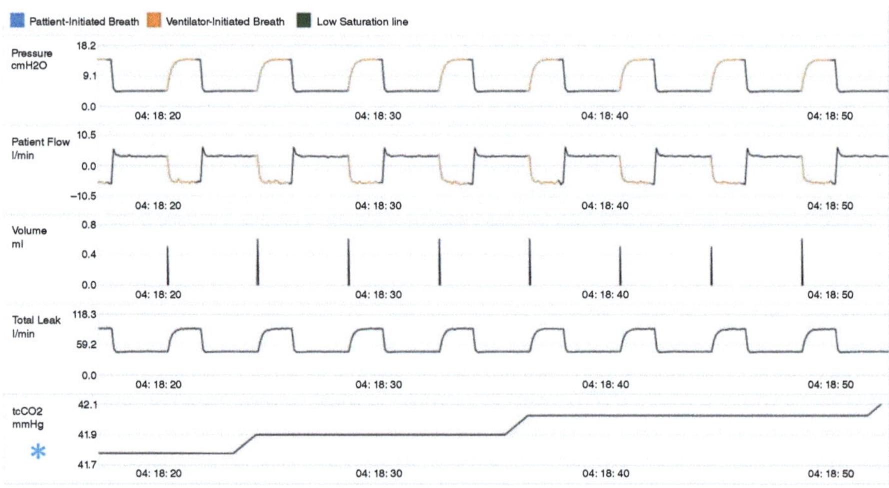

Fig. 6.7 Philips Respironics Care Orchestrator download of waveform data from a Trilogy Evo. The transcutaneous CO_2 data are shown in the bottom panel indicated by the blue asterisk. *tcCO₂* transcutaneous carbon dioxide

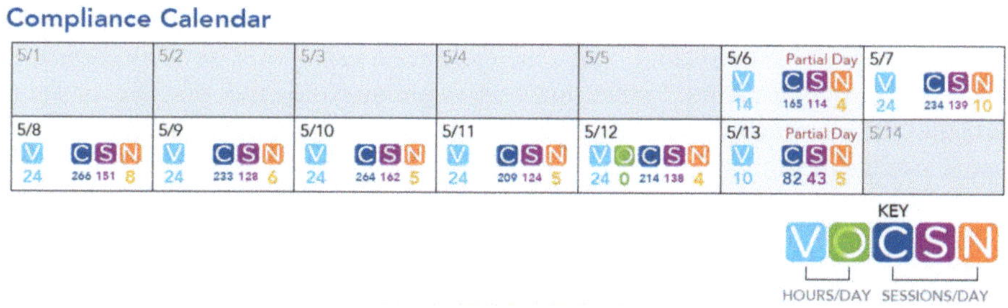

Compliance Calendar

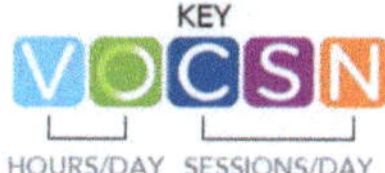

Fig. 6.8 Ventec Life Systems Multi-View data download from VOCSN multi-functional device between May 6th to May 13th. Data shown are daily usage of the ventilator (V), cough assist [C], suction (S), and nebulizer (N). Of note, the supplemental oxygen (O) was not used during this time interval

Breas

Breas ventilation devices such as the Vivo 45, 50, and 65 can upload data to the Breas proprietary platform, EveryWare. As of this writing, EveryWare is used sparingly in the United States and accessible only by DME companies. Advantages to EveryWare include integration of fraction of inspired oxygen, SpO_2, and transcutaneous CO_2 via connection to Sentec digital monitor.

Data Components, Reliability, and Accuracy

Remote ventilator data accuracy and reliability are paramount, especially for parameters such as tidal volume and minute ventilation that are calculated from directly measured flow and pressure profiles.

Leak

Noninvasive ventilation is subject to two types of leaks that make up the "total leak": unintentional and intentional leak. The type and amount of leak will depend on several factors, such as the circuit, mask type, mask fit, and integrity of equipment used.

Noninvasive ventilation involves three main types of circuits: (1) single limb passive, where exhaled air is released through a fixed exhalation valve in the system (usually via vented mask or inline passive exhalation valve); (2) single limb active, where a change in pressure or flow directs opening of an exhalation valve; or (3) dual-limb active circuit, where a secondary limb of tubing directs the exhaled air to a PEEP valve or back to the respiratory device. In single-limb passive and active circuits, the intentional leak can be built into a vented mask interface. If using an unvented mask or tracheostomy, then the exhalation valve must be incorporated in line with the circuit tubing. In dual-limb active circuits, the mask must be unvented and thus the intentional leak should be zero. The amount of intentional leak will be specific to the manufacturer of the mask or the exhalation port. When using pressure-targeted modes ventilators commonly employ "leak compensation" based on the intentional leak, which adjusts turbine airflow to the pressure set by the clinician.

Unintentional leak is a common culprit for insufficient or poorly tolerated NIV. The etiology may be multifactorial and can include poorly fit mask, body position, mouth opening, and/or excessive airway pressures interfering with mask seal. Unintentional leak will often vary throughout the night depending on sleep stage and phase of respiration.

An excessive unintentional leak will impair the ventilator's ability to report accurate ventilation parameters such as tidal volume or minute ventilation [10]. Patient-ventilator asynchrony may occur if the unintentional leak hinders the ventilator's ability to detect a change in airflow when a patient inspires for another breath. Therefore, reducing leak should generally take priority over other refinements.

Reliability of leak values and the level of "acceptable" intentional leak may depend on manufacturer of the respiratory device and mask interface. The components of reported "leak" by a device or monitoring report may vary by manufacturer, and could include total leak, unintentional leak, median leak, or average leak. A prior study found that at a set IPAP of 14 cm H_2O, seven different masks had unintentional leaks ranging from 30 to 45 L/min [11]. One study of devices across several brands found a bias in reported leak by as much as −25.9 L/min and range of limits of agreement up to 49 L/min [10]. A study of volume-targeted pressure support mode in six commercial ventilators with single-limb passive leak circuits found significant differences of tidal volume during both inspiration and exhalation [12]. Excess inspiratory leak, compared to no unintentional leak, caused a tidal volume decrease by 40% over 5 min. Acceptable ranges must be assessed on a case-by-case basis, as normal leak ranges may vary more between patients rather than within patients [13]. It is generally accepted that unintentional leaks above 40–50 L/min should be avoided and corrected [14]. While critical leak will vary by manufacturer, asynchrony tends to begin above a total leak of 30 L/min, but may be tolerated in certain devices up to ~55 L/min [15].

Tidal Volume

Tidal Volume can be reported as exhaled tidal volume (sometimes abbreviated as "Vte") or as inhaled tidal volume ("Vti"). Single limb circuits cause exhaled air to escape the system and therefore exhaled tidal volume (and therefore minute ventilation) must be estimated using dynamic flow measurements and proprietary algorithms.

The tidal volume can be influenced by several factors, including the rise time, inspiratory flow rate, magnitude of driving pressure, duration of inspiration, and leak (Fig. 6.9). Ventilator software heavily influences tidal volume accuracy, and prior work has found a consistent underestimation of tidal volume with an increasing bias at higher insufflation pressures (range 66–236 mL) and limits of agreement of 118–490 mL [10].

As mentioned above, the magnitude of leak can strongly influence estimated tidal volume and is heavily influenced by estimations made by proprietary algorithms. In a study by Luján et al. across several commercial ventilators, the highest leaks studied caused a meager immediate tidal volume fall of <10% [12]. Due to leak compensation, some devices have reported an increase in tidal volume immediately after introducing unintentional leak.

Airway Pressures

Ventilators contain a pneumotachograph, usually positioned where the air exits the device. As a ventilator delivers a specific pressure, the perceived pressure will drop proportionally to the resistance of the circuit. The reported pressure is interpreted as the difference between outgoing pressure and lost pressure from circuit resistance. Therefore, accurate pressure measurements require circuit calibration and inputting the correct circuit size and type into the machine [14].

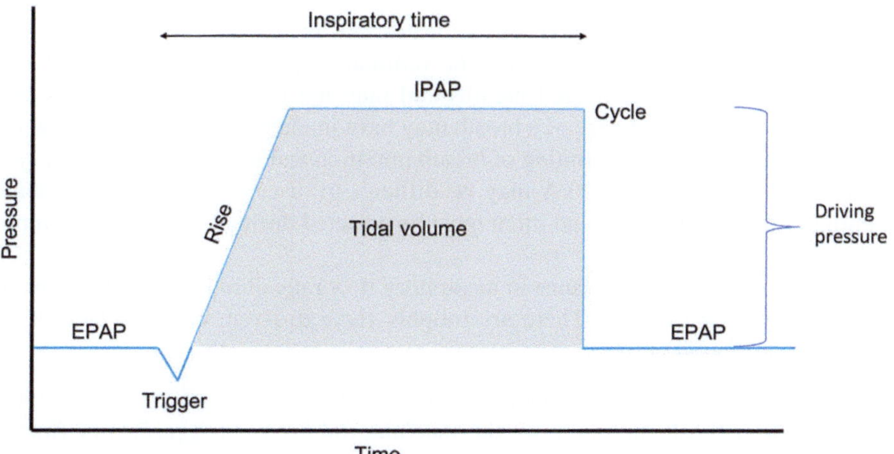

Fig. 6.9 Pressure-time curve associated with positive pressure ventilation. Notice that rise, driving pressure, and inspiratory time affect the area under the curve, which is directly proportional to the tidal volume. *IPAP* inspiratory positive airway pressure, *EPAP* expiratory positive airway pressure

Spontaneous Triggers and Cycles

The transition from exhalation to inhalation is referred to as the "trigger." This may be patient-initiated based on inspiratory efforts or initiated by the machine, as determined by the set backup respiratory rate.

Upper airway obstruction or leaks may hinder the ventilator's ability to detect inspiratory efforts and thus suggest a low percentage of patient-triggered breaths when in reality there is high patient-ventilator asynchrony.

The transition from inhalation to exhalation is referred to as the "cycle." Cycle behavior is highly dependent on the mode and may be determined by patient inspiratory effort or by the set inspiratory time.

In S/T mode and/or when a Ti minimum and maximum are set, a spontaneous cycle indicates that the patient's inspiratory effort reached the preset percentage of peak inspiratory flow. Spontaneous cycling can indicate that the patient's effort is sufficient to allow enough flow until a time period between the Ti minimum and maximum. However, a low percentage of spontaneous cycling indicates either (a) that the machine is cycling based on a set inspiratory time or (b) the patient's inspiratory flow effort is falling below the cycle threshold before the Ti minimum or (c) the inspiratory flow is above the cycle threshold until after the Ti maximum or (d) a system leak is inducing leak compensation to extend flow up to the Ti maximum.

Patient-Ventilator Asynchrony

Patient-ventilator asynchrony (PVA) indicates that breath delivery is out of sync with the patient's respiratory efforts. The ventilator reported respiratory rate is the frequency of machine-delivered breaths and may not represent the patient's true respiratory rate. The delivery of a breath may have inadequate or excessive flow for the patient. In addition, the timing of breath initiation and termination may not synchronize with the patient. PVA may be difficult to discern using standard home ventilator data monitoring, and often must be detected during a formal polysomnogram [16].

PVA represents a discordance in inspiratory flow rate, duration of inspiration, or breath frequency [17, 18]. There are roughly three different phases where asynchrony can occur [17]:

1. *Rate asynchrony* indicates that either (a) patient inspiratory efforts are not translating to a breath initiation by the machine (*ineffective triggering*) or (b) the machine rate exceeds the frequency of patient efforts (*auto-triggering, double-triggering, or uncoupling*).
2. *Flow asynchrony* suggests that the ventilator inspiratory flow either exceeds or undershoots the patient's inspiratory flow rate.
3. *Cycle asynchrony* occurs when the machine cycles either too early (*premature cycling*) or too late (*delayed cycling*) compared to the patient's natural cessation of inspiratory effort. Delayed cycling can occur due to high unintentional leaks.

There are several methods for detecting possible PVA outside of a polysomnography lab. One method includes comparing the patient's respiratory efforts to ventilator breath delivery while using the device in the office. Another method, also involving in-person observation of patient ventilator use, includes inspecting pressure and flow waveforms alongside tidal volume and leak outputs (Fig. 6.7). ResMed or Philips Respironics ventilators display real-time pressure and flow waveforms on the screen during device use. Using a USB device, the last 31 days of waveform data can be transferred from a Trilogy Evo to Care Orchestrator. Some Breas Vivo models can interpret data from thoracoabdominal effort belts [19], which can elucidate timing of patient inspiratory efforts. Accurate classification and troubleshooting will ultimately require a formal polysomnogram.

Respiratory Monitoring beyond the Ventilator

A thorough home ventilation monitoring program must consider methods of monitoring beyond ventilator data. There are several monitoring methods which can be particularly helpful prior to initiation of NIV. Clinicians should be aware of each method's advantages and limitations.

Spirometry

Telemonitoring of home spirometry may accelerate recognition of respiratory decline compared to waiting for an in-office assessment, particularly in rapidly progressive neuromuscular disease such as ALS [20]. Using Bluetooth and cloud-based monitoring, companies such as Medical International Research, NuvoAir, and Monitored Therapeutics Incorporated have developed handheld devices for performing home spirometry. Each company's proprietary software provides feedback on quality of maneuver. Data reports may be pushed by the patient to the clinician for review. Important limitations of spirometers include (a) variability in effort and consistency, (b) falsely low values in setting of bulbar weakness, and (c) static respiratory measurements as a surrogate for ventilation.

Pulse Oximetry

Home overnight pulse oximetry has wide dissemination and serves as an economical method for assessing nocturnal ventilation. The accuracy of pulse oximetry technology has been scrutinized recently, particularly in individuals with darkened skin pigment [21]. In the absence of pulmonary parenchymal, airways, or vascular disease, the primary mechanism for hypoxemia in neuromuscular disease includes hypoventilation. However, nocturnal pulse oximetry has been shown to be only 70% sensitive to nocturnal hypercapnia [22, 23]. Therefore, the absence of nocturnal hypoxemia may be falsely reassuring.

Noninvasive Measurement of Carbon Dioxide

The gold standard for assessing ventilation via partial pressure of carbon dioxide (PCO_2) is the arterial blood gas (ABG). Unfortunately, this is a largely impractical method for routine monitoring of home ventilation, particularly in the outpatient setting. Alternative, noninvasive means of assessing PCO_2 include sampling end-exhalation CO_2 ($PetCO_2$) or transcutaneous sensor measurements ($PtcCO_2$).

End-tidal estimates of carbon dioxide are most accurate in the setting of a closed system to ensure capture of all exhaled air. One example includes sampling $PetCO_2$ in-line with a ventilator circuit in a patient using invasive ventilation via tracheostomy. In noninvasive ventilation, $PetCO_2$ trends may be useful if the patient is spontaneously breathing without airflow obstruction. However, $PetCO_2$ often detects PCO_2 via nasal cannula, which can cause discomfort if used during NIV under a face mask.

Transcutaneous carbon dioxide assessments use a separate mechanism from pulse oximetry. The sensor heats the surface of the skin (typically ~42 °C) to dilate subcutaneous capillary beds to "arteriolize" the blood vessels. The vasodilation just under the skin facilitates gas diffusion to the skin surface. An electrolyte layer between the skin and the sensor membrane experiences a subsequent change in pH, which is converted by the monitor to a corresponding PCO_2. $PtcCO_2$ monitoring can be used as a brief assessment, for example, spot check over 15 min in the office (much like an additional vital sign) or as a continuous recording during NIV settings titrations or for overnight studies (Fig. 6.10). Compared to the ABG, a systematic review found that the $PtcCO_2$ has a low bias (+0.1 mmHg) and acceptable limits of agreement (±6 mmHg) [24].

$PtcCO_2$ monitoring has important limitations. Considering the mechanism of gas diffusion to the surface of the skin, the sensor placement should ideally target thin skin such as the forehead, cheek, or earlobe. Accuracy may be limited in areas of thickened skin or during states of low perfusion. Carbon dioxide drift can occur during prolonged monitoring sessions, which requires device calibration and drift correction at the end of the recording. Other limitations include air bubbles between the sensor and skin, sensor membrane damage, and an approximate 2-min delay in displayed CO_2 compared to real-time changes of $PaCO_2$ [14].

Home polysomnography offers methods for identifying early nocturnal hypoventilation in progressive neuromuscular disease. However, many home sleep test kits with sensor placement at the nose and mouth pose challenges when simultaneously using NIV or invasive ventilation. Some home sleep test kits only require wrist,

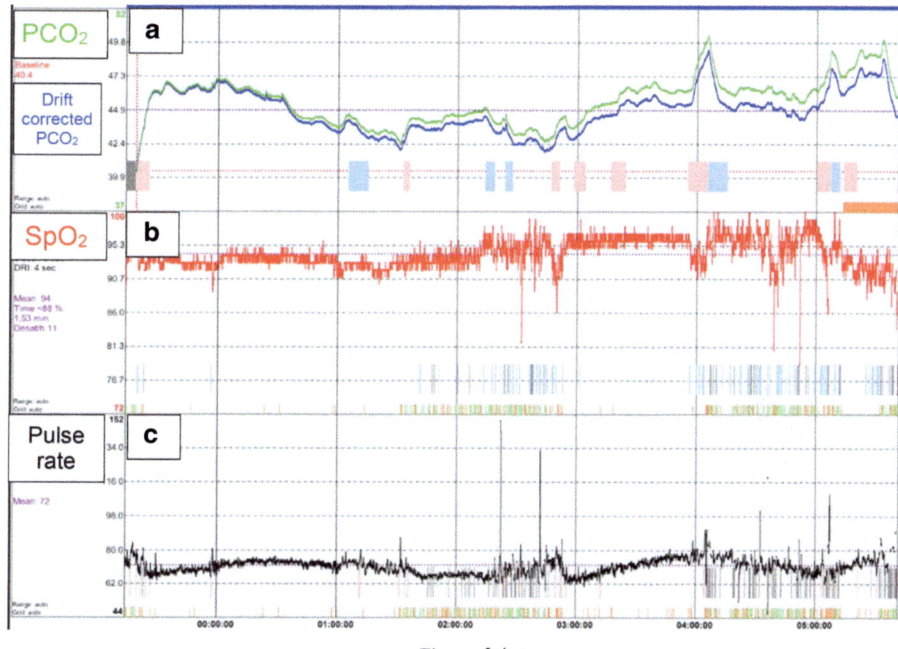

Fig. 6.10 Overnight Sentec tracing over 7 h showing (**a**) transcutaneous CO_2 (PCO_2) with original (green) and drift-corrected (blue) trend; (**b**) pulse oximetry (SpO_2); and (**c**) pulse rate

Fig. 6.11 Itamar Medical WatchPAT One device

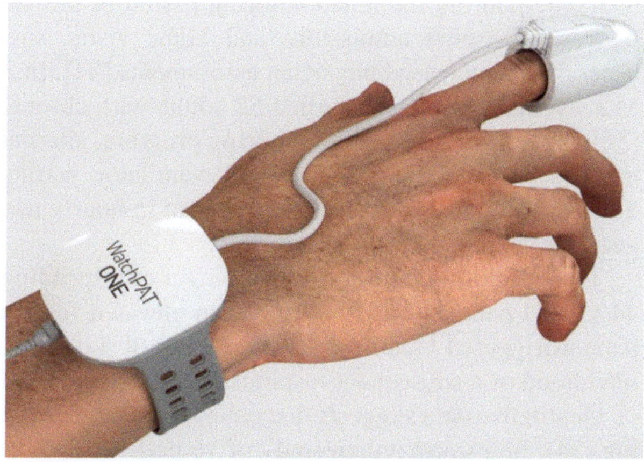

finger, and chest sensors, such as the WatchPAT series by Itamar Medical (Fig. 6.11). These devices utilize peripheral arterial signal, actigraphy, and chest sensors to estimate sleep duration, stage of sleep, and apnea/hypopnea events [25].

Evidence for Telemonitoring of Assisted Ventilation

Few studies have rigorously investigated the benefits of telemonitoring for home mechanical ventilation. Overall, there is a suggestion of potential benefit, but further research is necessary to identify the ideal patient populations, data sampling frequency, and NIV management strategies.

Prior work has demonstrated a survival benefit for ALS with NIV, and specifically for those with hourly usage of at least 4 h/day [26–28]. Pinto and colleagues performed a single-blinded controlled trial of weekly telemonitoring of NIV in ALS and found reduced hospital admissions and visits to the emergency room [29].

Vitacca and colleagues randomized 240 patients (36 with neuromuscular disease) with chronic respiratory failure to a 1-year telemonitoring program which included remote pulse oximetry and availability of a tele-assistance nurse or an on-call pulmonologist [30]. The intervention group experienced a reduction in hospitalizations by 36%, urgent physician calls by 65%, and acute exacerbations by 71%. Although, the authors comment that the majority of the beneficial signal was for the COPD group. In the TeleCRAFT trial of 68 patients with chronic respiratory failure (38 with COPD), Chatwin and colleagues performed a 6-month randomized crossover trial of telemonitoring to standard care [31]. The intervention consisted of telemonitoring NIV data, daily patient questionnaires, remote pulse oximetry, and a green/yellow/red light traffic system to alert the clinicians to patient status. Overall, telemonitoring was associated with no change in time to acute hospital admission or quality of life.

The increased data from telemonitoring does appear to "nudge" physicians to intervene. During the telemonitoring period in the TeleCRAFT trial, patients had increased hospital admissions and home visits, suggesting that telemonitoring necessitated increased physician assessments [31]. In 2018, a longitudinal study by Mansell and colleagues studied 52 adults with chronic hypercapnia on home NIV [32]. After initiating a telemonitoring program, alternative face masks were recommended in 79% of patients and ventilator settings were changed in 87%. Subsequently, there was an improvement in hourly usage per night and time at target tidal volume.

Telemonitoring may act as a harbinger of impending exacerbations. In a study of 44 COPD patients by Borel et al., an elevated respiratory rate and percentage of patient-triggered breaths on at least 2 out of 5 days was associated with increased likelihood of a subsequent respiratory exacerbation [33].

Qualitative data suggests that patients are supportive of cloud-based telemonitoring [34]. In a small Italian study of 16 patients on home ventilator telemonitoring, higher patient satisfaction was reported among those who adhered to therapy [35].

Several studies have estimated that telemonitoring of home ventilation is cost effective. Almeida and colleagues performed a prospective trial of telemonitoring in 40 ALS patients in Europe and estimated a cost savings of approximately €700 per patient per year for the United Kingdom National Health Service [36]. The aforementioned 1-year randomized trial of remote pulse oximetry by Vitacca et al. reported an estimated cost reduction of 33% per patient [30].

Despite the mixed signals in data thus far, the arc of outpatient management of chronic respiratory failure is bending toward increased telemonitoring in the wake of the COVID-19 pandemic. Eventually, telemonitoring of home mechanical ventilation may become standard of care, similar to management of sleep apnea [37]. As discussed later in this chapter, excitement for telemonitoring should be tempered by implications for physician time reimbursement and liability risk.

Clinical Applications of Noninvasive Ventilation Monitoring

Initial Setup

A clinician embarking on home ventilation initiation should aim to achieve the following goals, among others:

- Patient comfort to enable restorative sleep
- Improve gas exchange through minimizing atelectasis and dead space
- Increase time at target tidal volume and minute ventilation
- Maximize patient quality of life

For further detail on selecting device settings by disease physiology, see Chap. 4 of this text and a review by Selim et al. for a detailed guide [38]. Also, see a prior Respiratory Care article on a practical approach to long-term home ventilation [39].

Location of NIV setup could be influenced by a myriad of factors, including local resources, geography, clinician training background, and practice preferences. NIV may be initiated during an inpatient stay, within an in-lab polysomnography, in an outpatient clinic, or at home by a respiratory therapist.

The ideal location for NIV initiation is debatable and may be heavily influenced by local payer coverage determinations. It is not uncommon for clinicians in Europe to commence NIV over a 3–7-day inpatient stay [40]. Similar to the inpatient setting, in-lab polysomnography enables frequent review of ventilator data, gas exchange, and attendance to mask fit. A randomized trial consisting of mostly individuals with neuromuscular disease found that use of a sleep lab for titration of NIV settings led to improved device adherence and patient-device synchronization [41]. However, this study followed a protocol that is likely not generalizable to a sleep lab focused on obstructive sleep apnea rather than chronic respiratory failure. A case series of ALS patients with chronic hypercapnia described how inpatient admission enabled achievement of tolerable device settings, lowering of PCO_2, and patient adherence with device use >4 h/day [42].

In the United States, inpatient admission for initiation of NIV may not be covered for an otherwise stable patient. While an in-lab polysomnography would have benefits as mentioned above, the limited mobility of many individuals with neuromuscular disease may render in-lab studies infeasible. Thus, many patients begin NIV at home through services of a Durable Medical Equipment (DME) company. Typically, DMEs consist of respiratory therapists who visit patient's homes to provide the necessary supplies and settings adjustments in accordance with physician orders. Hazenberg and colleagues performed a single-center randomized trial of inpatient versus home NIV initiation in the Netherlands [43]. They found significantly lower median costs in the home group. In addition, the home group had a noninferior improvement in both $PaCO_2$ and quality of life. Regardless of NIV setup location, simultaneous monitoring of pulse oximetry (SpO_2) and $PtcCO_2$ can provide direct physiologic feedback for optimizing device settings.

Refinement of Initial Settings

During most office or home NIV titrations, initial settings chosen during the day while awake and sitting upright may not meet the needs of the patients' nocturnal respiratory drive and pulmonary compliance. Patients may experience significant changes in leak and minute ventilation overnight that may vary by stage of sleep and/or body position. The variability in ventilation efficacy may produce nocturnal alarms that were silent during a daytime titration. Therefore, it is strongly advised to begin home ventilator telemonitoring immediately upon NIV initiation. A review of ventilator data within 3–5 days after initial setup may enable early identification of issues.

The first few months after NIV initiation is a vulnerable period during which patients can experience significant discomfort, worsened quality of sleep, become discouraged, and rapidly lose trust in the device. After the initial encounter, it is prudent to schedule a return visit in 1–3 weeks for telemonitoring data review, adjustment of device settings, and changing of face mask, as appropriate. Achieving optimal settings and mask selection may require several iterative visits over a 3–6-month period.

Troubleshooting and Long-Term Monitoring

The ideal ventilator telemonitoring strategy remains undetermined. As of this writing, there are no society guidelines on rate of data sampling, thresholds for intervention, or algorithms for settings adjustments. For now, recommendations for approaches to remote monitoring rely on expert opinion [5–8, 10].

Broadly speaking, responding to telemonitoring can follow a reactive or proactive approach. Reactive monitoring occurs when a patient or caregiver notifies a clinician office about device discomfort or worsening respiratory symptoms. An organized approach to troubleshooting issues may enable rapid correction, potentially staving off further decompensation or the need for emergency care.

Alternatively, a systemic approach to proactively identify issues may act as an "early warning system." One method for doing this, although time consuming and laborious, includes surveying patient ventilator data on a regular basis (e.g., every 2–4 weeks). The frequency of data review should be tailored to the patient's underlying disorder and the severity of the patient's condition, as recently ill patients may require data survey every few days, while more stable patients only require a survey every 4–6 months. Customizable alerts are available with most cloud-based monitoring software, which can assist with proactive monitoring. A proactive data review approach demonstrated benefit in a multicenter case control study of 48 pediatric patients, where daily ventilator data pushes reduced hospitalizations, emergency room visits, and shortened median hospital length of stay [44].

Troubleshooting Scenarios

Low Adherence

Telemonitoring allows for an objective assessment of a patient's true adherence. Even the most well-meaning patients may incorrectly report their daily hourly usage. Persistent daytime hypercapnia or daytime fatigue may be due to low hourly usage rather than an issue with inadequate NIV settings.

The ideal daily "dose" of NIV hourly usage is debated. There are data for ALS suggesting that usage $\geq$4 h/day provides mortality benefit [26, 28]. The ideal duration of use may depend on stage of disease, with necessary hourly usage increasing over time. In general, usage <4 h is considered inadequate and often may be flagged as "nonadherent" by insurance companies in the United States.

The etiology for low hourly use may be multifactorial. If the patient is new to the device and experiencing claustrophobia, one can implement a slow process for acclimation. Patients are encouraged to begin wearing their mask during the day at home without connection to the ventilator, usually starting at a goal of 15–30 min, then slowly up titrating their daily usage as tolerated. Once patients complete 1–2 h of wearing only a mask during the day, then they are encouraged to connect their mask to the ventilator until they can tolerate 1–2 h awake. At that point, they are ready to try ventilation through the mask at night, again slowly increasing duration of use time. Addressing insomnia with pharmacotherapy should be done with caution in the neuromuscular population.

Patients often struggle to tolerate their mask or settings. They should be asked about their comfort with their current mask, any skin breakdown, and the presence of discernible leaks overnight. After addressing mask fit, attention should be diverted to ventilator settings. A careful history throughout each stage of the breath can elucidate which settings should be changed (Table 6.1).

Patients may reduce duration of device usage if they are awakened frequently throughout the night by ventilator alarms. They may hesitate to report this as an

Table 6.1 Patient interview questions and corresponding ventilator settings for adjustment

Question	Ventilator setting
Q1. Do you have any difficulty starting a breath?	• Trigger • Respiratory rate
Q2. Does the air rush in too quickly or too slowly?	• Rise
Q3. Do you feel like your lungs fill with enough air?	• Tidal volume • Inspiratory pressure
Q4. Does the breath end when you want it to?	• Cycle • Inspiratory time

issue assuming that alarms are a normal side effect of ventilator use. A careful history and review of the alarm log on telemonitoring reports can elucidate frequency and type of alarms. Patients using nocturnal-only NIV who are well-attended to by a caregiver can often afford to silence most alarms while leaving one or two critical ones (e.g., circuit disconnect and/or low minute ventilation) active. The ideal alarm settings will depend on the patient's stage of disease and the presence of home care attendants.

Other sources of low adherence include bed partners and humidifiers. A bed partner can be a source of low adherence if the noise from the machine disturbs sleep for anyone nearby. Partners may have to wear earplugs or sleep in separate rooms. Depending on the setting, humidifiers may run out of water overnight and alert the patient to refill the reservoir. Some DME companies can configure a setup that includes a hanging intravenous bag administering water to the reservoir all night. The Fisher & Paykel Healthcare MR 810 humidifier is compatible with heated wire circuits, which lessens the chance of circuit condensation.

High Leak

Excessive mask leak is one of the most common issues noted on telemonitoring data [45, 46]. When troubleshooting inefficacious NIV, addressing leak should take precedence over addressing other ventilator parameters.

While thresholds may vary by manufacturer, it is well-accepted that the upper limit of *total leak* should be kept under 50–60 L/min [15]. Before deciding on whether a leak is pathological, it is vital to check whether the monitoring data are reporting *total* leak (a composite of unintentional and intentional leak) or *unintentional* leak (the leak in excess of what would be expected for using the interface specified in the device settings). Leak source can come from any equipment piece between the ventilator and the patient's mask. The most common cause of a high leak is either a poorly fit mask or poorly adjusted straps. Common methods for addressing this includes education on mask adjustments, modifying strap tension, or substituting to a new mask. Occasionally, excessive facial hair can contribute to inadequate mask fit. Excessive head movement can cause migration of the mask overnight. A solution for the latter cause includes obtaining a mask interface with an additional contact point on the forehead such as the Fisher & Paykel Healthcare Vitera full face mask or ResMed Mirage series nasal mask (Figs 6.12a, b).

If the leak at the mask interface is not obvious, then check the security of all connections between (a) the mask and circuit, (b) circuit to any inline devices, and (c) circuit to filter/ventilator. Occasionally, cracks in the corrugated tubing may be the primary cause.

If the mask and circuitry fit well, then attention should focus on mouth opening during the night. Leak in a sawtooth pattern (Fig. 6.13) indicates recurrent jaw relaxation overnight with partial awakenings that cause loss of contact with the mask.

There are several approaches to troubleshooting mouth opening. First, address any overnight nasal obstruction. If using a nasal mask, consider switching to an oronasal mask, keeping in mind that the sawtooth leak can occur with either type of mask. If an oronasal mask fitting over the bridge of the nose is riding upward at night-time leading to mouth leak, convert to an oronasal mask that fits under the nose such as the ResMed AirFit F30i or Philips Respironics DreamWear full-face mask (Fig. 6.14). If the jaw is still pulling away from the mask at night, then

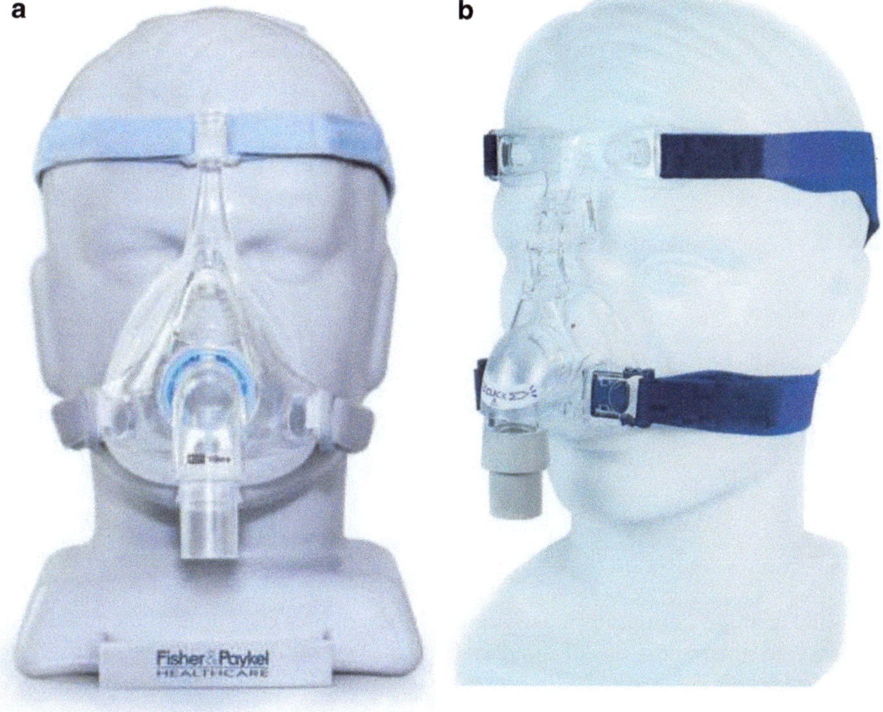

Fig. 6.12 Masks with forehead stabilizers. (**a**) Fisher & Paykel Healthcare Vitera full face mask, (**b**) ResMed Ultra Mirage II

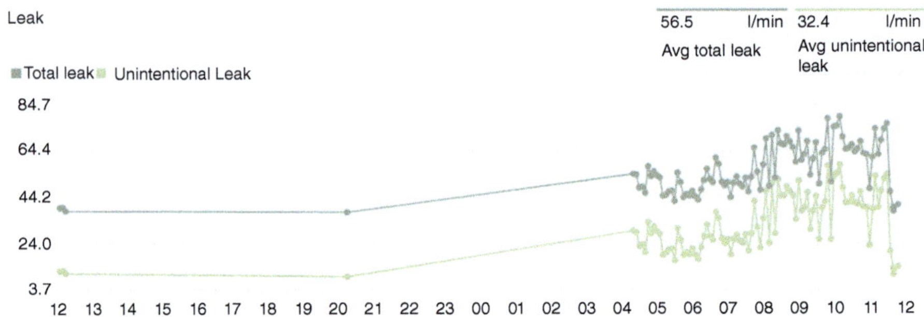

Fig. 6.13 Philips Respironics Care Orchestrator recoding showing saw-tooth pattern to leak suggestive of intermittent mouth opening

Fig. 6.14 ResMed AirFit F30i mask, an example of an oronasal interface that includes a nasal port that runs under the bridge of the nose

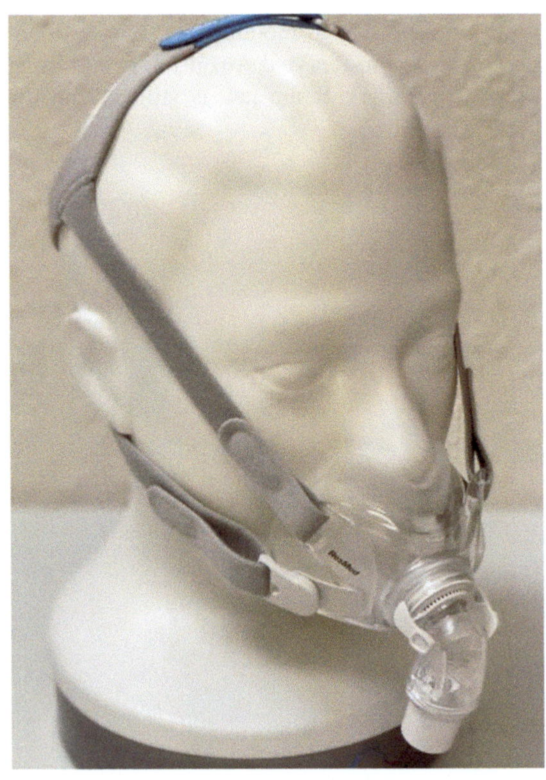

consider using a chin strap. Lastly, many patients find chin straps uncomfortable, but may be open to the use of mouth or lip tape such as Wallzon Mouth Bow Strips or Chin-Up strips.

Inadequate Tidal Volume

A common issue in pressure-targeted or volume-targeted modes with auto-adjusting inspiratory pressure (e.g., VAPS) is failure to achieve goal tidal volumes. A structured algorithmic approach should include the following assessments, generally in the following order:

1. Daily adherence
2. Leak
3. Mode
4. Inspiratory time and cycling control
5. Inspiratory airway pressure
6. Obstructive events

Daily Adherence

Daily adherence may affect average tidal volumes, or the source of low adherence is related to small tidal volumes. Target daily hourly usage goals will vary depending on the severity of disease, the patient lifestyle, and the overall goals of care. Identifying adherence issues should prompt detailed questioning about reasons and motivations behind the patient's low hourly usage. Please see the aforementioned section on "Low Adherence" for further details on addressing adherence.

Leak

As mentioned above, leak above a certain threshold can cause a significant fall in tidal volumes by as much as 40% [12]. In an auto-adjusting mode like VAPS, significant leak will cause the device algorithm to make adjustments based on misleading information. Please see the aforementioned section on "High Leak" for further details on addressing leaks.

Mode

Insufficient tidal volume can be related to incorrect mode selection, depending on the stage of the disease and/or the level of neuromuscular respiratory muscle weakness. Patients with more mild weakness may maintain a well-preserved inspiratory drive enough to prefer the ability to vary breath sizes. Such patients may be more comfortable in S/T mode as it allows for tidal volume augmentation by altering inspiratory flow. However, once inspiratory drive weakens and flow rates are more difficult to maintain, then improperly set S/T settings can predispose to rapid shallow breathing. Switching to pressure control mode may be more comfortable as it ensures a consistent inspiratory time regardless of inspiratory flow strength. ResMed devices and the Trilogy Evo enable an inspiratory time minimum feature that can be used to minimize this drawback of S/T mode with advancing disease.

Inspiratory Time and Cycling Control

Adequate inspiratory time is a critical component of the area under the pressure-time curve and thus the tidal volume (Fig. 6.9). After ensuring the patient is in the right mode, clinicians should direct their attention to inspiratory time control. Many of the manufacturer defaults include an inspiratory time of ~0.3–0.4 s. A patient with purely restrictive physiology with neuromuscular disease often requires an inspiratory time of around 1.0 s or greater for adequate, satisfying tidal volumes. Many patients with ALS often request very long inspiratory times of approximately 1.5 s or more. Patients with quadriplegia or cervical spinal cord injury may feel more comfortable at very high (>10 cc/kg) tidal volumes [47].

In S/T mode (including AVAPS-AE), the flow cycle sensitivity setting determines the inspiratory time anytime the patient is over-breathing the back-up rate. A high cycle sensitivity (e.g., >50%) can be detrimental to the tidal volumes of a patient with neuromuscular disease and weak inspiratory flows as it will cause the breath to terminate relatively early and thus cause small tidal volumes. To protect against premature cycling, a relatively low cycle sensitivity, such as 20–25% can be a good starting point. The clinician can titrate the sensitivity based on careful questioning during a ventilator titration session. Most manufacturers allow you to set the cycle sensitivity as low as 5–10%.

Inspiratory Airway Pressure

The inspiratory pressure should only be assessed after addressing the aforementioned variables. Focusing only on adjusting inspiratory pressure may not significantly improve tidal volumes and comfort unless the patient has a well-controlled leak, is in the correct mode, and has adequate inspiratory time control.

If adherence, leak, mode, and inspiratory time control are suitable, then the clinician should focus on level of driving pressure (difference between inspiratory and expiratory pressures). Often, low driving pressure or inadequately set inspiratory pressure window (e.g., low IPAP maximum) may be to blame. In an auto-titrating (e.g., VAPS) mode, low tidal volumes can occur if the maximum inspiratory pressure is set too low, which appears as the pressure tracing "flat-lining" for most of the night at the upper bounds of the inspiratory pressure setting (Fig. 6.15). In this scenario, the IPAP range should be shifted upward. The IPAP maximum should be increased by a few cm H_2O while concurrently the IPAP minimum should be increased to 1–2 cm H_2O below the previous IPAP maximum. Increasing the IPAP maximum without increasing the minimum may cause an IPAP minimum that is far lower than the effective IPAP, which can predispose to hypoventilation. Upon turning on the device, the software may start the IPAP at the lower end or middle of the

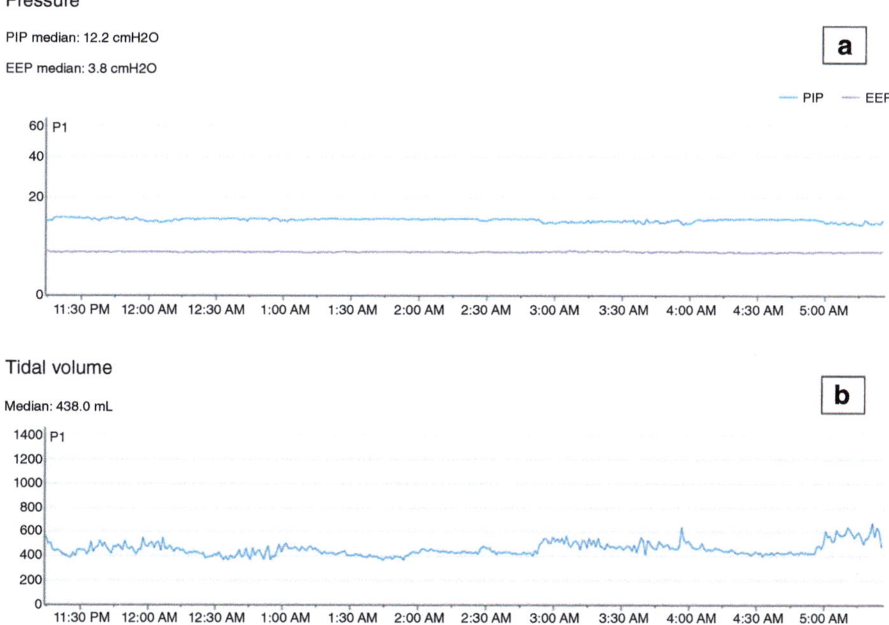

Fig. 6.15 Pressure support "pinned" at maximum setting. This ResMed Astral data is for a man with Becker muscular dystrophy. The mode is PS with safety tidal volume of 500 cc. The EPAP is set to 4 cm H_2O with PS min—max window set to 6–8 cm H_2O. (**a**) notice the pressure remains "pinned" at 12 cm H_2O for most of the night, (**b**) notice that the tidal volume is below target. Not shown is a well-controlled median leak of 18 L/min

IPAP window. This may lead to a delay in effective driving pressure and ineffective ventilation for the initial part of the night.

Obstructive Events

Many patients with neuromuscular disease, particularly those with bulbar weakness in ALS, may experience issues with glottic closure while using NIV. Some devices collect apnea-hypopnea index (AHI), such as ResMed AirView. Outside of a sleep lab, it can be difficult to determine what makes up an elevated AHI. Several home ventilators have an auto-adjusting EPAP setting. During apneas, the auto-EPAP algorithm may use a flow-response or forced oscillation to determine the presence of airway obstruction. During hypopneas, the algorithm responds to a change in minute ventilation or flow characteristics.

An elevated AHI in neuromuscular disease could be related to (a) pseudo-obstruction of the upper airway as in central apnea, (b) hypopnea, (c) transient hypoventilation, or (d) glottic closure. The latter does not improve with auto-adjusting EPAP. One entity known as upper airway obstruction with decreased central drive (ODCD) is characterized by expiratory vocal fold closure accompanied by central apnea, and has been associated with reduced survival in ALS [48, 49].

Lack of Telemonitoring Data

Telemonitoring reports require several key components for data acquisition and transfer (Fig. 6.16). First, the device itself must be collecting data (Fig 6.16a). For example, Trilogy Legacy series ventilators require an SD card for data collection. The absence of an SD card can go unnoticed until the SD card compartment is opened.

Second, the ventilator needs to be connected to a device with capability of data transfer via cellular signal (Fig. 6.16b). For ResMed, the AirCurve has a built-in modem with cellular capability. ResMed ventilators (i.e., Astral) require wired connection to a modem. Philips Respironics has Bluetooth technology that can communicate wirelessly with a hub plugged into a wall outlet. This hub is about the size of a deck of cards and must come within a certain distance (~50 ft) of the device to transfer data. Any data saved on the device while it is out of range can be uploaded the next time the two devices are in proximity with one another. Third, both the modem and Bluetooth hub must be connected to an active power outlet (Fig 6.16c).

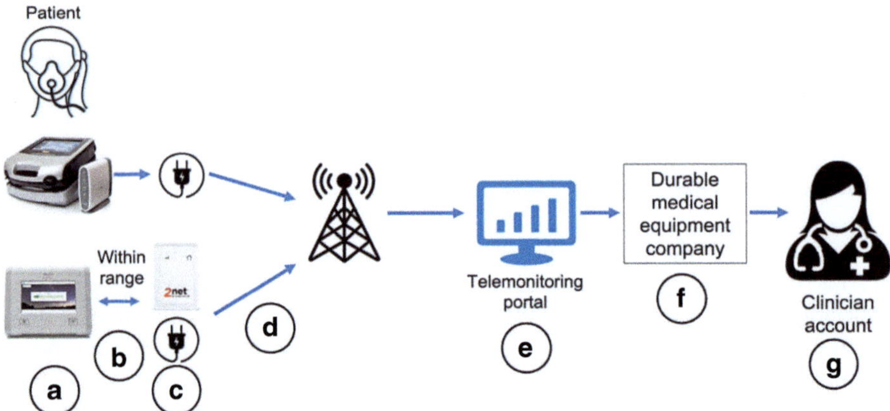

Fig. 6.16 Schematic of necessary connections for successful telemonitoring of home ventilator. (**a**) The patient must be using a device which collects data, which may require a SD card present. (**b**) The data is sent to connected wired modem or wirelessly to a Bluetooth hub which are connected to a power outlet (**c**). (**d**) The data are transmitted to a cellular tower with adequate signal. (**e**) The cellular data reach a web server connected to an online telemonitoring portal. (**f**) The DME company sets up a personalized account for the patient's data collection. (**g**) The patient's account must be connected to the physician's telemonitoring portal account

Fourth, the data transfer requires an adequate cellular signal (Fig 6.16d). Patients living in remote areas with poor cellular service may struggle to have successful data uploads.

Fifth, the data must reach the proper telemonitoring portal (Fig 6.16e). Sixth, the DME must set up a personalized portal account for collecting the patients' data (Fig 6.16f). Seventh, DME must link the patient's data to the clinician's account (Fig 6.16g). Often, DMEs may monitor their own patient's usage without connecting a physician unless they are requested to do so. If the patient has more than one ventilator, the DME must connect the patient's account to the serial numbers of both machines.

Daytime Hypercapnia

Daytime hypercapnia can be secondary to either (a) inadequate nocturnal support causing nocturnal hypercapnia with secondary daytime hypoventilation or (b) inadequate daytime support despite well-controlled nocturnal PCO_2.

The first step in addressing daytime hypercapnia is to ensure that nocturnal ventilation is optimized. Following the aforementioned troubleshooting approach, one should explore reasons why nocturnal support has been inadequate and address accordingly. An in-lab polysomnogram with transcutaneous CO_2 testing may be necessary to assess nocturnal hypoventilation. If available, a nocturnal transcutaneous CO_2 report can provide valuable complementary insights alongside ventilator performance data (Fig. 6.10). The Philips Respironics Trilogy Evo and Breas Vivo 45 enable direct connection to a Sentec Digital Monitoring System for integration of PCO_2 alongside typical ventilator parameters (see Fig. 6.7).

Once nocturnal ventilation has been addressed, then the patient's daytime PCO_2 should be reevaluated. If daytime hypercapnia persists despite adequate nocturnal support, then daytime ventilator assistance is necessary. For some patients, this may be as simple as extending nocturnal ventilator usage for a few hours in the morning or scheduling a session for a few hours in the afternoon. However, some patients may have advanced respiratory symptoms of daytime fatigue and dyspnea with eating and prolonged talking. Assisted ventilation requirements may exceed 12–14 h/day. Such a scenario may benefit from having mouthpiece ventilation as a secondary preset on their machine. See Chap. 4, for further details on setting up mouthpiece ventilation.

Legal and Ethical Issues with Telemonitoring

As ventilator telemonitoring has gained traction in recent years, it has outpaced formal society guidelines for best practices. Consequently, gaps remain on the legal and ethical responsibilities of all parties involved in creating a cohesive, safe, and effective telemonitoring system.

Fertile ground for legal risks extends beyond the typical physician–patient relationship. Additional elements of the system include the DME company, the ventilator, modem transfer, cellular signal strength, and the data monitoring software. Each element creates multifaceted relationships that contribute to potential system vulnerabilities. A limited list of examples includes data inaccuracy, modem failure, lack of physician competency with a specific manufacturer's telemonitoring software, delays in clinician office response, among other weaknesses commonly associated with telemedicine [50, 51]. Telemonitoring is particularly advantageous for the care of individuals with neuromuscular disease given their limited mobility; however, it should not replace critical in-person visits.

Ethical concerns hang over such a system with frequent data transfer. Under most scenarios, cloud-based data monitoring collects data at least once daily—far more frequent than physician practices can typically review. With such an abundance of data and a high noise-to-signal ratio, there is an increased likelihood of occult issues that raise questions such as (a) how frequently should a clinician review a patient's data?; (b) whose primary responsibility is it to relay an issue—the DME, the patient, or the physician?; and (c) how quickly should a physician respond to abnormalities in the ventilator data? For the aforementioned reasons and many others, telemonitoring should only be instituted after informed consent and documenting that the patient understands the various risks involved [52].

Reimbursement

Implementing ventilator telemonitoring as standard of care for all chronic respiratory failure patients can amount to a time-consuming endeavor. Much of the data review, response, troubleshooting, and communication often falls on time between office visits.

The American Medical Association and Centers for Medicare and Medicaid Services (CMS) have implemented codes for capturing care coordination for prolonged office visits and non-face-to-face time [53]. Current Procedural and Terminology (CPT) codes pertinent to outpatient billing are shown in Table 6.2. For same-day face-to-face visits, the CPT code G2212 can capture additional care coordination time for both new patient and established patient visits if time extends beyond specific thresholds.

Multiple CPT codes permit billing for care between office visits under specific criteria. Care coordination between office visits, or non-face-to-face time, can be billed using 99358/9 for services requiring >30 min on a separate calendar day prior to or subsequent to an office visit. Clinicians can also bill for care coordination related to remote physiologic monitoring (such as ventilator data) using 99457/8 and 99091 depending on the length of time spent, staff involved, and complexity of the patient interaction. A useful guide for remote physiologic telemonitoring codes has been created by ResMed [54].

Table 6.2 Medicare Physician Fee Schedule billable services for prolonged care time and remote physiologic monitoring [53]

Code	Location	Service	Description
Prolonged care time services			
99358[a] 99359[a]	Between office visits	Prolonged non-face-to-face service on a different calendar day as a face-to-face office visit	Captures care related to E/M services occurring on any day preceding or following an office visit. Use 99358 after the first 30 min (threshold >29 min), and 99359 for each additional 30 min beyond the first hour (threshold >74 min)[b]
G2212[c]	Outpatient face-to-face visit	Prolonged care on same calendar day of office visit	Add on for each additional 15 min of care coordination beyond 55 min for 99215 or 75 min for 99205
Remote physiologic monitoring services			
99457 99458	Between office visits	Remote physiologic monitoring management services	Remote physiologic monitoring management services, clinical staff/physician/other qualified healthcare professional time requiring interactive communication with an established patient/caregiver during the month. Use 99457 the first 20 min, and 99458 each additional 20 min once in a calendar month
99091	Between office visits	Collection and interpretation of transmitted physiologic data	Collection and interpretation of physiologic data digitally stored and/or transmitted by the patient and/or caregiver to the physician or other qualified healthcare professional, requiring a minimum of 30 min of time within a calendar month

E/M evaluation and management

[a] As of 1/1/2023, CMS has designated that they will not pay for these codes. Individual payers will determine their own reimbursement strategy

[b] Cannot be billed for services performed on the same day as an office visit due to G2212 guidelines

[c] 99417 is the American Medical Association Current Procedural Terminology code that is analogous to G2212

Future Considerations for Telemonitoring

Remote ventilator telemonitoring has spread rapidly across several countries as an important tool for improving the outpatient delivery of home-assisted ventilation. A competent clinical team coupled with a proactive DME company offers promise for optimizing outpatient NIV, improving quality of life, and reducing burden of acute care inpatient admissions.

Employing widespread use of home ventilation telemonitoring will require traversing a gap between the limits of possibility and what is commonly delivered as standard of respiratory care for individuals with neuromuscular disease [55]. Suggested focus areas for improving care include incorporating home ventilation into pulmonary/sleep fellowship education, broadening eligibility for neurology-focused clinical research grants to include respiratory investigations, garnering financial support for a multidisciplinary approach to neuromuscular disease, and employing an iterative approach to NIV settings adjustments to maximize treatment benefit to all who qualify [55].

Remote telemonitoring of ventilator usage across multiple manufacturers has created enormous repositories of data. The breadth of information across a large variety of diseases, geographic regions, and time span creates incredible potential for examining data beyond one-on-one patient interactions. The next phase of advancing the outpatient respiratory care of individuals with chronic respiratory failure will involve multicenter clinical trials and patient registries focused on optimizing strategies for improving ventilation efficacy and patient outcomes.

References

1. Mehta S, Hill NS. Noninvasive ventilation. Am J Resp Crit Care. 2001;163(2):540–77.
2. Lobato SD, Alises SM. Modern non-invasive mechanical ventilation turns 25. Arch Bronconeumol Engl Ed. 2013;49(11):475–9.
3. Hind M, Polkey MI, Simonds AK. AJRCCM: 100-year anniversary. Homeward bound: a centenary of home mechanical ventilation. Am J Resp Crit Care. 2017;195(9):1140–9.
4. Ambrosino N, Vitacca M, Dreher M, Isetta V, Montserrat JM, Tonia T, et al. Tele-monitoring of ventilator-dependent patients: a European Respiratory Society statement. Eur Respir J. 2016;48(3):648–63. https://www.ncbi.nlm.nih.gov/pubmed/27390283.
5. Borel J, Palot A, Patout M. Technological advances in home non-invasive ventilation monitoring: reliability of data and effect on patient outcomes. Respirology. 2019;24(12):1143–51.
6. Canal JMM, Suárez-Girón M, Egea C, Embid C, Matute-Villacís M, Martínez LM, et al. Posicionamiento de la Sociedad Española de Neumología y Cirugía Torácica en el uso del la telemedicina en los trastornos respiratorios del sueño y ventilación mecánica. Arch Bronconeumol. 2021;57(4):281–90.
7. Janssens JP, Cantero C, Pasquina P, Georges M, Rabec C. Monitoring long term noninvasive ventilation: benefits, caveats and perspectives. Front Med. 2022;9:874523.
8. Ackrivo J, Elman L, Hansen-Flaschen J. Telemonitoring for home-assisted ventilation: a narrative review. Ann Am Thorac Soc. 2021;18(11):1761–72.
9. Lehner WE, Ballard IM, Figueroa WG, Woodruff DS. Home care utilizing a ventilator in a patient with amyotrophic lateral sclerosis. J Fam Pract. 1980;10(1):39–42.
10. Contal O, Vignaux L, Combescure C, Pepin JL, Jolliet P, Janssens JP. Monitoring of non-invasive ventilation by built-in software of home bilevel ventilators a bench study. Chest. 2012;141(2):469–76.
11. Borel JC, Sabil A, Janssens JP, Couteau M, Boulon L, Lévy P, et al. Intentional leaks in industrial masks have a significant impact on efficacy of bilevel noninvasive ventilation: a bench test study. Chest. 2009;135(3):669–77.
12. Luján M, Sogo A, Grimau C, Pomares X, Blanch L, Monsó E. Influence of dynamic leaks in volume-targeted pressure support noninvasive ventilation: a bench study. Respir Care. 2015;60(2):191–200.
13. Jeganathan V, Rautela L, Conti S, Saravanan K, Rigoni A, Graco M, et al. Typical within and between person variability in non-invasive ventilator derived variables among clinically stable, long-term users. BMJ Open Respir Res. 2021;8(1):e000824.
14. Arnal JM, Oranger M, Gonzalez-Bermejo J. Monitoring systems in home ventilation. J Clin Med. 2023;12(6):2163.
15. Zhu K, Rabec C, Gonzalez-Bermejo J, Hardy S, Aouf S, Escourrou P, et al. Combined effects of leaks, respiratory system properties and upper airway patency on the performance of home ventilators: a bench study. BMC Pulm Med. 2017;17(1):145.

16. Fanfulla F, Taurino AE, Lupo ND, Trentin R, D'Ambrosio C, Nava S. Effect of sleep on patient/ventilator asynchrony in patients undergoing chronic non-invasive mechanical ventilation. Respir Med. 2007;101(8):1702–7.
17. Gonzalez-Bermejo J, Janssens JP, Rabec C, Perrin C, Lofaso F, Langevin B, et al. Framework for patient-ventilator asynchrony during long-term non-invasive ventilation. Thorax. 2019;74(7):715.
18. Ramsay M. Patient ventilator asynchrony and sleep disruption during non-invasive ventilation. J Thorac Dis. 2018;10(1):S80–5.
19. M L. Usefulness of effort belts: usefulness of effort belts as monitoring tool during non-invasive positive pressure ventilation. 2016 [cited 2023 Mar 14]. https://breas.com/wp-content/uploads/2019/05/Usefulness-of-Effort-Belts-during-NIV.pdf.
20. Geronimo A, Simmons Z. Evaluation of remote pulmonary function testing in motor neuron disease. Amyotroph Lateral Scler Frontotemporal Degener. 2019;20(5–6):348–55.
21. Sjoding MW, Dickson RP, Iwashyna TJ, Gay SE, Valley TS. Racial bias in pulse oximetry measurement. N Engl J Med. 2020;383(25):2477–8.
22. Georges M, Nguyen-Baranoff D, Griffon L, Foignot C, Bonniaud P, Camus P, et al. Usefulness of transcutaneous PCO_2 to assess nocturnal hypoventilation in restrictive lung disorders: diagnosis of nocturnal hypoventilation. Respirology. 2016;21(7):1300–6.
23. Boentert M, Glatz C, Helmle C, Okegwo A, Young P. Prevalence of sleep apnoea and capnographic detection of nocturnal hypoventilation in amyotrophic lateral sclerosis. J Neurol Neurosurg Psychiatry. 2018;89(4):418.
24. Conway A, Tipton E, Liu WH, Conway Z, Soalheira K, Sutherland J, et al. Accuracy and precision of transcutaneous carbon dioxide monitoring: a systematic review and meta-analysis. Thorax. 2019;74(2):157.
25. Yalamanchali S, Farajian V, Hamilton C, Pott TR, Samuelson CG, Friedman M. Diagnosis of obstructive sleep apnea by peripheral arterial tonometry: meta-analysis. JAMA Otolaryngol Head Neck Surg. 2013;139(12):1343–50.
26. Berlowitz DJ, Howard ME, Fiore JF, Hoorn SV, O'Donoghue FJ, Westlake J, et al. Identifying who will benefit from non-invasive ventilation in amyotrophic lateral sclerosis/motor neurone disease in a clinical cohort. J Neurol Neurosurg Psychiatry. 2016;87(3):280–6.
27. Kleopa KA, Sherman M, Neal B, Romano GJ, Heiman-Patterson T. Bipap improves survival and rate of pulmonary function decline in patients with ALS. J Neurol Sci. 1999;164(1):82–8.
28. Ackrivo J, Hsu JY, Hansen-Flaschen J, Elman L, Kawut SM. Non-invasive ventilation use is associated with better survival in amyotrophic lateral sclerosis. Ann Am Thorac Soc. 2021;18:486.
29. Pinto A, Almeida JP, Pinto S, Pereira J, Oliveira AG, de Carvalho M. Home telemonitoring of non-invasive ventilation decreases healthcare utilisation in a prospective controlled trial of patients with amyotrophic lateral sclerosis. J Neurol Neurosurg Psychiatry. 2010;81(11):1238–42.
30. Vitacca M, Bianchi L, Guerra A, Fracchia C, Spanevello A, Balbi B, et al. Tele-assistance in chronic respiratory failure patients: a randomised clinical trial. Eur Respir J. 2009;33(2):411–8.
31. Chatwin M, Hawkins G, Panicchia L, Woods A, Hanak A, Lucas R, et al. Randomised crossover trial of telemonitoring in chronic respiratory patients (TeleCRAFT trial). Thorax. 2016;71(4):305–11.
32. Mansell SK, Cutts S, Hackney I, Wood MJ, Hawksworth K, Creer DD, et al. Using domiciliary non-invasive ventilator data downloads to inform clinical decision-making to optimise ventilation delivery and patient compliance. BMJ Open Respir Res. 2018;5(1):e000238.
33. Borel JC, Pelletier J, Taleux N, Briault A, Arnol N, Pison C, et al. Parameters recorded by software of non-invasive ventilators predict COPD exacerbation: a proof-of-concept study. Thorax. 2015;70(3):284–5.
34. Mansell SK, Kilbride C, Wood MJ, Gowing F, Mandal S. Experiences and views of patients, carers and healthcare professionals on using modems in domiciliary non-invasive ventilation (NIV): a qualitative study. BMJ Open Respir Res. 2020;7(1):e000510.

35. Bertini S, Picariello M, Gorini M, Renda T, Augustynen A, Villella G, et al. Telemonitoring in chronic ventilatory failure: a new model of survellaince, a pilot study. Monaldi Arch Chest Dis. 2012;77(2):57–66.

36. de Almeida JPL, Pinto A, Pinto S, Ohana B, de Carvalho M. Economic cost of home-telemonitoring care for BiPAP-assisted ALS individuals. Amyotroph Lateral Scler. 2012;13(6):533–7.

37. Schwab RJ, Badr SM, Epstein LJ, Gay PC, Gozal D, Kohler M, et al. An official American Thoracic Society statement: continuous positive airway pressure adherence tracking systems. The optimal monitoring strategies and outcome measures in adults. Am J Resp Crit Care. 2013;188(5):613–20.

38. Selim BJ, Wolfe L, Coleman JM, Dewan NA. Initiation of noninvasive ventilation for sleep related hypoventilation disorders advanced modes and devices. Chest. 2018;153(1):251–65.

39. Hansen-Flaschen J, Ackrivo J. Practical guide to management of long-term noninvasive ventilation for adults with chronic neuromuscular disease. Respir Care. 2023;68(8):1123.

40. Georges M, Perez T, Rabec C, Jacquin L, Finet-Monnier A, Ramos C, et al. Proposals from a French expert panel for respiratory care in ALS patients. Respir Med Res. 2022;81:100901.

41. Hannan LM, Rautela L, Berlowitz DJ, McDonald CF, Cori JM, Sheers N, et al. Randomised controlled trial of polysomnographic titration of noninvasive ventilation. Eur Respir J. 2019;53(5):1802118.

42. Quigg KH, Wilson MW, Choi PJ. Transcutaneous CO_2 monitoring as indication for inpatient non-invasive ventilation initiation in patients with amyotrophic lateral sclerosis. Muscle Nerve. 2021;65(4):444–7.

43. Hazenberg A, Kerstjens HAM, Prins SCL, Vermeulen KM, Wijkstra PJ. Initiation of home mechanical ventilation at home: a randomised controlled trial of efficacy, feasibility and costs. Respir Med. 2014;108(9):1387–95.

44. Trucco F, Pedemonte M, Racca F, Falsaperla R, Romano C, Wenzel A, et al. Tele-monitoring in paediatric and young home-ventilated neuromuscular patients: a multicentre case-control trial. J Telemed Telecare. 2018;25(7):414–24.

45. Alvarez RF, Cuadrado GR, Jerez FR, Garcia AG, Menendez PR, Clara PC. Home mechanical ventilation through mask: monitoring leakage and nocturnal oxygenation at home. Respiration. 2013;85(2):132–6.

46. Gonzalez J, Sharshar T, Hart N, Chadda K, Raphaël JC, Lofaso F. Air leaks during mechanical ventilation as a cause of persistent hypercapnia in neuromuscular disorders. Intensive Care Med. 2003;29(4):596–602.

47. Vázquez RG, Sedes PR, Fariña MM, Marqués AM, Velasco MEF. Respiratory management in the patient with spinal cord injury. Biomed Res Int. 2013;2013:168757.

48. Sancho J, Burés E, Ferrer S, Ferrando A, Bañuls P, Servera E. Unstable control of breathing can lead to ineffective noninvasive ventilation in amyotrophic lateral sclerosis. ERJ Open Res. 2019;5(3):00099-2019.

49. Georges M, Attali V, Golmard JL, Morélot-Panzini C, Crevier-Buchman L, Collet JM, et al. Reduced survival in patients with ALS with upper airway obstructive events on non-invasive ventilation. J Neurol Neurosurg Psychiatry. 2016;87(10):1045.

50. Stanberry B. Legal and ethical aspects of telemedicine. J Telemed Telecare. 2006;12(4):166–75.

51. Greene J, Yellowlees PM. Electronic and remote prescribing: administrative, regulatory, technical, and clinical standards and guidelines, April 2013. Telemed J E Health. 2013;20(1):63–74.

52. Bauer KA. The ethical and social dimensions of home-based telemedicine. Crit Rev Biomed Eng. 2000;28(3–4):541–4.

53. Peters SG. New billing rules for outpatient office visit codes. Chest. 2020;158(1):298–302.

54. ResMed quick reference guide: assisting healthcare professionals with information about remote patient monitoring billing codes. [cited 2023 Apr 17]. https://www.resmed.com/us/dam/documents/articles/1013491_Reimbursement_FF_downloads.pdf.

55. Ackrivo J. Pulmonary care for ALS: progress, gaps, and paths forward. Muscle Nerve. 2023;67(5):341–53.

Chapter 7
Approach to the Pediatric Patient with Respiratory Complications of Neuromuscular Disease

Jon Maniaci and Howard B. Panitch

Introduction

Childhood neuromuscular disorders are heterogeneous in terms of age of onset and rate of progression [1]. Nevertheless, their effects on the respiratory system are somewhat predictable [2]. Weakness of inspiratory, bulbar, or expiratory muscles impairs coughing, compromises swallowing, and leads to impaired clearance of secretions. Secretion retention, in turn, predisposes to atelectasis and pneumonia, which then cause a reduction in lung compliance and an increase in resistance that contribute to an increased load on the respiratory muscles. As work exceeds the maximal output of the chest wall and respiratory muscles, respiratory failure ensues. Symptoms of respiratory failure first present during sleep, with sleep disruption, poor sleep quality, daytime fatigue, and poor school performance. As the imbalance between respiratory pump output and load worsens, nocturnal hypoventilation develops, and eventually extends to diurnal hypercapnia.

The impacts of neuromuscular weakness on respiratory system function in children are generally similar to those of adults, but maturational differences of the respiratory system of children can exacerbate those effects. The growing spine, chest wall, and airways lack the structural stiffness to withstand deformation as well as mature structures do, exacerbating both restrictive and obstructive processes of

J. Maniaci
Division of Pulmonary and Sleep Medicine, The Children's Hospital of Philadelphia, Philadelphia, PA, USA
e-mail: maniacij@chop.edu

H. B. Panitch (✉)
Division of Pulmonary and Sleep Medicine, The Children's Hospital of Philadelphia, Philadelphia, PA, USA

14523 HUB for Clinical Collaboration, Philadelphia, PA, USA
e-mail: PANITCH@chop.edu

N. Lechtzin (ed.), *Pulmonary Complications of Neuromuscular Disease*, Respiratory Medicine, https://doi.org/10.1007/978-3-031-65335-3_7

the underlying disorder. Those characteristics also require different strategies for intervention from those used in adults. In this chapter, we will review the common respiratory complications of pediatric neuromuscular disease (NMD), with a focus on the unique features that must be considered in the assessment and care of children with chronic neuromuscular weakness.

Epidemiology

Most of the progressive disorders that cause neuromuscular weakness in children are inherited, but occasionally they result from metabolic conditions, toxic or infectious exposures, trauma, or inflammatory or collagen-vascular disorders [3]. The most common inherited childhood NMD is Duchenne muscular dystrophy (DMD), an X-linked recessive disorder with a prevalence of 15.9–19.5 cases per 100,000 live male births [4], although female carriers can also be affected. It is caused by mutations in the dystrophin gene, resulting in absent or nonfunctional protein. In its absence, recurrent injury to muscle fibers leads to chronic inflammation, and replacement of muscle tissue with fibrotic and fatty tissue [5]. Ensuing weakness begins in the preschool years, and without intervention boys with DMD commonly become non-ambulant by 10–12 years of age and require assisted ventilation to treat sleep-disordered breathing or diurnal hypercapnia in adolescence [6]. Diaphragm weakness is the principal cause of inspiratory muscle weakness, and it may precede intercostal muscle involvement [7]. Boys with DMD can also have macroglossia, which, along with reduced tone in oropharyngeal muscles, contributes to problems with obstructive sleep apnea in younger subjects [8]. Cardiac muscle is also involved in patients with DMD, and dysrhythmias and cardiomyopathy frequently develop [4].

Spinal muscular atrophy (SMA) affects approximately 1 in 11,000 live births [9]. It was previously considered the most common inherited cause of mortality in infancy, but since its inclusion in newborn screening and with the introduction of disease-modifying therapies, that is no longer true. It is caused by a mutation in the Survival Motor Neuron 1 (SMN1) gene, leading to degeneration of alpha motor neurons in the spinal column and progressive muscle atrophy, weakness, and paralysis [9]. Different phenotypes are classified into groups based on the age at onset of symptoms and the maximum motor function achieved: Group 1 patients demonstrate hypotonia and diffuse weakness by 6 months of age and cannot sit independently; those with Type 2 disease develop weakness between 6 and 18 months and can sit but not stand independently; and those with Type 3 disease present after 18 months, often with an abnormal gait [10]. Before disease-modifying therapies were available, infants with Type 1 SMA had a life expectancy of <2 years if untreated, while those with Type 2 disease could survive into their third decade. Type 3 patients were expected to have a normal life expectancy. The principal cause of death in Types 1 and 2 SMA is progressive respiratory failure. Unlike patients with DMD, those with SMA demonstrate relative sparing of diaphragm function but marked weakness of intercostal musculature [11].

Less common are congenital muscular dystrophies (CMDs), a group of disorders that present within the first 2 years of life. Although epidemiologic data are sparse, among European populations approximately 1 in 100,000 individuals are affected [12]. The CMDs are subdivided into three main categories: (1) collagenopathies or collagen VI (COL-VI)-related myopathies, (2) merosinopathies or merosin-deficient myopathies, and (3) dystroglycanopathies or α-dystroglycan-related MDs [12]. There is phenotypic heterogeneity among the different subgroups of CMDs as well as overlap with congenital myopathies (CMs), but these disorders usually present with hypotonia and weakness. Respiratory muscle involvement is variable in terms of severity and rate of progression, as well as in the groups of respiratory muscles affected: those with COL-VI-related dystrophy and selenoprotein N (SEPN) myopathy can have primarily diaphragm weakness, whereas in other CMDs and CMs accessory or expiratory muscles are primarily affected [13]. Furthermore, the decline in respiratory muscle strength may not be mirrored in peripheral muscle weakness in diseases like SEPN myopathy or multiminicore myopathy [13, 14].

Myotonic dystrophy (DM1) is the most common muscular dystrophy seen in adults [14], although it occurs in infancy and childhood as well [15]. There is a broad range in its severity, but its most severe form occurs congenitally with an incidence of 1 in 47,619 live births [16]. Inheritance is autosomal dominant and results from a mutation in the DMPK (dystrophia myotonica protein kinase) gene, which causes a trinucleotide repeat expansion; a greater number of repeats is associated with more severe disease [17]. The clinical course of infants with congenital DM1 can be bimodal with a neonatal course characterized by reduced fetal movements, polyhydramnios, swallowing dysfunction, weakness and hypotonia, arthrogryposis, scoliosis, and respiratory failure. If the infant can be supported through the neonatal period, however, there may be some improvement in symptoms before adult symptoms appear later in life [15]. About 40% of neonates with congenital DM1 experience respiratory failure, but it is much less common in the infantile and juvenile forms of the disease [18]. Approximately 50% of children with DM1 experience excessive daytime somnolence that does not necessarily correlate with the presence of sleep-disordered breathing [19].

Some causes of neuromuscular weakness in children are static. These include traumatic spinal cord injury and nontraumatic spinal cord dysfunction. Nontraumatic lesions can be congenital (spina bifida, Chiari malformation), infectious, inflammatory, malignant or benign tumors, vascular lesions, or metabolic abnormalities. The approximate annual incidence of traumatic spinal cord injury among US children is 1.99 per 100,000, of whom 95% are adolescents and predominantly male [20]. In addition, >80% of traumatic spinal cord lesions in children are cervical [21]. Spinal cord dysfunction or injury can be proximal to the anterior horn cells (upper motor neuron) and associated with hyperreflexia and spasticity, or distal to the anterior horn cells (lower motor neuron), and result in flaccidity, muscle atrophy, and absent deep tendon reflexes. Those lesions involving the upper cervical region (C1–C5) can interrupt phrenic nerve function and result in diaphragm weakness or paralysis [22]. Concomitant loss of phonation can affect communication skills depending on the age of the child, and add to significant psychosocial impairment [23]. Brainstem lesions can affect control of breathing, while upper thoracic lesions can affect accessory muscles of inspiration and abdominal muscles, thus impairing airway clearance in addition to ventilation.

Pathophysiology

Developmental differences in the normal respiratory system magnify the effects of processes that increase respiratory load in children relative to adults. Thus, early onset of NMDs can increase the risk of respiratory failure, and perhaps even affect the normal growth of the respiratory system.

Pediatric Airway

The pediatric airway, from nares to respiratory bronchioles, is narrower than the adult airway. In infancy, the total cross-sectional area of the trachea and main bronchi are only about 8–13% of their adult size [24]. Central airway diameter rapidly increases during the first 3 years of life, slows during school-aged years, and increases rapidly again during adolescence to reach the final adult size [24]. Given the inverse relationship between airway size and resistance, even small changes in airway radius, for example, from airway wall edema, has greater effects in an infant compared with an adult: a 1 mm reduction in airway diameter could lead to a 16-fold increase in airflow resistance in an infant when compared to the same degree of airway narrowing in an adult [25]. In addition, central and peripheral airways resistances are evenly divided in children under 5 years of age, while in older children and adults the central airways comprise 90% of total resistance and small airways contribute only 10% [26]. Therefore, any process that affects small airways will have a greater impact on younger patients and can result in profound respiratory distress.

Additionally, the pediatric airway is more compliant than its adult counterpart [27]. Although its cartilaginous framework is developed by the 25th week of gestation, there is an age-dependent reduction in water and proteoglycan content, resulting in progressive airway stiffening with age [28]. As a result, the infant airway is prone to collapse under conditions of increased transmural pressure. This can result in a further decrease in airway diameter, increasing airflow resistance [29].

Finally, collateral ventilation can minimize the effects of distal airway mucus impaction in adults [30]. However, interalveolar pores of Kohn, alveolar-bronchiole channels of Lambert and interbronchiolar channels of Martin are not present at birth, and likely do not develop until at least 4 years of age [30, 31]. When present, collateral channels can serve as alternative pathways to bypass obstructed airways and prevent atelectasis. However, this is not the case in young children, placing them at greater risk for atelectasis when secretions are increased [30, 32].

Pediatric Chest Wall

The orientation and composition of the pediatric chest wall and respiratory muscles place them at a mechanical disadvantage. In infancy, the ribs lie in a horizontal orientation [25, 33]. It is not until about 3 years of age, in part due to the effects of gravity as children obtain an upright posture, that the ribs become caudally declined [33] (Fig. 7.1). Prior to this change, the external intercostals are at a biomechanical disadvantage. The external intercostal muscles increase the thoracic volume by elevating and widening the rib cage during inspiration [34]. The near vertical angle of insertion of the external intercostals on each inferior rib of the immature rib cage, however, reduces the torque generated by muscles and minimizes elevation of the ribs during their contraction. It is not until the ribs assume a sloped orientation that the angle of muscle insertion becomes advantageous so that the muscle can generate effective torque. Simultaneously, the rib cage begins to change from a round structure in infancy to a more elliptical one throughout childhood [35]. This geometrical change results in the "bucket-handle" effect of the intercostals as their contraction results in outward and upward displacement of the thorax, adding to the expansion of the lungs [34].

Until this change in chest shape occurs, nearly the entire tidal volume is dependent on the function of the diaphragm. Yet, during infancy, the diaphragm is also poorly adapted. Like the rib cage, it too assumes a horizontal position [25, 36, 37]. As a result, the diaphragm has a reduced ability to displace the abdominal contents caudally, minimizing the resulting increase in thoracic volume upon inspiration. Furthermore, the horizontal orientation of the diaphragm results in a decreased area of apposition with the lower rib cage, reducing its ability to displace the ribs laterally [36, 37]. For these reasons, the tidal volume in young children is relatively fixed, so that in times of respiratory distress the child must increase respiratory rate to maintain minute ventilation, exerting excess energy to do so.

The anatomic disadvantages of the developing respiratory pump are compounded by its mechanical properties. At birth, the rib cage is composed primarily of cartilage, and ossifies with age. As a result, the neonatal chest wall is particularly compliant. Within the first 2 years of life, it is up to three times as compliant as the developing lung, reversing the mature balance between the inward recoil of the lung and the outward pull of the chest wall [38]. During inspiration, negative intrathoracic pressure therefore draws the ribcage inward, so that intercostal muscle contraction is required to defend against the loss of tidal volume. Additionally, the reduced outward recoil of the more compliant chest wall causes infants to have a lower relaxed functional residual capacity (FRC) [38, 39] and so they must maintain a dynamically elevated end expiratory lung volume above the resting FRC [40]. As the chest wall stiffens over time, less energy is required to stabilize it, as the increased outward recoil results in establishment of a relaxed FRC with age [38–40].

The respiratory muscles of neonates are primarily comprised of type II muscle fibers, which are fast-twitch, low oxidative, and fatigue-susceptible [41]. In

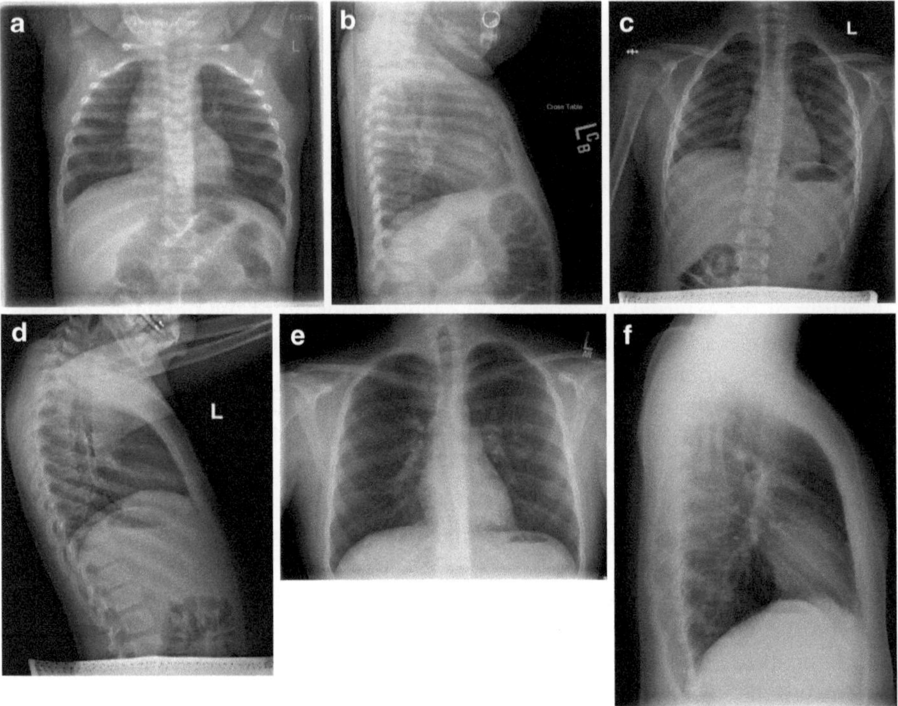

Fig. 7.1 Frontal and lateral chest radiographs demonstrating the gradual change in rib configuration with age, at 5 months (**a**, **b**), 8 years (**c**, **d**), and 16 years (**e**, **f**), from horizontal to caudal declination

contrast, type I fibers, which are slow-twitch, high oxidative, and fatigue-resistant, predominate in older children and adults.

In summary, infants and young children must overcome increased airway resistance from narrow airways which are prone to dynamic collapse, with fatigue-susceptible respiratory muscles that are placed in a suboptimal configuration. As a result, even healthy children can rapidly develop respiratory failure when challenged. That risk is amplified in children whose neuromuscular disease presents prenatally through early childhood.

Airway Clearance Impairment

Most children with neuromuscular weakness do not have underlying pulmonary parenchymal pathology at the onset of their disease. However, as weakness ensues, patients follow a stereotypical progression of respiratory involvement, beginning with impairment of airway clearance [42]. Functional airway clearance is essential to rid the airways of pollutants and infectious organisms, and is primarily comprised of two mechanisms: the mucociliary escalator and cough [42]. The mucociliary escalator is responsible for clearing the peripheral airways, while an effective cough clears the central airways and pharynx [43].

The mucociliary escalator is the primary innate defense mechanism of the lung. The cilia beat in a synchronized fashion to generate a wave that propels mucus and entrapped particulate matter in the cephalad direction [44]. Chronic breathing at low tidal volumes results in a decreased cephalad airflow bias that reduces expiratory airflow velocity and decreases the effectiveness of mucociliary clearance [42]. However, the primary factor that impairs airway clearance in NMD is an ineffective cough.

Impairment in either the inspiratory, compressive, or expiratory phases of cough results in a reduced ability to clear the airway of secretions. Yet in NMDs, owing to inspiratory and expiratory muscle weakness as well as bulbar dysfunction, all three phases of cough can be affected. The mechanics of an effective cough in children are no different from those of adults [42], but the pressures and flows generated for an effective cough are not well studied in children. As with other measures of lung function, the cough peak flow (CPF) is dependent on size and age, as well as respiratory muscle strength [45]. Thus, healthy younger children with smaller airways and lungs and reduced elastic recoil have a lower CPF than adults. While guidelines for cough assistance, based on small numbers of adults with NMD, are available [46, 47], no such guidelines are available for prepubertal children.

Bulbar Dysfunction, Dysphagia, and Sialorrhea

Involvement of the bulbar muscles commonly occurs in patients with NMDs and leads to challenges with dysphagia, dysarthria, impaired cough, and aspiration of oral secretions and/or gastric contents. Safe and effective swallowing requires adequate strength, intact sensation, and complex coordination of the oral, facial, and pharyngeal muscles [48]. A pooled study of pediatric patients with NMDs estimated the prevalence of dysphagia to be 47%, though the actual prevalence varies greatly based on age and severity of muscle weakness [49]. As a consequence of delayed swallow, pharyngeal residue, and oftentimes poor dentition, patients can produce excessive saliva, frequently exceeding 0.5 L/day [48]. This can be burdensome for the patient and further complicates the clearance of oral contents. Additionally, common viral respiratory infections will lead to additional production and thickening of secretions, while compromising overall muscle strength, thus increasing the prevalence of dysphagia during times of illness [50]. These challenges predispose patients with neuromuscular weakness to aspiration of saliva, upper airway secretions, and gastric contents. Subsequently, uncontested aspiration can develop into aspiration pneumonia.

Parenchymal Lung Disease and Hypoxemia

With disease progression, patients are at risk for the development of both hypoxemic and hypercarbic respiratory failure. Hypoxemic respiratory failure reflects lung parenchymal disease and develops as a consequence of impaired airway clearance and/or recurrent aspiration, leading to recurrent lower respiratory tract infections. Additionally, children are particularly susceptible to atelectasis because of their smaller airways and lack of collateral ventilation. In turn, chronic mucus impaction and atelectasis lead to further infection and chronic inflammation that result in bronchiectasis. The prevalence of parenchymal lung disease varies based on the severity of underlying weakness and presence of risk factors such as aspiration or gastroesophageal reflux [51]. For example, bronchiectasis was present in 33% of patients with SMA1, compared to only 15% of patients with SMA2 and SMA3 [51].

Hypercarbic Respiratory Failure

Chest Wall Restriction

Hypercarbic respiratory failure is far more common than hypoxemic respiratory failure in children with NMD and results from an imbalance between the output of the respiratory pump and the load against which it must operate. The respiratory pump is comprised of the chest wall, inspiratory muscles, and central controller [52]. As noted above, the unique orientation of the developing ribcage and diaphragm reduce maximal pump output. Additionally, the increased compliance of the pediatric chest leads to thoracoabdominal asynchrony with paradoxical inward chest wall motion during inspiration. Over time, deformation in chest wall shape exacerbates chest wall restriction, impeding thoracic expansion and limiting ventilation. For example, infants with congenital neuromuscular weakness develop a bell-shaped chest from lack of expansion of the upper rib cage, and acquired pectus excavatum occurs frequently in infants with SMA1 [53]. In children with SMA2, progressive inward collapse of the ribcage with exaggerated caudal declination of the ribs can develop as a result of weakness of the intercostal muscles and has been coined the "collapsing parasol" deformity [54] (Fig. 7.2). These deformities are associated with impaired pulmonary function in children old enough to perform spirometry [54]. Additionally, scoliosis further impairs chest wall expansion and respiratory mechanics. It results from an imbalance between truncal muscle strength and tone. Scoliosis is more common in hypotonic NMDs; it is present in over 60% of children with SMA and over 80% of children with DMD, but it is readily seen in hypertonic conditions as well [55].

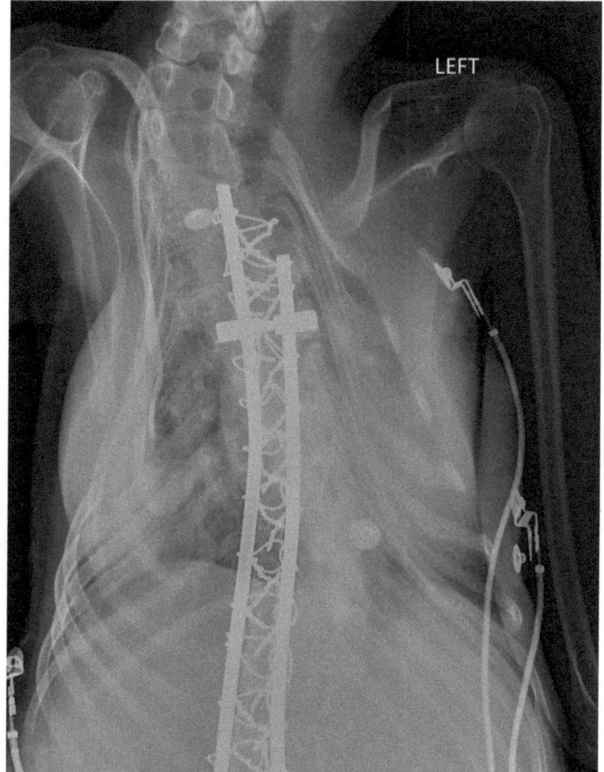

Fig. 7.2 "Collapsing parasol" deformity in a 12-year-old girl with SMA2 and spinal instrumentation for scoliosis

Hypoventilation

As respiratory muscle weakness progresses, respiratory pump output becomes insufficient for the imposed load, and periods of elevated pCO_2 develop. Hypoventilation is initially seen during sleep as a result of a reduction in tidal volume from inspiratory muscle relaxation during rapid eye movement (REM) sleep [42, 56]. Frequent arousals from sleep occur as a protective mechanism from rising CO_2, altering the sleep state to recruit previously atonic inspiratory muscles to return the body to a eucapnic state [2]. Although arousals temporarily alleviate prolonged hypercapnia and minimize hypoxemia, over time this sleep fragmentation leads to poor sleep quality, daytime fatigue, and reduced quality of life [57]. Recurrent cycles of hypoventilation and arousal ultimately lead to blunting of the chemoreceptor response to hypercapnia, resulting in more profound and prolonged CO_2 retention [58]. Eventually, hypercapnia will persist beyond sleep, resulting in diurnal hypercapnic respiratory failure. Symptomatic diurnal hypercapnia developed within 12–24 months of nocturnal hypoventilation in patients with various forms of congenital NMD (mean age, 18 years) [59]. Consequences of untreated diurnal hypercapnia are grave, as mean life expectancy was <10 months in patients with DMD after onset of diurnal hypoventilation in the absence of intervention [60].

Sleep-Disordered Breathing

Sleep-disordered breathing (SDB) in NMDs refers not only to hypoventilation, but also to hypoxemia, central and obstructive hypopneas and apneas, sleep fragmentation and frequent arousals, poor sleep efficiency, and seizures [42]. Obstructive sleep apnea (OSA) resulting from weakness of the pharyngeal dilator muscles, particularly the genioglossus, occurs frequently in all types of NMD. It is especially common in children with primary upper respiratory muscle involvement, as seen in cerebral palsy, traumatic brain injuries, and motor neuropathies like Charcot–Marie–Tooth disease [61]. Some NMDs have associated craniofacial abnormalities like retrognathia, flattening of the malar eminences, or macroglossia that predispose to obstructive sleep apnea [62]. Both patient age and natural history of muscle involvement in the NMD can affect the type of SDB seen: in a study of 34 boys with DMD, 10 had polysomnographic evidence of OSA between 1 and 14 years of age (median 8 years), but over the ensuing 5-year observation period, 11 demonstrated sleep hypoventilation [8]. The authors speculated that their observed bimodal distribution of types of SDB was the result of age and disease-specific muscle involvement. In the younger boys with relatively preserved diaphragm function, findings of OSA predominated. As the boys aged and diaphragm weakness progressed, they would not be able to generate enough intrathoracic negative pressure to cause upper airway obstruction, and evidence of hypoventilation would predominate [8]. Treatment of the underlying disease can also influence the type of SDB seen. Corticosteroid treatment of boys with DMD is associated with excessive weight gain, and the degree of OSA in boys with DMD is strongly correlated with increased body mass index [63].

Central apnea is also a concern in certain conditions. Children with myotonic dystrophy have impairment of neurons in the medullary respiratory centers, increasing the potential for central apnea [64]. Central apnea is also commonly present in children with myelomeningocele associated with Arnold–Chiari malformation, as downward displacement of the medulla results in impingement of the central respiratory centers [65]. The prevalence of SDB in children with NMD is estimated between 27% and 62%, depending on age and underlying diagnosis [61]. Regardless, the actual prevalence is markedly higher than the 3% reported in otherwise healthy children [61].

Challenges of Respiratory Assessments in Children

Symptoms of respiratory insufficiency and SDB are often insidious and subtle in children with NMD, making assessment difficult. Infants and young children do not have the verbal skills to describe increasing dyspnea, and older children may not recognize fatigue related to respiratory muscle weakness, instead ascribing symptoms to progression of more generalized weakness. Detection of SDB in children can be hampered by reliance on observations of parents or other caregivers who may not be aware of alterations in the child's sleep pattern [66]. Both documented evidence of diurnal hypercapnia and the presence of recurrent episodes of pneumonia are considered indicators for assisted airway clearance and assisted ventilatory support [67, 68]. Significant problems with sleep fragmentation, nocturnal hypoxemia and hypercapnia, daytime fatigue, and poor school performance, however, typically precede those indications and can contribute to poorer quality of life when left untreated. Thus, practitioners must have a high index of suspicion to assess respiratory function and intervene early.

Measurements that change with growth, like anthropometrics or lung function, rely on data sets from healthy populations to determine normal and abnormal values. These, however, may be inaccurate or nonexistent for some children with NMDs. For instance, growth patterns of ambulant boys with DMD differ from those of the general male population, with DMD males being shorter, at the extremes of weight, and with a higher body mass index [69]. Typical weight-for-age curves do not account for muscle wasting, so children whose disease starts early in life are often well below the normal range [70]. Thus, standard growth curves do not reflect the population of children with NMD and may be insensitive for early detection of respiratory-related compromised growth. For some lung function measurements like CPF, scarce normative data in children exist [45]. The cutoff values of CPF or maximal expiratory pressure (MEP) used to determine need for airway clearance assistance [71, 72] are not appropriate for younger children, and no such cutoff values exist for them. In those younger children with NMD, the finding of recurrent lower respiratory illness or qualitative assessment of a "weak cough" by caregivers are usually the indicators to begin assisted airway clearance [73].

Volitional tests of lung function rely on patient effort and cooperation. Young children and those with intellectual disability, therefore, may not be able to cooperate with such testing. Investigators have used techniques like stimulating a cry or obstructing the airway for several breaths to measure inspiratory and expiratory muscle strength in infants [74, 75]. Tests of flow (peak expiratory flow, CPF) and of volume (VC) cannot be reliably assessed in preschool children, but such testing can be accomplished in children by 5 or 6 years of age [76]. Maneuvers like a sniff nasal inspiratory pressure (SNIP) may be easier to perform and therefore better suited to younger children [77]. Measurement of SNIP is not interchangeable with a static maximal inspiratory pressure (MIP) measurement; rather, the two provide complementary information [77].

Indications for Testing

Historical clues that should prompt assessment for the need for cough assistance include recurrent pneumonias, coughing or choking with feedings, and a weak cry. Before disease-modifying therapies for SMA were available, the diagnosis of SMA Type 1 was enough to initiate cough assistance without the need for testing, but similar considerations should be given to other NMDs that clearly can be anticipated to include impaired cough like cervical spinal cord injury or congenital myotonic dystrophy. Indicators of SDB, when present, could include poor school performance, frequent morning headache, poor sleep quality, and late day fatigue. Assessments for SDB are recommended for any child with SMA who has symptoms of SDB [78]. Guidelines for patients with DMD recommend annual sleep studies for nonambulant subjects with symptoms of SDB [79]. Other NMD guidelines suggest SDB assessment at least annually for children with a VC of <60% predicted, those who have become nonambulant or never attained the ability to walk, any infant with weakness, weak children with symptoms of OSA or hypoventilation, children with obvious diaphragmatic weakness, and those with rigid spine syndromes [68]. Children whose rate of progression of the underlying disease is uncertain, those who experience frequent lower respiratory infections, or those who develop new onset symptoms of SDB may require more frequent assessments [68]. A trend of weight loss or sustained lack of weight gain in the presence of adequate caloric intake should also prompt additional testing for abnormalities of gas exchange.

Some physical examination findings increase the suspicion for respiratory compromise. Paradoxical movement between the rib cage and abdomen during quiet inspiration causes increased respiratory work, in part because of loss of tidal volume in either the rib cage or abdominal compartment. The breathing pattern points to the more affected muscle group: the abdomen moves in while the rib cage moves out in those with primarily diaphragm weakness, whereas the rib cage sinks in as the abdomen expands in those with primarily intercostal muscle weakness. Such abnormalities in breathing patterns can be analyzed and quantified using respiratory inductance plethysmography or optoelectronic plethysmography [80, 81]. A bell-shaped chest and acquired pectus excavatum deformity reflect longstanding intercostal muscle weakness, as seen in infants with SMA.

Laboratory Testing

Tests are available to measure adequacy of gas exchange, strength and endurance of respiratory muscles, and changes in fractional lung volumes associated with disease progression (Table 7.1). Several tests of muscle and lung function are volitional and require patient effort and cooperation. Tests of gas exchange and of sleep quality are non-volitional, allowing the subject to be passive in the measurement process.

Gas Exchange

Arterial blood gas determinations are considered the gold standard in assessing adequacy of ventilation as reflected in the $PaCO_2$, but repeated arterial puncture or use of an indwelling arterial catheter is not feasible, given that the procedure itself

Table 7.1 Select tests of respiratory function

	Volitional/ nonvolitional	Comments
Gas exchange		
ABG, CBG	NV	Can use to calculate A-a gradient (hypoventilation); pain can cause immediate hyperventilation; repeated/frequent measurements not feasible
$ETCO_2$	NV	May be artificially low as weakness increases and breathing becomes more shallower
$TcCO_2$	NV	Technology for unobserved overnight $TcCO_2$ monitoring requires more investigation in children; may be artificially high secondary to drift artifact
SpO_2	NV	Readily available; does not directly assess degree of hypoventilation, but there is a unique pattern of desaturation in patients with NMD and SDB
Respiratory strength/chest wall characteristics		
RIP	NV	Must differentiate paradox secondary to muscle weakness from upper airway obstruction
Optoelectric plethysmography	NV	Similar to RIP but less widely available
Lung volumes		
VC	V	Can perform forced, slow, or inspiratory, usually after ~5 years of age; longitudinal monitoring provides information about disease progression; "integrative"—Reflects chest wall, inspiratory and expiratory muscles
RV	V	Reflects expiratory muscles and chest wall characteristics
Muscle strength		
MIP	V	May be difficult to sustain static inspiratory pressure; can predict clinical outcomes
MEP	V	Used as threshold for cough assistance in older children and adults
SNIP	V	Easier to perform than MIP; usually higher than MIP; can use to track disease progression
Crying mouth P	V	Used in infants; no data to track disease progression
PEFR/CPF	V	Primarily test of expiratory muscles, but influenced by inspiratory effort; CPF thresholds for older children and adults used as threshold for cough assistance
TTmus/TTdi	V	Reflects endurance of inspiratory muscles; TTmus noninvasive, TTdi-invasive
Polysomnogram	NV	Can detect abnormalities of gas exchange as well as sleep disruption; availability limited and work-intensive

ABG arterial blood gas, *CBG* capillary blood gas, *ETCO₂* end-tidal CO_2, *TcCO₂* transcutaneous CO_2, *SpO₂* oxyhemoglobin saturation, *RIP* respiratory inductance plethysmography, *VC* vital capacity, *RV* residual volume, *MIP* maximal inspiratory pressure, *MEP* maximal expiratory pressure, *SNIP* sniff nasal inspiratory pressure, *PEFR* peak expiratory flow rate, *CPF* cough peak flow, *TTmus* tension-time index of the respiratory muscles, *TTdi* tension-time index of the diaphragm is disruptive of sleep, and the pain from the procedure can cause hyperventilation that significantly lowers $PaCO_2$ [82]. As a result, capillary blood gases are recommended for use in children [83], but these can be inaccurate if perfusion of the site being tested is poor or if the child hyperventilates during the procedure. To bypass these problems, noninvasive methods to determine CO_2 levels have been tested in children and adults with NMD, with mixed results [82, 84, 85]. Continuous monitoring of $ETCO_2$ was compared with $PaCO_2$ levels obtained during sleep at 23:00, 03:00, and 07:00 in 21 children with NMD who were 6–18 years old (mean 10.55 ± 5 years) [84]. There was generally good concordance between the two measures, with an intraclass correlation coefficient of 0.791 (95% CI 0.517–0.843) between mean $ETCO_2$ and the 07:00 $PaCO_2$.

Measurements of $ETCO_2$ could be artificially low when a person with NMD sleeps, due to failure to capture end-tidal air as breathing becomes shallower or because of leakage of air through the mouth. To avoid that issue, other investigators have assessed the accuracy of home overnight transcutaneous CO_2 ($TcCO_2$) monitoring. Among 24 ventilator-assisted adults with NMD, there was good correlation between home overnight $TcCO_2$, $ETCO_2$, and morning arterial blood gases [86]. Among 39 children with NMD 11 months to 16 years old, however, ambulatory $TcCO_2$ monitoring lacked diagnostic accuracy when compared to polysomnography conducted in a monitored sleep laboratory [85]. While the cause of this discrepancy is unclear, routine use of home $TcCO_2$ measurements to detect nocturnal hypoventilation in children cannot be recommended without additional evaluation. Daytime measurement of serum bicarbonate could be another possible screening tool. In a small retrospective study, it was elevated in children with NMD and nocturnal hypoventilation, even when daytime hypoventilation was absent [87].

Polysomnography in a monitored sleep laboratory remains the benchmark for diagnosing nocturnal hypoventilation and SDB in children [83]. The sleep laboratory must be capable of monitoring carbon dioxide, be compliant with access requirements as set forth in the Americans with Disabilities Act of 1990, provide adequate room for a caregiver, and have capabilities of performing airway clearance for patients who might require it. The number of facilities able to do such testing in children is limited. One study from Canada suggested that there was at least a 7.5-fold greater demand for diagnostic polysomnograms in children than available capacity [88]. The polysomnogram can detect both obstructive apnea and hypoventilation, and it also provides information about sleep disruption and arousals. There are specific criteria for diagnosing hypoventilation in children, but in 2018, additional refinements were proposed to enhance the detection of hypoventilation in patients with DMD. These include an $ETCO_2$ or $TcCO_2$ >50 mmHg for at least 2% of sleep time, an increase in $ETCO_2$ or $TcCO_2$ during sleep of 10 mmHg above the awake baseline for at least 2% of sleep time, an SpO_2 $\leq$88% for at least 2% of sleep time or for at least 5 min continuously, or an apnea-hypopnea index of 5 events/h or more [79]. When compared to the standard criteria established by the American Academy of Sleep Medicine for the diagnosis of SDB in children <18 years old, sleep hypoventilation was diagnosed more frequently using these disease-specific criteria in a cohort of 105 pediatric patients with DMD [89].

Measurement of pulse oximetry, with or without $TcCO_2$ measurements, has been suggested to screen for nocturnal hypoventilation in children with NMD when full polysomnography is not readily available [68, 84]. Investigators described a unique pattern of baseline lower oxyhemoglobin saturation (SpO_2) with frequent desaturations dispersed throughout the night in 12 children with NMD and symptoms of SDB, when compared with children with Prader Willi syndrome, obstructive sleep apnea, or normal controls [90]. Monitoring of oximetry alone may not detect all children with significant episodes of hypoventilation [87, 91], but British Thoracic Society guidelines note that in asymptomatic children with NMD, a technically adequate overnight pulse oximetry study in which the SpO_2 remains $\geq 93\%$ is adequate to rule out significant nocturnal hypoventilation [68]. Any child with an abnormal oximetry study, however, should undergo more detailed testing [68].

Tests of Respiratory Muscle Strength and Endurance

A recent clinical practice guideline recommended periodic testing of maximal inspiratory pressure (MIP) or maximal expiratory pressure (MEP), SNIP, or CPF in patients with NMD, as these tests (as well as the VC) are considered predictors of clinical outcomes [83]. All are volitional and require patient cooperation, limiting their applicability in young children or those with intellectual impairment. As noted above, lack of normative data in children under 12 years of age limits the predictive ability of CPF to determine the need for airway clearance assistance. Similarly, while a MEP <60 cm H_2O has been associated with the need for assisted airway clearance in adults [72], no such cutoff value has been established for children. Nevertheless, both MIP and MEP have been shown to correlate with measurements of VC in several studies [68]. In contrast, a longitudinal study of boys with DMD showed that the youngest boys studied in the nontreatment group, between 7 and 7.9 years of age, had percent predicted values of MIP and MEP that were abnormally low while the FVC and peak expiratory flow rate were still within the normal range [92]. In boys <10 years of age, the greatest impairment relative to normative values was reflected in the MIP and MEP. There is also poor test-retest reliability for these tests [93], and the young age at which patients with DMD reached "floor" values of MIP and MEP make them less valuable as outcome predictors [92]. The SNIP is a more natural maneuver to perform and is usually higher than the MIP [94]. It correlates well with MIP and also with FVC in children with NMD, however, and it is easier to perform than an FVC maneuver; thus, it is considered a useful measure to track the clinical course of children with NMD [76, 77, 93, 95].

Tests of respiratory muscle endurance reflect different characteristics of the muscles from tests that measure their strength. The tension-time index of the respiratory muscles (TTmus) is a noninvasive measurement that provides a dimensionless number used to predict the time to respiratory muscle fatigue [96]. The TTmus assesses the fraction of maximal effort generated by the inspiratory muscles along with the amount of time they are contracted during an inspiration, and the value is the product of two ratios: the mean inspiratory pressure/MIP and the inspiratory time/total respiratory cycle time. In adults, a TTmus of 0.33 defines the fatigue threshold [96]; values of TTmus above that threshold are associated with fatiguability of the respiratory muscles, so that the higher the value of TTmus, the sooner fatigue will set in. In children with NMD, elevation of the TTmus is primarily the result of a reduction of MIP relative to the mean inspiratory pressure [97]. Measurements of TTmus and the tension-time index of the diaphragm (TTdi) can be successfully measured throughout childhood, even in infants with NMD [74]. Although age-related differences in the TTmus have not been described throughout childhood, respiratory muscle endurance increases because of pubertal changes [98]. In a cohort of boys with DMD whose lung functions were studied longitudinally, the TTdi increased over time but it became abnormally high later than other abnormalities in lung function occurred [99]. An elevated TTmus is a strong predictor of respiratory failure in patients with NMD, and it is inversely correlated with the inspiratory VC or MIP [100].

Lung Volumes

The VC represents an integrated test that assesses both inspiratory and expiratory muscles, as well as characteristics of the chest wall itself. Respiratory muscle weakness causes a unique pattern of reduction in fractional lung volumes, in which the total lung capacity, VC, and expiratory reserve volumes are all decreased, but the residual volume and FRC are elevated. This is the result of the inability of the expiratory muscles to deform the chest wall below its resting volume. While a forced VC (FVC) maneuver is required to provide information about the rate of emptying of the lung in obstructive disorders, it is not necessary to provide information about respiratory function in patients with neuromuscular weakness. A slow VC may be an easier maneuver for weak patients to perform, and other studies have used the inspiratory VC in children to predict complications of disease like chest infections or SDB [101, 102].

Serial determinations of VC provide objective information about progression of respiratory muscle weakness in a variety of progressive childhood NMDs [92, 99, 103, 104]. The decrease in VC occurs not only because of loss of respiratory muscle strength, but also because of ankylosis of costovertebral joints after prolonged low tidal volume breathing, replacement of muscle with fibrotic tissue, and the development of microatelectasis that increases the respiratory load [2]. A decrease in VC of 25% or more between maneuvers performed in the supine versus the upright position reflects diaphragm weakness [105]. Reduction in upright VC is associated with the development of hypoventilation; in young males with DMD, for every 10% decline in the percent predicted FVC, the odds of hypoventilation increased 20% (OR 0.8, 95% CI 0.74–0.87, $p = 0.001$) [63]. Once the VC has fallen to <1 L, there is an increase in 5-year mortality among patients with DMD [106], and an overall 4.1-fold increase in mortality [92].

Use of the VC has helped determine which patients would benefit from manual assisted coughing and which would require other techniques like mechanical in-exsufflation [107]. The ability of the VC to predict which patients require assisted ventilation during sleep is less straightforward. The risk of SDB was not associated with a fall in the supine FVC among 21 males with DMD [108]. Others have shown poor correlation between the VC and the presence of SDB in children with a variety of NMDs [8, 108–110]. In contrast, some investigations have found an association between the percent predicted VC and findings of SDB in children with NMDs [102, 111–113]. In those studies, nocturnal hypoventilation was associated with threshold values of FVC <70% predicted (sensitivity 71.4%, specificity 64.1%) [112], an FVC z score of −3.24 (sensitivity 78%, specificity 73%) or FVC <60% predicted (sensitivity 78%, specificity 73%) [111], an FVC <50% predicted (sensitivity 73%, specificity 86%), or an inspiratory VC <40% predicted (sensitivity 96%, specificity 88%) [102]. Such findings have led to the recommendations that noninvasive ventilation should be initiated in males with DMD once the VC is <50% predicted [79, 114], and that testing for SDB should be performed no less than annually for children whose VC is <60% predicted [68].

Treatment

Early and aggressive treatment of the respiratory complications of NMDs reduces healthcare utilization, improves quality of life, and prolongs survival [115, 116]. Treatment guidelines for the most common NMDs primarily focus on augmenting airway clearance and assisting ventilation [68, 78, 79]. However, there is no consensus regarding recommendations for several adjunctive interventions, and the effects of novel therapeutics, which may alter the clinical course of several progressive NMDs, are yet to be determined.

Lung Volume Recruitment

Clinicians use lung volume recruitment (LVR) (i.e., "hyperexpansion therapy"; "breath-stacking") to maximize total lung capacity, reduce atelectasis, and slow the rate of lung volume decline. It is often the first intervention implemented in attempt to preserve lung function. In its simplest form, LVR is performed with a manual resuscitation bag to deliver positive pressure via a facemask and one-way valve. Repetitive insufflations are administered until maximum chest wall expansion is achieved. While this method is inexpensive and readily available, young children often do not have the ability to cooperate and complete the technique [117]. Expansions can also be performed utilizing intermittent positive pressure ventilation via noninvasive ventilation (NIV) set in a Volume Control mode, or through the insufflation phase of a mechanical in-exsufflator. However, these methods are more expensive and may not be readily available in resource-limited settings. In one prospective study, 18 patients (mean age 15 years) with a variety of NMDs were empirically prescribed daily manual LVR [118]. They had improvements in CPF, though there was no change in FVC after 6 months [118]. In separate retrospective studies, LVR use was associated with decreased ER visits, hospitalizations, and length of stay [119, 120]. However, in these studies, LVR was performed via combined mechanical in-exsufflation (MI-E), and the utility of hyperexpansion therapy alone is therefore less certain.

Some DMD guidelines recommend that LVR be initiated when FVC falls below 60% predicted [79]. In a retrospective study of 16 adolescents and young adults with DMD and advanced lung disease, the rate of decline in FVC % predicted fell significantly from −4.5 percentage points/year before initiation of LVR to −0.5/year following its use [121]. In contrast, in a randomized controlled prospective study involving 66 boys aged 6–16 years with DMD who had relatively normal lung function at the beginning of the study, there was no difference in decline of FVC % predicted between those boys who used LVR twice daily and those who did not [122]. Thus, some reduction in lung function may be required before the onset of LVR use to appreciate the effects of the intervention, and premature use of LVR could lead to treatment burden without benefit.

Airway Clearance

Cough Augmentation: Manually Assisted Cough

The two most common methods of cough augmentation are manually assisted cough and MI-E. Manually assisted cough (MAC) is performed by a caregiver who delivers synchronized thrusts of the chest and abdominal wall as the patient coughs, thereby augmenting the patient's expiratory muscle function to increase expiratory airflow [123]. Since the initial phase of a physiologic cough is a deep inspiration, MAC is often preceded by a manual or mechanical insufflation to enhance elastic recoil during the expiratory phase. In a study of 61 young men with DMD (mean age 22 years; range 12–36 years), CPF increased from 138 L/min (unassisted) to 204 L/min with MAC, and increased further still to 302 L/min utilizing a combination of LVR and MAC [71]. While this combination may be effective in adults and older children, young children or those with developmental delays often cannot cooperate to perform MAC effectively. Kan et al. evaluated the effectiveness of a training program to teach MAC to caregivers of 28 children with a variety of NMDs (mean age 12 years) [124]. At the conclusion of the program, there was no change in CPF. The investigators concluded that MAC was challenging to implement in this age group and that further training or alternative treatment should be considered. In addition, MAC requires a significant amount of active participation and physical effort from a caregiver and may not be sustainable during acute illnesses when the frequency of treatment must be increased.

Cough Augmentation: Mechanical Insufflation-Exsufflation

Mechanical insufflation-exsufflation (MI-E) devices cycle positive (insufflation) and negative (exsufflation) pressures to the airway. The rapid pressure swings compensate for both inspiratory and expiratory muscle weakness and help generate airflow shifts that mimic a normal cough [123]. Insufflation and exsufflation pressures, as well as inspiratory and expiratory times, can be individualized to patient comfort as well as to achieve optimal chest rise and secretion clearance. A longer inspiratory time with a shorter expiratory time is most likely to enhance inspiratory volume and expiratory flow [125]. Striegl and colleagues used an infant lung model to assess the effect of various pressure settings on maximum expiratory flow. They found that a more negative exsufflation pressure correlated with improved expiratory flows [126]. There is no consensus regarding optimal settings, however, and each patient should be reassessed frequently to ensure treatments are tolerated and efficacious. Because of the particularly compliant airways of young children, large pressure swings can cause central airway collapse, negating any treatment benefit. Additionally, patients with bulbar dysfunction can also experience upper airway collapse during treatments [127]. Under these circumstances, patients may benefit from lower pressures and/or longer delivery times.

In a small qualitative study, parents and children with NMDs reported that MI-E overall provided a positive impact on their quality of life by enabling them to manage some respiratory illnesses and acute emergencies without leaving home [128]. Given its overall ease of use, MI-E has become first-line therapy in children with NMD [129]. The main limitations of MI-E are its cost, estimated to be around US$4000–$6000 [42], and tolerance of very young children to application of a face mask for its use.

Although there are several retrospective, observational studies demonstrating decreased frequency of hospital admissions for respiratory tract infections, decreased length of stay, and improved patient satisfaction with MI-E use [119, 120, 130, 131], a recent Cochrane review concluded that there is insufficient evidence regarding the safety and efficacy of MAC and MI-E [132]. This conclusion was based on a paucity of randomized controlled trials evaluating the effect of MI-E use on healthcare utilization. These therapies, however, have become standard of care in the management of NMD, and loss of equipoise makes withholding them for research purposes untenable. Furthermore, these treatments are often implemented concurrently with other interventions such as NIV. Therefore, it is difficult to evaluate the isolated effect of cough augmentation.

Mucus Mobilization

While cough augmentation assists in clearing the central airway, secretions in the distal airways are cleared by mucociliary transport. Mucus mobilization techniques have been devised to move secretions proximally, so they can subsequently be cleared by cough. While there is a variety of treatments that can accomplish this goal, several (i.e., positive expiratory pressure [PEP], oscillatory PEP) are not appropriate for children with NMDs, as active participation is required and this population typically cannot generate sufficient expiratory flow for them to be effective [123]. The three main therapies used in children with NMD are chest physiotherapy (CPT), high-frequency chest wall compression (HFCWC), and intrapulmonary percussive ventilation (IPV).

Chest Physiotherapy

When combined with patient positioning to exploit gravitational forces, CPT consists of manual percussion of designated areas of the thorax to promote postural drainage of secretions. Advantages of CPT include its universal availability and its ease of administration in infants due to their small size and ease of positioning. In contrast, CPT is labor-intensive, with treatments lasting 20–30 min (6 areas per lung, 2 min per area). Additionally, CPT may not be feasible in larger patients or patients with scoliosis, as they are more difficult to position, and treatment may not be delivered in the necessary location. There is a lack of evidence regarding the efficacy of prophylactic CPT in children with NMD, but it has been shown to reduce atelectasis following extubation in the inpatient setting [133].

High-Frequency Chest Wall Compressions

This therapy is administered by fitting an inflating vest over the thorax. An air pressure generator rapidly pulses air via tubing to the vest, producing chest compressions at a prescribed frequency, typically between 5 and 15 Hz [123]. High-frequency airflow oscillations create shearing forces at the air-mucus interface and an expiratory flow bias draws the secretions centrally [42]. Treatments are approximately 15 min in duration, and do not require active participation by the patient or the caregiver. Further, the use of a form fitting vest facilitates treatment for children with chest wall deformities. However, HFCWC devices are expensive, with an estimated cost of $13,000 [134]. Infants are also not candidates for their use, as vests are not designed for their size and there is potential for chest wall trauma. Randomized trials are lacking, but observational studies have demonstrated reduced healthcare utilization in children with NMDs following implementation of HFCWC therapy. Fitzgerald et al. retrospectively analyzed 22 children with a variety of NMDs (mean age 9 years), most of whom had cerebral palsy [135]. They found that 45% of children required hospital admission in the 2 years prior to initiation of HFCWC therapy, whereas only 13% did at 2 years' follow-up ($p = 0.002$). Lechtzin et al. reviewed a much larger cohort of 426 patients, 43.9% of whom were aged 0–18 years, and reported a 20.2% reduction in hospital admissions and an 18.1% reduction in diagnosis of pneumonia in the 6 months following the initiation of HFCWC therapy compared to the 6 months prior [136]. While a diagnosis of NMD historically did not qualify a patient to receive reimbursement for HFCWC therapy, insurance policies have recently extended the qualifying criteria to include patients with NMDs who have failed or are "intolerant" of standard airway clearance therapies (i.e., chest physiotherapy) [137].

Intrapulmonary Percussive Ventilation

Intrapulmonary percussive ventilation consists of intermittent bursts of positive pressure (10–40 cm H_2O) at a frequency of 1–10 Hz, delivered by a pneumatic device via a mouthpiece, face mask, or artificial airway [42, 123]. The low-amplitude, high-frequency bursts create internal percussions of the airways, loosening secretions and aiding in lung recruitment. As with HFCWC, inspiratory time is lengthened to create an expiratory flow bias, ensuring that secretions move centrally. The oscillatory vibrations are superimposed on the patient's spontaneous or assisted breathing. The technique also allows for simultaneous delivery of inhaled medications such as bronchodilators or mucolytics. However, cost and access to care remain significant barriers to widespread implementation. Studies regarding pediatric use of IPV in the ambulatory setting are limited. Bidiwala et al. retrospectively compared healthcare utilization in eight tracheostomy-dependent children with NMD, half of whom used IPV while the other half used HFCWC for airway clearance [138]. They found a significant reduction in hospital admissions, length of stay, antibiotic use, and bronchodilator use in the cohort utilizing IPV. More commonly, IPV is utilized in the inpatient setting, where it has reduced atelectasis and decreased length of stay during acute respiratory illnesses [139].

In sum, the optimal clearance regimen would include a method of mucus mobilization for peripheral airway clearance, followed by cough augmentation to remove mobilized secretions from the central airways. However, it is often challenging to procure one, yet alone two, airway clearance devices approved by insurance companies. Newer MI-E devices have an optional oscillation feature, superimposing high-frequency pressure shifts on the prescribed insufflation and exsufflation pressures, mimicking IPV [140]. While this is promising and potentially alleviates the necessity for multiple devices, there have yet to be any studies demonstrating its efficacy [140].

Ventilatory Assistance

The goals of ventilatory assistance for children with NMD include reversal of hypercapnia, offloading respiratory muscle work, relief of dyspnea, correction of SDB, improvement of daytime functioning, aiding growth and development, and ultimately, prolonging survival. Noninvasive ventilation improves quality of life [59, 141]. Several studies have also demonstrated the beneficial effect of ventilatory support on life expectancy in children with NMD. A study of 835 patients with DMD, placed in cohorts by birth decade (1960–2006), demonstrated improved survival over the period of observation, attributed to increased availability and use of ventilator support [142]. In that cohort, mean life expectancy of young men without ventilator assistance was 17.7 years, but it improved to 27.9 years for those who used chronic ventilator support [142]. Similarly, a birth cohort study involving 143 infants with SMA1 born between 1980 and 2006 demonstrated that life expectancy increased from 7.5 months in those born prior to 1994 to 24.0 months in children born in 1995 or later, following the widespread implementation of NIV in that patient population [143].

Noninvasive Ventilation

Children with NMD who require ventilatory assistance for chronic respiratory failure usually begin with noninvasive support. While a small number of children use a cuirass or chest shell to receive negative pressure ventilation, most are supported by noninvasive positive pressure ventilation via a nasal, oronasal, or full-face mask interface. In most instances, children with NMD who require ventilatory assistance also benefit from offloading inspiratory muscle demands with positive pressure breaths, so continuous positive airway pressure (CPAP) alone is not recommended [78, 79]. Clinicians should adjust the difference in inspiratory (IPAP) and expiratory (EPAP) pressures to target a size-appropriate tidal volume (8–10 mL/kg). This can typically be achieved using relatively low pressures given the greater compliance of the pediatric chest wall, although the presence of chest wall abnormalities or advanced disease will necessitate higher settings. Children may not be able to generate sufficient inspiratory muscle force to trigger some ventilators and small children can also have difficulty cycling pressure-supported breaths, leading to both trigger and cycle asynchronies [144]. The difficulty is magnified when large leaks between the interface and face exist. Therefore, use of a backup rate close to the child's physiologic rate or a mode of ventilation that provides a fixed inspiratory time can limit energy expenditure from spontaneous respirations while also enhancing patient comfort and tolerance [11].

There are also challenges and special considerations regarding the implementation of NIV in the pediatric population. Fitting a child with an appropriately sized headgear and interface is critical to maximize patient comfort and minimize leak. However, for small infants, well-fitting headgear and masks often do not exist, and creative modifications are sometimes necessary [145]. Additionally, interfaces that cover the mouth should be used with caution, as young children or those with advanced muscular weakness who are unable to remove the mask in the event of emesis or increased oral secretions will be at increased risk of asphyxiation [145]. Of note, the pressure applied to a child's midface from chronic NIV use can compromise midface growth and development. Consequently, midface flattening and maxillary retrusion have been reported in up to two-thirds of children with chronic NIV use [146]. This can result in further upper airway obstruction, potentially necessitating facial reconstruction surgery.

Diurnal Ventilatory Support

As respiratory muscle failure progresses, patients with NMD will require diurnal respiratory assistance. This can be achieved noninvasively using mouthpiece ventilation during the day, and nasal ventilation during sleep. A mouthpiece is placed within easy reach of the child's mouth and delivers positive pressure on demand. Newer ventilators with dedicated mouthpiece ventilation settings require only a light touch on the mouthpiece to trigger a breath. While this modality is commonly used in teenaged patients, it is often difficult to implement in younger children who may not grasp the concept, or in children with advanced bulbar weakness, as they may not be able to form a proper seal around the mouthpiece [147]. Nasal ventilation, using varying and preferably less intrusive interfaces, is another noninvasive option for delivering daytime ventilatory support. For example, NIV delivered through nasal prongs was shown to treat hypercarbia and reduce dyspnea effectively in a cohort of 19 pediatric patients, including patients with progressive NMDs [148].

Tracheostomy

As progressive respiratory muscle weakness leads to a requirement for continuous ventilatory support, discussions should be held with the patient and family regarding tracheostomy placement. Long-term survival was shown to be equivalent in DMD and SMA patients whether they received daytime ventilation invasively or noninvasively [149, 150]. Therefore, patient and family preferences must be considered when making this decision. Some patients may regard tracheostomy to be preferable, as it relieves the face from what they perceive to be bulky and uncomfortable mask interfaces. However, others may be dissuaded by the increasing complexity of care and predisposition to infection associated with tracheostomy [150]. Factors favoring tracheostomy placement include an inability to provide adequate ventilation noninvasively, bulbar involvement with pharyngeal collapse, or an inability of the child to control secretions. In contrast, if the child is well supported noninvasively, there is no imperative to advance to tracheostomy placement over time.

Ancillary Treatments in Neuromuscular Disorders

Sialorrhea Management

Sialorrhea and the inability to manage oral secretions can lead to aspiration of saliva and the development of aspiration pneumonia. Pharmacologic or surgical approaches can be used to reduce the production of saliva to minimize this risk. Anticholinergic medications act as anti-sialagogues by blocking parasympathetic innervation of the salivary glands. Glycopyrrolate is the only FDA approved anticholinergic medication for the management of sialorrhea in children, but transdermal scopolamine, sublingual atropine, benztropine, and trihexyphenidyl have also been studied [151]. While they have all been shown subjectively to reduce drooling [151], there are no published data regarding their impact on frequency of respiratory infections or long-term pulmonary outcomes. Further, these medications can lead to undesirable side effects like constipation, urinary retention, visual disturbance, behavioral changes, and thickening of respiratory secretions. They should be used with caution in select patients for whom benefits outweigh risks, and when other modes of secretion control are not available.

Injection of botulinum toxin A (BT-A) into the salivary glands recently gained FDA approval for the treatment of sialorrhea in children and is an alternative to anticholinergic therapy. It directly targets the source of oral secretions, potentially minimizing systemic side effects. Small, retrospective studies in adults have demonstrated the safety and efficacy of salivary BT-A injection in reducing drooling in patients with a variety of progressive NMDs [152]. However, the use of BT-A in children has mostly been studied in those with static neurologic diseases (i.e., cerebral palsy). Among 22 children with severe neurologic dysfunction, parotid and submandibular gland BT-A injections decreased the quantity of saliva over 24 h, from 510.62 to 101.25 mL ($p = 0.001$), and were associated with a decrease in hospital admissions for respiratory illnesses to 6.54/year in the year following treatment compared to 8.09/year in the year prior ($p = 0.017$) [153]. A case series of BT-A use in four children with SMA1 reported that all demonstrated improvement in drooling frequency without adverse events [154]. The drug must be administered with caution, as there has also been a case report of systemic intoxication leading to severe hypotonia, profound dysphagia, and impaired airway clearance in a 17-month-old child with SMA1 [155].

For patients with refractory sialorrhea despite conservative treatment, several surgical interventions are available. These include salivary duct ligation, submandibular duct rerouting with or without sublingual gland excision, and submandibular gland excision with or without parotid duct ligation or rerouting [156]. While success of these procedures is generally good, potential complications include recurrence of drooling, xerostomia, altered dental health, and mucous plugging in patients with tracheostomies [156].

Dysphagia Management

Swallowing dysfunction leading to aspiration "from above" or severe gastroesophageal reflux leading to aspiration "from below" can result in aspiration pneumonia, development of parenchymal lung disease, and bronchiectasis [157]. Thus, an integral part of routine multidisciplinary care should include evaluation by a nutritionist, speech-language pathologist, and gastroenterologist in this patient population [4, 9, 158].

Children with central nervous system injury like cerebral palsy can develop dysphagia because of poorly coordinated swallowing function and are at risk for aspiration of liquids. In contrast, those with neuromuscular weakness have intact swallowing reflexes but progressive weakness of oropharyngeal musculature, placing them at greater risk for aspiration of solids [159]. For the former, thickening of liquids or shifting from liquid to purees or solid oral intake represents an initial intervention. For those with neuromuscular weakness, however, the mealtime modifications would include cutting food into smaller pieces, smaller but more frequent meals, or adjusting the consistency of feeds toward a soft or pureed diet. Should concern or evidence of aspiration persist, however, enteral feeding by nasogastric tube or gastrostomy placement should be considered. Among 72 children with SMA2, 15% used an NG tube and 33% had undergone gastrostomy tube placement with or without fundoplication [160]. In that group, body mass index improved in 84% of patients after enteral tube feeding initiation and parental reports of recurrent chest infections decreased by 80% [160]. In patients with severe gastroesophageal reflux, fundoplication should be considered to minimize soiling of the pulmonary parenchyma.

Management of Chest Wall Deformities

Prevention or correction of chest wall deformities can lessen chest wall restriction. Pectus excavatum can arise if respiratory muscle insufficiency occurs in infancy and young childhood when the chest wall is highly compliant, especially in those children with thoracoabdominal paradox [53]. In this setting, application of positive pressure during assisted ventilation and with mechanical insufflation can reverse the deformation [53, 161]. Among 13 infants with SMA1 treated with NIV (mean age at presentation, 7.5 months; mean age at NIV initiation, 11 months), none who had a normal chest wall at the onset of positive pressure ventilation developed a pectus excavatum, while a 12-month old with a pectus excavatum deformity at the time of presentation demonstrated resolution of the deformity 6 months after NIV initiation [161].

Scoliosis develops in the majority of patients with DMD and SMA, although the age of onset differs between the two [55]. Severe scoliosis distorts chest wall shape and limits thoracic expansion, resulting in a decreased VC and impaired airway clearance [162]. Minimally invasive interventions include bracing and serial casting, which can slow the progression of scoliosis and delay the need for surgical intervention by several years [163]. These approaches, however, have the potential to limit chest wall expansion, resulting in reduced tidal volume and VC, increased respiratory rate, and acceleration in the rate of advancement of scoliosis [55, 164]. Spinal fusion is the definitive treatment to arrest progression of scoliosis, but scoliosis in some NMDs begins well before puberty. Spinal fusion before a child attains adult height would have the deleterious effect of limiting thoracic (and therefore lung) growth. To address this problem, other newer surgical options have been developed to stabilize the chest wall but still allow for growth. These include placement of growth, telescoping, and titanium expandable rods, which can be lengthened as the child grows to allow for continued vertical thoracic growth [55]. This approach is used as a bridge until the child completes linear growth and then can undergo spinal fusion. Correction of scoliosis does not lead to improved lung function [68, 165–167] or reduction in frequency of pulmonary infections [168]. But it can arrest or slow the decline in lung function and lessen pelvic obliquity so that it is more comfortable for a patient to sit [55]. The decision to proceed with surgical treatment of scoliosis should be based on patient preference, comfort, and quality of life [68].

Novel Therapeutics

There have been tremendous pharmacotherapeutic advances over the past decade that can alter the natural history of children born with genetic NMDs. Thanks to disease-modifying therapies and newborn screening, children with SMA are now surviving what was once the most common genetic cause of infant death [169]. The first disease-modifying therapy to become approved for the treatment of SMA was nusinersen (Spinraza), in 2016. Nusinersen, an antisense oligonucleotide administered intrathecally, functions by modulating the splicing of survival motor neuron 2 (SMN2) mRNA to increase the production of full length, functional SMN protein [170]. The initial phase 3 trial (ENDEAR) included 121 symptomatic infants with SMA1 randomized 2: 1 to receive nusinersen or sham control (mean age at first dose, 161 days) [170]. Death or need for permanent ($\geq$ 16 h/day) assisted ventilation occurred in 68% of controls compared to only 39% in the treatment group at 1-year follow-up. Subanalyses of the ENDEAR trial suggested that early treatment is critical for improved outcomes. In a phase 2 open label multicenter study of nusinersen in 25 presymptomatic infants with SMA1 and SMA2 (NURTURE trial; mean age at first dose, 22 days), all children were alive and did not require permanent ventilatory support at 2-year follow-up [171]. In contrast, death or need for continuous ventilation would have been expected by 13.5 months in treatment-naïve historical controls [171].

Risdiplam (Evrysdi), FDA approved in 2020, is a daily oral medication with similar mechanism of action to nusinersen. Data from the largest ongoing open-label trial of risdiplam (FIREFISH) involving 41 infants with SMA1 (mean age at enrollment, 5.3 months) after 24 months of treatment showed that 80% of children were receiving chronic ventilatory assistance at the time of follow-up, although only 10% required permanent ventilation [172]. Additionally, only three patients (7%) had died.

Onasemnogene abeparvovec (Zolgensma) is a one-time intravenous infusion of the SMN1 gene delivered by a recombinant adeno-associated viral vector. It was FDA-approved in 2019 and is the only treatment providing replacement of the previously nonexistent SMN1. The SMN1 gene incorporates into the nucleus of motor neurons, where transcription and translation into functional SMN protein can occur. The initial trial included symptomatic patients with SMA1 (START trial; mean age at first dose = 3 months), with all 15 patients still alive and without permanent ventilator support at 2-year follow-up [173]. Five years following treatment, all patients who received treatment dosing were still alive, with no progression of their respiratory support needs [173]. Furthermore, 60% did not require any mechanical ventilatory support, while 40% utilized NIV overnight, which had constituted their baseline support prior to treatment [173].

There have also been remarkable advancements in the treatment of DMD. Corticosteroids were the first pharmacologic therapy to change the natural progression of the disease [92], and they have become standard of care in DMD management. Treatment with prednisone or deflazacort delays the loss of ambulation, improves pulmonary function, reduces the need for mechanical ventilation and prolongs survival [174, 175]. Adverse effects of chronic steroids include weight gain, behavior changes, bone demineralization, and glucose intolerance.

Gene editing via exon skipping agents can modestly increase the expression of functional dystrophin. Antisense oligonucleotides locate and excise a problematic exon where a mutation previously resulted in a truncated or nonfunctional protein [176]. To date, four drugs directed at mutations in specific exons have been approved: these include eteplirsen (exon 51), casimerson (exon 45), golodirsen (exon 53), and viltolarsen (exon 53). Eteplirsen was the first to gain FDA approval in 2016, and has been shown to improve the 6-min walk test and attenuate the annual rate of decline in FVC, from 6% to 2–4% [177]. Long-term pulmonary outcomes using the newer agents have not been widely reported, but since they all result in a similar increase in dystrophin expression (1–6%) [176], outcomes are expected to be comparable. Unfortunately, only about 30% of DMD patients are currently eligible for treatment with these drugs based on their mutations [176]. Gene transfer therapy would potentially allow for the delivery of a functional dystrophin gene, but that approach has its challenges. The dystrophin gene is the largest gene in the human genome. Therefore, it has been difficult to find a vector that can accommodate a gene of this size [178]. Instead, alternative approaches to gene therapy, including microdystrophin gene transfer using adeno-associated vectors, as well as genome editing utilizing CRISPR-Cas technology, are currently under investigation [179].

Breakthrough scientific advancements have not been isolated to SMA and DMD, as novel therapeutics have been developed for rarer NMDs as well. Fortnightly enzyme replacement therapy with alglucosidase alfa in infantile onset Pompe disease led to a 79% reduction in death and 58% reduction in risk for need of invasive ventilation at 2-year follow-up (mean age at first dose, 15.7 months) [180]. In patients with X-linked myotubular myopathy (XLMTM), initial studies of gene transfer therapy utilizing an adeno-associated vector showed initial promise [181]. Patients were ventilator-dependent prior to the start of the trial, and all seven were able to achieve ventilator independence following treatment. However, four of these children subsequently died from fatal hepatic dysfunction and sepsis [181]. While it is uncertain if these deaths were secondary to the underlying disease process or adverse effects from treatment, the trial has been suspended pending further investigation.

Although preliminary data for most of these disease-modifying therapies have been encouraging, the deaths in the XLMTM study serve as a cautionary tale. These therapies have only been available for a short time, and longer periods of observation will be required to understand fully their long-term benefits on pulmonary function, morbidity, and survival, as well as potential adverse treatment effects. In addition, novel therapeutics are expensive and may not be available in resource-limited settings, introducing a source of healthcare disparities. Finally, while they offer hope of attenuating the typical decline in motor and respiratory function seen in NMDs, no treatment to date has provided a definitive cure. Until that occurs, respiratory specialists must continue to play an active role in the multidisciplinary care of these patients, with an emphasis on optimizing airway clearance and ventilation, to reduce pulmonary-related morbidity and mortality.

Transitioning to Adult Care

The interventions mentioned in this chapter and improvements in care of children with NMDs have allowed many to live well into adulthood. Improved survival of children with NMDs has highlighted the need for specialized programs staffed by practitioners of adult medicine and organized and careful transitional care from pediatric programs to ensure continuity of care and patient safety [182]. One of the unique challenges in the NMD population is that as adolescent patients are expected to assume more autonomy and self-direction, their disease processes rob them of the physical ability to do that and make them even more dependent on caregivers. Identified barriers to transition to adult care include a relative dearth of adult providers familiar with diseases that formerly were within the purview of pediatric practitioners, changes in health insurance between pediatric and adult healthcare systems, absence of formal transition preparation, and patient and family insecurity with a new healthcare system [183]. These obstacles are surmountable, but require effort and special attention of both pediatric and internal medicine providers.

Summary

Processes that lead to morbidity and mortality in children with NMD are similar to those seen in adults. Maturational changes in the respiratory system, however, can augment the effects of NMD in younger children, predisposing them to chronic respiratory failure. As in adults, the mainstays of therapy in childhood NMDs include assistance with airway clearance and ventilation, but assessments for timing of those interventions may be hampered by inability of the child to cooperate, or lack of age-appropriate normative and threshold data upon which to make decisions. Thus, caregivers must have a high index of suspicion for respiratory compromise based on the natural history of the particular NMD coupled with a few tests that broadly point to increased risk. Novel therapies can modulate the course of some NMDs and represent new challenges in anticipating the respiratory needs of children who receive them. Nevertheless, survival has improved for children with NMD over the last several decades, necessitating strategies for the careful transitioning of their medical care to adult programs.

References

1. Borrelli M, Terrone G, Evangelisti R, Fedele F, Corcione A, Santamaria F. Respiratory phenotypes of neuromuscular diseases: a challenging issue for pediatricians. Pediatr Neonatol. 2023;64(2):109–18. https://doi.org/10.1016/j.pedneo.2022.09.016.
2. Perrin C, Unterborn JN, Ambrosio CD, Hill NS. Pulmonary complications of chronic neuromuscular diseases and their management. Muscle Nerve. 2004;29(1):5–27. https://doi.org/10.1002/mus.10487.
3. Leon-Astudillo C, Okorie CUA, McCown MY, Dy FJ, Puranik S, Prero M, et al. ATS Core Curriculum 2022. Pediatric pulmonary medicine: updates in pediatric neuromuscular disease. Pediatr Pulmonol. 2023;58(7):1866–74. https://doi.org/10.1002/ppul.26448.
4. Birnkrant DJ, Bushby K, Bann CM, Apkon SD, Blackwell A, Brumbaugh D, et al. Diagnosis and management of Duchenne muscular dystrophy, part 1: diagnosis, and neuromuscular, rehabilitation, endocrine, and gastrointestinal and nutritional management. Lancet Neurol. 2018;17(3):251–67. https://doi.org/10.1016/S1474-4422(18)30024-3.
5. Blake DJ, Weir A, Newey SE, Davies KE. Function and genetics of dystrophin and dystrophin-related proteins in muscle. Physiol Rev. 2002;82(2):291–329. https://doi.org/10.1152/physrev.00028.2001.
6. Duan D, Goemans N, Takeda S, Mercuri E, Aartsma-Rus A. Duchenne muscular dystrophy. Nat Rev Dis Primers. 2021;7(1):13. https://doi.org/10.1038/s41572-021-00248-3.
7. Barnard AM, Lott DJ, Batra A, Triplett WT, Forbes SC, Riehl SL, et al. Imaging respiratory muscle quality and function in Duchenne muscular dystrophy. J Neurol. 2019;266(11):2752–63. https://doi.org/10.1007/s00415-019-09481-z.
8. Suresh S, Wales P, Dakin C, Harris MA, Cooper DG. Sleep-related breathing disorder in Duchenne muscular dystrophy: disease spectrum in the paediatric population. J Paediatr Child Health. 2005;41(9–10):500–3. https://doi.org/10.1111/j.1440-1754.2005.00691.x.
9. Mercuri E, Finkel RS, Muntoni F, Wirth B, Montes J, Main M, et al. Diagnosis and management of spinal muscular atrophy: part 1: recommendations for diagnosis, rehabilitation, orthopedic and nutritional care. Neuromuscul Disord. 2018;28(2):103–15. https://doi.org/10.1016/j.nmd.2017.11.005.
10. Schroth MK. Special considerations in the respiratory management of spinal muscular atrophy. Pediatrics. 2009;123(Suppl 4):S245–9. https://doi.org/10.1542/peds.2008-2952K.
11. Fauroux B, Griffon L, Amaddeo A, Stremler N, Mazenq J, Khirani S, et al. Respiratory management of children with spinal muscular atrophy (SMA). Arch Pediatr. 2020;27(7S):7S29–34. https://doi.org/10.1016/S0929-693X(20)30274-8.
12. Kang PB, Morrison L, Iannaccone ST, Graham RJ, Bonnemann CG, Rutkowski A, et al. Evidence-based guideline summary: evaluation, diagnosis, and management of congenital muscular dystrophy: report of the guideline development subcommittee of the American Academy of Neurology and the practice issues review panel of the American Association of Neuromuscular & Electrodiagnostic Medicine. Neurology. 2015;84(13):1369–78. https://doi.org/10.1212/WNL.0000000000001416.
13. Fauroux B, Amaddeo A, Quijano-Roy S, Barnerias C, Desguerre I, Khirani S. Respiratory insight to congenital muscular dystrophies and congenital myopathies and its relation to clinical trial. Neuromuscul Disord. 2018;28(9):731–40. https://doi.org/10.1016/j.nmd.2018.06.013.
14. Shahrizaila N, Kinnear WJ, Wills AJ. Respiratory involvement in inherited primary muscle conditions. J Neurol Neurosurg Psychiatry. 2006;77(10):1108–15. https://doi.org/10.1136/jnnp.2005.078881.
15. Ho G, Widger J, Cardamone M, Farrar MA. Quality of life and excessive daytime sleepiness in children and adolescents with myotonic dystrophy type 1. Sleep Med. 2017;32:92–6. https://doi.org/10.1016/j.sleep.2016.12.005.
16. Jain A, Al Khalili Y. Congenital myotonic dystrophy. Treasure Island, FL: StatPearls; 2023.

17. Turner C, Hilton-Jones D. Myotonic dystrophy: diagnosis, management and new therapies. Curr Opin Neurol. 2014;27(5):599–606. https://doi.org/10.1097/WCO.0000000000000128.
18. Lagrue E, Dogan C, De Antonio M, Audic F, Bach N, Barnerias C, et al. A large multicenter study of pediatric myotonic dystrophy type 1 for evidence-based management. Neurology. 2019;92(8):e852–e65. https://doi.org/10.1212/WNL.0000000000006948.
19. Quera Salva MA, Blumen M, Jacquette A, Durand MC, Andre S, De Villiers M, et al. Sleep disorders in childhood-onset myotonic dystrophy type 1. Neuromuscul Disord. 2006;16(9–10):564–70. https://doi.org/10.1016/j.nmd.2006.06.007.
20. Davidson LT, Evans MC. Congenital and acquired spinal cord injury and dysfunction. Pediatr Clin N Am. 2023;70(3):461–81. https://doi.org/10.1016/j.pcl.2023.01.017.
21. Benmelouka A, Shamseldin LS, Nourelden AZ, Negida A. A review on the etiology and management of pediatric traumatic spinal cord injuries. Adv J Emerg Med. 2020;4(2):e28. https://doi.org/10.22114/ajem.v0i0.256.
22. Brown R, DiMarco AF, Hoit JD, Garshick E. Respiratory dysfunction and management in spinal cord injury. Respir Care. 2006;51(8):853–68;discussion 69–70.
23. Harness J, Pierce J, Malas N. Psychiatric evaluation and management in pediatric spinal cord injuries: a review. Curr Psychiatry Rep. 2021;23(7):40. https://doi.org/10.1007/s11920-021-01256-6.
24. Luscan R, Leboulanger N, Fayoux P, Kerner G, Belhous K, Couloigner V, et al. Developmental changes of upper airway dimensions in children. Paediatr Anaesth. 2020;30(4):435–45. https://doi.org/10.1111/pan.13832.
25. Di Cicco M, Kantar A, Masini B, Nuzzi G, Ragazzo V, Peroni D. Structural and functional development in airways throughout childhood: children are not small adults. Pediatr Pulmonol. 2021;56(1):240–51. https://doi.org/10.1002/ppul.25169.
26. Hogg JC, Williams J, Richardson JB, Macklem PT, Thurlbeck WM. Age as a factor in the distribution of lower-airway conductance and in the pathologic anatomy of obstructive lung disease. N Engl J Med. 1970;282(23):1283–7. https://doi.org/10.1056/NEJM197006042822302.
27. Trachsel D, Erb TO, Hammer J, von Ungern-Sternberg BS. Developmental respiratory physiology. Paediatr Anaesth. 2022;32(2):108–17. https://doi.org/10.1111/pan.14362.
28. Rains JK, Bert JL, Roberts CR, Pare PD. Mechanical properties of human tracheal cartilage. J Appl Physiol (1985). 1992;72(1):219–225. doi: https://doi.org/10.1152/jappl.1992.72.1.219.
29. Safshekan F, Tafazzoli-Shadpour M, Abdouss M, Behgam Shadmehr M, Ghorbani F. Investigation of the mechanical properties of the human tracheal cartilage. Tanaffos. 2017;16(2):107–14.
30. Terry PB, Traystman RJ. The clinical significance of collateral ventilation. Ann Am Thorac Soc. 2016;13(12):2251–7. https://doi.org/10.1513/AnnalsATS.201606-448FR.
31. Rosenberg DE, Lyons HA. Collateral ventilation in excised human lungs. Respiration. 1979;37(3):125–34. https://doi.org/10.1159/000194018.
32. Inners CR, Terry PB, Traystman RJ, Menkes HA. Collateral ventilation and the middle lobe syndrome. Am Rev Respir Dis. 1978;118(2):305–10. https://doi.org/10.1164/arrd.1978.118.2.305.
33. Bastir M, Garcia Martinez D, Recheis W, Barash A, Coquerelle M, Rios L, et al. Differential growth and development of the upper and lower human thorax. PLoS One. 2013;8(9):e75128. https://doi.org/10.1371/journal.pone.0075128.
34. De Troyer A, Kirkwood PA, Wilson TA. Respiratory action of the intercostal muscles. Physiol Rev. 2005;85(2):717–56. https://doi.org/10.1152/physrev.00007.2004.
35. Openshaw P, Edwards S, Helms P. Changes in rib cage geometry during childhood. Thorax. 1984;39(8):624–7. https://doi.org/10.1136/thx.39.8.624.
36. Devlieger H, Daniels H, Marchal G, Moerman P, Casaer P, Eggermont E. The diaphragm of the newborn infant: anatomical and ultrasonographic studies. J Dev Physiol. 1991;16(6):321–9.
37. Greenspan JS, Miller TL, Shaffer TH. The neonatal respiratory pump: a developmental challenge with physiologic limitations. Neonatal Netw. 2005;24(5):15–22. https://doi.org/10.1891/0730-0832.24.5.15.

38. Papastamelos C, Panitch HB, England SE, Allen JL. Developmental changes in chest wall compliance in infancy and early childhood. J Appl Physiol (1985). 1995;78(1):179–84. https://doi.org/10.1152/jappl.1995.78.1.179.
39. Thorsteinsson A, Jonmarker C, Larsson A, Vilstrup C, Werner O. Functional residual capacity in anesthetized children: normal values and values in children with cardiac anomalies. Anesthesiology. 1990;73(5):876–81. https://doi.org/10.1097/00000542-199011000-00014.
40. Colin AA, Wohl ME, Mead J, Ratjen FA, Glass G, Stark AR. Transition from dynamically maintained to relaxed end-expiratory volume in human infants. J Appl Physiol (1985). 1989;67(5):2107–11. https://doi.org/10.1152/jappl.1989.67.5.2107.
41. Keens TG, Bryan AC, Levison H, Ianuzzo CD. Developmental pattern of muscle fiber types in human ventilatory muscles. J Appl Physiol Respir Environ Exerc Physiol. 1978;44(6):909–13. https://doi.org/10.1152/jappl.1978.44.6.909.
42. Panitch HB. Respiratory implications of pediatric neuromuscular disease. Respir Care. 2017;62(6):826–48. https://doi.org/10.4187/respcare.05250.
43. Fink JB. Forced expiratory technique, directed cough, and autogenic drainage. Respir Care. 2007;52(9):1210–21; discussion 21–3.
44. Bustamante-Marin XM, Ostrowski LE. Cilia and mucociliary clearance. Cold Spring Harb Perspect Biol. 2017;9(4):a028241. https://doi.org/10.1101/cshperspect.a028241.
45. Bianchi C, Baiardi P. Cough peak flows: standard values for children and adolescents. Am J Phys Med Rehabil. 2008;87(6):461–7. https://doi.org/10.1097/PHM.0b013e318174e4c7.
46. Bach JR, Ishikawa Y, Kim H. Prevention of pulmonary morbidity for patients with Duchenne muscular dystrophy. Chest. 1997;112(4):1024–8. https://doi.org/10.1378/chest.112.4.1024.
47. Bach JR, Saporito LR. Criteria for extubation and tracheostomy tube removal for patients with ventilatory failure. A different approach to weaning. Chest. 1996;110(6):1566–71. https://doi.org/10.1378/chest.110.6.1566.
48. Britton D, Karam C, Schindler JS. Swallowing and secretion management in neuromuscular disease. Clin Chest Med. 2018;39(2):449–57. https://doi.org/10.1016/j.ccm.2018.01.007.
49. Kooi-van Es M, Erasmus CE, de Swart BJM, Voet NBM, van der Wees PJ, de Groot IJM, et al. Dysphagia and dysarthria in children with neuromuscular diseases, a prevalence study. J Neuromuscul Dis. 2020;7(3):287–95. https://doi.org/10.3233/JND-190436.
50. Cherchi C, Chiarini Testa MB, Deriu D, Schiavino A, Petreschi F, Ullmann N, et al. All you need is evidence: what we know about pneumonia in children with neuromuscular diseases. Front Pediatr. 2021;9:625751. https://doi.org/10.3389/fped.2021.625751.
51. Chacko A, Marshall J, Taylor O, McEniery J, Sly PD, Gauld LM. Dysphagia and lung disease in children with spinal muscular atrophy treated with disease-modifying agents. Neurology. 2023;100(19):914–20. https://doi.org/10.1212/WNL.0000000000206826.
52. Roussos C, Macklem PT. The respiratory muscles. N Engl J Med. 1982;307(13):786–97. https://doi.org/10.1056/nejm198209233071304.
53. Bach JR, Bianchi C. Prevention of pectus excavatum for children with spinal muscular atrophy type 1. Am J Phys Med Rehabil. 2003;82(10):815–9. https://doi.org/10.1097/01.PHM.0000083669.22483.04.
54. Johnson MA, Galagedera N, Ho S, Hilmara D, Campbell RM, Anari JB, et al. Correlation of pulmonary function to novel radiographic parameters of collapsing parasol deformity in spinal muscular atrophy. Orthopedics. 2021;44(2):e287–93. https://doi.org/10.3928/01477447-20201216-05.
55. Mayer OH. Scoliosis and the impact in neuromuscular disease. Paediatr Respir Rev. 2015;16(1):35–42. https://doi.org/10.1016/j.prrv.2014.10.013.
56. Katz SL. Assessment of sleep-disordered breathing in pediatric neuromuscular diseases. Pediatrics. 2009;123(Suppl 4):S222–5. https://doi.org/10.1542/peds.2008-2952E.
57. O'Brien LM. The neurocognitive effects of sleep disruption in children and adolescents. Child Adolesc Psychiatr Clin N Am. 2009;18(4):813–23. https://doi.org/10.1016/j.chc.2009.04.008.

58. Piper A. Sleep abnormalities associated with neuromuscular disease: pathophysiology and evaluation. Semin Respir Crit Care Med. 2002;23(3):211–9. https://doi.org/10.1055/s-2002-33029.
59. Ward S, Chatwin M, Heather S, Simonds AK. Randomised controlled trial of non-invasive ventilation (NIV) for nocturnal hypoventilation in neuromuscular and chest wall disease patients with daytime normocapnia. Thorax. 2005;60(12):1019–24. https://doi.org/10.1136/thx.2004.037424.
60. Vianello A, Bevilacqua M, Salvador V, Cardaioli C, Vincenti E. Long-term nasal intermittent positive pressure ventilation in advanced Duchenne's muscular dystrophy. Chest. 1994;105(2):445–8. https://doi.org/10.1378/chest.105.2.445.
61. Arens R, Muzumdar H. Sleep, sleep disordered breathing, and nocturnal hypoventilation in children with neuromuscular diseases. Paediatr Respir Rev. 2010;11(1):24–30. https://doi.org/10.1016/j.prrv.2009.10.003.
62. Aboussouan LS, Mireles-Cabodevila E. Sleep-disordered breathing in neuromuscular disease: diagnostic and therapeutic challenges. Chest. 2017;152(4):880–92. https://doi.org/10.1016/j.chest.2017.03.023.
63. Sawnani H, Thampratankul L, Szczesniak RD, Fenchel MC, Simakajornboon N. Sleep disordered breathing in young boys with Duchenne muscular dystrophy. J Pediatr. 2015;166(3):640–5 e1. https://doi.org/10.1016/j.jpeds.2014.12.006.
64. Ono S, Takahashi K, Jinnai K, Kanda F, Fukuoka Y, Kurisaki H, et al. Loss of catecholaminergic neurons in the medullary reticular formation in myotonic dystrophy. Neurology. 1998;51(4):1121–4. https://doi.org/10.1212/wnl.51.4.1121.
65. Rocque BG, Maddox MH, Hopson BD, Shamblin IC, Aban I, Arynchyna AA, et al. Prevalence of sleep disordered breathing in children with myelomeningocele. Neurosurgery. 2021;88(4):785–90. https://doi.org/10.1093/neuros/nyaa507.
66. Fauroux B, Khirani S, Griffon L, Teng T, Lanzeray A, Amaddeo A. Non-invasive ventilation in children with neuromuscular disease. Front Pediatr. 2020;8:482. https://doi.org/10.3389/fped.2020.00482.
67. Finder JD, Birnkrant D, Carl J, Farber HJ, Gozal D, Iannaccone ST, et al. Respiratory care of the patient with Duchenne muscular dystrophy: ATS consensus statement. Am J Respir Crit Care Med. 2004;170(4):456–65. https://doi.org/10.1164/rccm.200307-885ST.
68. Hull J, Aniapravan R, Chan E, Chatwin M, Forton J, Gallagher J, et al. British Thoracic Society guideline for respiratory management of children with neuromuscular weakness. Thorax. 2012;67(Suppl 1):i1–40. https://doi.org/10.1136/thoraxjnl-2012-201964.
69. West NA, Yang ML, Weitzenkamp DA, Andrews J, Meaney FJ, Oleszek J, et al. Patterns of growth in ambulatory males with Duchenne muscular dystrophy. J Pediatr. 2013;163(6):1759–63 e1. https://doi.org/10.1016/j.jpeds.2013.08.004.
70. Messina S, Pane M, De Rose P, Vasta I, Sorleti D, Aloysius A, et al. Feeding problems and malnutrition in spinal muscular atrophy type II. Neuromuscul Disord. 2008;18(5):389–93. https://doi.org/10.1016/j.nmd.2008.02.008.
71. Ishikawa Y, Bach JR, Komaroff E, Miura T, Jackson-Parekh R. Cough augmentation in Duchenne muscular dystrophy. Am J Phys Med Rehabil. 2008;87(9):726–30. https://doi.org/10.1097/PHM.0b013e31817f99a8.
72. Szeinberg A, Tabachnik E, Rashed N, McLaughlin FJ, England S, Bryan CA, et al. Cough capacity in patients with muscular dystrophy. Chest. 1988;94(6):1232–5. https://doi.org/10.1378/chest.94.6.1232.
73. Wang CH, Finkel RS, Bertini ES, Schroth M, Simonds A, Wong B, et al. Consensus statement for standard of care in spinal muscular atrophy. J Child Neurol. 2007;22(8):1027–49. https://doi.org/10.1177/0883073807305788.
74. Finkel RS, Weiner DJ, Mayer OH, McDonough JM, Panitch HB. Respiratory muscle function in infants with spinal muscular atrophy type I. Pediatr Pulmonol. 2014;49(12):1234–42. https://doi.org/10.1002/ppul.22997.

75. Shardonofsky FR, Perez-Chada D, Milic-Emili J. Airway pressures during crying: an index of respiratory muscle strength in infants with neuromuscular disease. Pediatr Pulmonol. 1991;10(3):172–7. https://doi.org/10.1002/ppul.1950100307.
76. Miller K, Mayer OH. Pulmonary function testing in patients with neuromuscular disease. Pediatr Pulmonol. 2021;56(4):693–9. https://doi.org/10.1002/ppul.25182.
77. Fauroux B, Quijano-Roy S, Desguerre I, Khirani S. The value of respiratory muscle testing in children with neuromuscular disease. Chest. 2015;147(2):552–9. https://doi.org/10.1378/chest.14-0819.
78. Finkel RS, Mercuri E, Meyer OH, Simonds AK, Schroth MK, Graham RJ, et al. Diagnosis and management of spinal muscular atrophy: part 2: pulmonary and acute care; medications, supplements and immunizations; other organ systems; and ethics. Neuromuscul Disord. 2018;28(3):197–207. https://doi.org/10.1016/j.nmd.2017.11.004.
79. Birnkrant DJ, Bushby K, Bann CM, Alman BA, Apkon SD, Blackwell A, et al. Diagnosis and management of Duchenne muscular dystrophy, part 2: respiratory, cardiac, bone health, and orthopaedic management. Lancet Neurol. 2018;17(4):347–61. https://doi.org/10.1016/S1474-4422(18)30025-5.
80. Diaz CE, Deoras KS, Allen JL. Chest wall motion before and during mechanical ventilation in children with neuromuscular disease. Pediatr Pulmonol. 1993;16(2):89–95. https://doi.org/10.1002/ppul.1950160203.
81. Lissoni A, Aliverti A, Tzeng AC, Bach JR. Kinematic analysis of patients with spinal muscular atrophy during spontaneous breathing and mechanical ventilation. Am J Phys Med Rehabil. 1998;77(3):188–92. https://doi.org/10.1097/00002060-199805000-00002.
82. Won YH, Choi WA, Lee JW, Bach JR, Park J, Kang SW. Sleep transcutaneous vs. end-tidal CO_2 monitoring for patients with neuromuscular disease. Am J Phys Med Rehabil. 2016;95(2):91–5. https://doi.org/10.1097/PHM.0000000000000345.
83. Khan A, Frazer-Green L, Amin R, Wolfe L, Faulkner G, Casey K, et al. Respiratory management of patients with neuromuscular weakness: an American College of Chest Physicians clinical practice guideline and expert panel report. Chest. 2023;164(2):394–413. https://doi.org/10.1016/j.chest.2023.03.011.
84. Ayhan Y, Yuksel Karatoprak E, Onay ZR, Can Oksay S, Girit S. Assessment of nocturnal hypoventilation by different methods and definitions in children with neuromuscular disease: oxycapnography and blood gas analysis. Medeni Med J. 2021;36(2):106–16. https://doi.org/10.5222/MMJ.2021.42385.
85. Shi J, Chiang J, Ambreen M, Snow N, Mocanu C, McAdam L, et al. Ambulatory transcutaneous carbon dioxide monitoring for children with neuromuscular disease. Sleep Med. 2023;101:221–7. https://doi.org/10.1016/j.sleep.2022.10.028.
86. Orlikowski D, Prigent H, Ambrosi X, Vaugier I, Pottier S, Annane D, et al. Comparison of ventilator-integrated end-tidal CO_2 and transcutaneous CO_2 monitoring in home-ventilated neuromuscular patients. Respir Med. 2016;117:7–13. https://doi.org/10.1016/j.rmed.2016.05.022.
87. Trucco F, Pedemonte M, Fiorillo C, Tan HL, Carlucci A, Brisca G, et al. Detection of early nocturnal hypoventilation in neuromuscular disorders. J Int Med Res. 2018;46(3):1153–61. https://doi.org/10.1177/0300060517728857.
88. Katz SL, Witmans M, Barrowman N, Hoey L, Su S, Reddy D, et al. Paediatric sleep resources in Canada: the scope of the problem. Paediatr Child Health. 2014;19(7):367–72. https://doi.org/10.1093/pch/19.7.367.
89. Hurvitz MS, Sunkonkit K, Massicotte C, Li R, Bhattacharjee R, Amin R. Characterization of sleep-disordered breathing in children with Duchenne muscular dystrophy by the American Academy of Sleep Medicine criteria vs disease-specific criteria: what are the differences? J Clin Sleep Med. 2022;18(2):609–16. https://doi.org/10.5664/jcsm.9678.
90. Kaditis AG, Polytarchou A, Moudaki A, Panaghiotopoulou-Gartagani P, Kanaka-Gantenbein C. Measures of nocturnal oxyhemoglobin desaturation in children with neuromuscular

disease or Prader-Willi syndrome. Pediatr Pulmonol. 2020;55(8):2089–96. https://doi.org/10.1002/ppul.24899.

91. Paiva R, Krivec U, Aubertin G, Cohen E, Clement A, Fauroux B. Carbon dioxide monitoring during long-term noninvasive respiratory support in children. Intensive Care Med. 2009;35(6):1068–74. https://doi.org/10.1007/s00134-009-1408-5.

92. McDonald CM, Gordish-Dressman H, Henricson EK, Duong T, Joyce NC, Jhawar S, et al. Longitudinal pulmonary function testing outcome measures in Duchenne muscular dystrophy: long-term natural history with and without glucocorticoids. Neuromuscul Disord. 2018;28(11):897–909. https://doi.org/10.1016/j.nmd.2018.07.004.

93. Meier T, Rummey C, Leinonen M, Spagnolo P, Mayer OH, Buyse GM, et al. Characterization of pulmonary function in 10-18 year old patients with Duchenne muscular dystrophy. Neuromuscul Disord. 2017;27(4):307–14. https://doi.org/10.1016/j.nmd.2016.12.014.

94. Rafferty GF, Leech S, Knight L, Moxham J, Greenough A. Sniff nasal inspiratory pressure in children. Pediatr Pulmonol. 2000;29(6):468–75. https://doi.org/10.1002/(sici)1099-0496(200006)29:6<468::aid-ppul9>3.0.co;2-2.

95. Chiang J, Mehta K, Amin R. Respiratory diagnostic tools in neuromuscular disease. Children (Basel). 2018;5(6):78. https://doi.org/10.3390/children5060078.

96. Ramonatxo M, Boulard P, Prefaut C. Validation of a noninvasive tension-time index of inspiratory muscles. J Appl Physiol (1985). 1995;78(2):646–53. https://doi.org/10.1152/jappl.1995.78.2.646.

97. Mulreany LT, Weiner DJ, McDonough JM, Panitch HB, Allen JL. Noninvasive measurement of the tension-time index in children with neuromuscular disease. J Appl Physiol (1985). 2003;95(3):931–7. https://doi.org/10.1152/japplphysiol.01087.2002.

98. Koechlin C, Matecki S, Jaber S, Soulier N, Prefaut C, Ramonatxo M. Changes in respiratory muscle endurance during puberty. Pediatr Pulmonol. 2005;40(3):197–204. https://doi.org/10.1002/ppul.20271.

99. Khirani S, Ramirez A, Aubertin G, Boule M, Chemouny C, Forin V, et al. Respiratory muscle decline in Duchenne muscular dystrophy. Pediatr Pulmonol. 2014;49(5):473–81. https://doi.org/10.1002/ppul.22847.

100. Mellies U, Stehling F, Dohna-Schwake C. Normal values for inspiratory muscle function in children. Physiol Meas. 2014;35(10):1975–81. https://doi.org/10.1088/0967-3334/35/10/1975.

101. Dohna-Schwake C, Ragette R, Teschler H, Voit T, Mellies U. Predictors of severe chest infections in pediatric neuromuscular disorders. Neuromuscul Disord. 2006;16(5):325–8. https://doi.org/10.1016/j.nmd.2006.02.003.

102. Mellies U, Ragette R, Schwake C, Boehm H, Voit T, Teschler H. Daytime predictors of sleep disordered breathing in children and adolescents with neuromuscular disorders. Neuromuscul Disord. 2003;13(2):123–8. https://doi.org/10.1016/s0960-8966(02)00219-5.

103. Foley AR, Quijano-Roy S, Collins J, Straub V, McCallum M, Deconinck N, et al. Natural history of pulmonary function in collagen VI-related myopathies. Brain. 2013;136(Pt 12):3625–33. https://doi.org/10.1093/brain/awt284.

104. Khirani S, Colella M, Caldarelli V, Aubertin G, Boule M, Forin V, et al. Longitudinal course of lung function and respiratory muscle strength in spinal muscular atrophy type 2 and 3. Eur J Paediatr Neurol. 2013;17(6):552–60. https://doi.org/10.1016/j.ejpn.2013.04.004.

105. Fromageot C, Lofaso F, Annane D, Falaize L, Lejaille M, Clair B, et al. Supine fall in lung volumes in the assessment of diaphragmatic weakness in neuromuscular disorders. Arch Phys Med Rehabil. 2001;82(1):123–8. https://doi.org/10.1053/apmr.2001.18053.

106. Phillips MF, Quinlivan RC, Edwards RH, Calverley PM. Changes in spirometry over time as a prognostic marker in patients with Duchenne muscular dystrophy. Am J Respir Crit Care Med. 2001;164(12):2191–4. https://doi.org/10.1164/ajrccm.164.12.2103052.

107. Toussaint M, Boitano LJ, Gathot V, Steens M, Soudon P. Limits of effective cough-augmentation techniques in patients with neuromuscular disease. Respir Care. 2009;54(3):359–66.

108. Khan Y, Heckmatt JZ. Obstructive apnoeas in Duchenne muscular dystrophy. Thorax. 1994;49(2):157–61. https://doi.org/10.1136/thx.49.2.157.
109. Katzberg HD, Vajsar J, Vezina K, Qashqari H, Selvadurai S, Chrestian N, et al. Respiratory dysfunction and sleep-disordered breathing in children with myasthenia gravis. J Child Neurol. 2020;35(9):600–6. https://doi.org/10.1177/0883073820924213.
110. Pinard JM, Azabou E, Essid N, Quijano-Roy S, Haddad S, Cheliout-Heraut F. Sleep-disordered breathing in children with congenital muscular dystrophies. Eur J Paediatr Neurol. 2012;16(6):619–24. https://doi.org/10.1016/j.ejpn.2012.02.009.
111. Frohlich M, Widger J, Thambipillay G, Teng A, Farrar M, Chuang S. Daytime predictors of nocturnal hypercapnic hypoventilation in children with neuromuscular disorders. Pediatr Pulmonol. 2022;57(6):1497–504. https://doi.org/10.1002/ppul.25890.
112. Katz SL, Gaboury I, Keilty K, Banwell B, Vajsar J, Anderson P, et al. Nocturnal hypoventilation: predictors and outcomes in childhood progressive neuromuscular disease. Arch Dis Child. 2010;95(12):998–1003. https://doi.org/10.1136/adc.2010.182709.
113. Zambon AA, Trucco F, Laverty A, Riley M, Ridout D, Manzur AY, et al. Respiratory function and sleep disordered breathing in pediatric Duchenne muscular dystrophy. Neurology. 2022;99(12):e1216–26. https://doi.org/10.1212/WNL.0000000000200932.
114. Sheehan DW, Birnkrant DJ, Benditt JO, Eagle M, Finder JD, Kissel J, et al. Respiratory management of the patient with Duchenne muscular dystrophy. Pediatrics. 2018;142(Suppl 2):S62–71. https://doi.org/10.1542/peds.2018-0333H.
115. Bach JR, Martinez D. Duchenne muscular dystrophy: continuous noninvasive ventilatory support prolongs survival. Respir Care. 2011;56(6):744–50. https://doi.org/10.4187/respcare.00831.
116. Tzeng AC, Bach JR. Prevention of pulmonary morbidity for patients with neuromuscular disease. Chest. 2000;118(5):1390–6. https://doi.org/10.1378/chest.118.5.1390.
117. Jenkins HM, Stocki A, Kriellaars D, Pasterkamp H. Breath stacking in children with neuromuscular disorders. Pediatr Pulmonol. 2014;49(6):544–53. https://doi.org/10.1002/ppul.22865.
118. Marques TB, Neves Jde C, Portes LA, Salge JM, Zanoteli E, Reed UC. Air stacking: effects on pulmonary function in patients with spinal muscular atrophy and in patients with congenital muscular dystrophy. J Bras Pneumol. 2014;40(5):528–34. https://doi.org/10.1590/s1806-37132014000500009.
119. Mahede T, Davis G, Rutkay A, Baxendale S, Sun W, Dawkins HJ, et al. Use of mechanical airway clearance devices in the home by people with neuromuscular disorders: effects on health service use and lifestyle benefits. Orphanet J Rare Dis. 2015;10:54. https://doi.org/10.1186/s13023-015-0267-0.
120. Moran FC, Spittle A, Delany C, Robertson CF, Massie J. Effect of home mechanical in-exsufflation on hospitalisation and life-style in neuromuscular disease: a pilot study. J Paediatr Child Health. 2013;49(3):233–7. https://doi.org/10.1111/jpc.12111.
121. Katz SL, Barrowman N, Monsour A, Su S, Hoey L, McKim D. Long-term effects of lung volume recruitment on maximal inspiratory capacity and vital capacity in Duchenne muscular dystrophy. Ann Am Thorac Soc. 2016;13(2):217–22. https://doi.org/10.1513/AnnalsATS.201507-475BC.
122. Katz SL, Mah JK, McMillan HJ, Campbell C, Bijelic V, Barrowman N, et al. Routine lung volume recruitment in boys with Duchenne muscular dystrophy: a randomised clinical trial. Thorax. 2022;77(8):805–11. https://doi.org/10.1136/thoraxjnl-2021-218196.
123. Chatwin M, Toussaint M, Goncalves MR, Sheers N, Mellies U, Gonzales-Bermejo J, et al. Airway clearance techniques in neuromuscular disorders: a state of the art review. Respir Med. 2018;136:98–110. https://doi.org/10.1016/j.rmed.2018.01.012.
124. Kan AF, Butler JM, Hutchence M, Jones K, Widger J, Doumit MA. Teaching manually assisted cough to caregivers of children with neuromuscular disease. Respir Care. 2018;63(12):1520–7. https://doi.org/10.4187/respcare.06213.

125. Gomez-Merino E, Sancho J, Marin J, Servera E, Blasco ML, Belda FJ, et al. Mechanical insufflation-exsufflation: pressure, volume, and flow relationships and the adequacy of the manufacturer's guidelines. Am J Phys Med Rehabil. 2002;81(8):579–83. https://doi.org/10.1097/00002060-200208000-00004.

126. Striegl AM, Redding GJ, Diblasi R, Crotwell D, Salyer J, Carter ER. Use of a lung model to assess mechanical in-exsufflator therapy in infants with tracheostomy. Pediatr Pulmonol. 2011;46(3):211–7. https://doi.org/10.1002/ppul.21353.

127. Andersen TM, Hov B, Halvorsen T, Roksund OD, Vollsaeter M. Upper airway assessment and responses during mechanically assisted cough. Respir Care. 2021;66(7):1196–213. https://doi.org/10.4187/respcare.08960.

128. Moran FC, Spittle AJ, Delany C. Lifestyle implications of home mechanical insufflation-exsufflation for children with neuromuscular disease and their families. Respir Care. 2015;60(7):967–74. https://doi.org/10.4187/respcare.03641.

129. Sterni LM, Collaco JM, Baker CD, Carroll JL, Sharma GD, Brozek JL, et al. An official American Thoracic Society clinical practice guideline: pediatric chronic home invasive ventilation. Am J Respir Crit Care Med. 2016;193(8):e16–35. https://doi.org/10.1164/rccm.201602-0276ST.

130. Hov B, Andersen T, Toussaint M, Mikalsen IB, Vollsaeter M, Markussen H, et al. User-perceived impact of long-term mechanical assisted cough in paediatric neurodisability. Dev Med Child Neurol. 2023;65(5):655–63. https://doi.org/10.1111/dmcn.15543.

131. Veldhoen ES, Verweij-van den Oudenrijn LP, Ros LA, Hulzebos EH, Papazova DA, van der Ent CK, et al. Effect of mechanical insufflation-exsufflation in children with neuromuscular weakness. Pediatr Pulmonol. 2020;55(2):510–3. https://doi.org/10.1002/ppul.24614.

132. Morrow B, Argent A, Zampoli M, Human A, Corten L, Toussaint M. Cough augmentation techniques for people with chronic neuromuscular disorders. Cochrane Database Syst Rev. 2021;4(4):CD013170. https://doi.org/10.1002/14651858.CD013170.pub2.

133. Bilan N, Poorshiri B. The role of chest physiotherapy in prevention of postextubation atelectasis in pediatric patients with neuromuscular diseases. Iran J Child Neurol. 2013;7(1):21–4.

134. Ansaripour A, Roehrich K, Mashayekhi A, Wanjala M, Noel S, Hemami MR, et al. Budget impact of the vest high frequency chest wall oscillation system for managing airway clearance in patients with complex neurological disorders: a US healthcare payers' perspective analysis. Pharmacoecon Open. 2022;6(2):169–78. https://doi.org/10.1007/s41669-021-00299-y.

135. Fitzgerald K, Dugre J, Pagala S, Homel P, Marcus M, Kazachkov M. High-frequency chest wall compression therapy in neurologically impaired children. Respir Care. 2014;59(1):107–12. https://doi.org/10.4187/respcare.02446.

136. Lechtzin N, Wolfe LF, Frick KD. The impact of high-frequency chest wall oscillation on healthcare use in patients with neuromuscular diseases. Ann Am Thorac Soc. 2016;13(6):904–9. https://doi.org/10.1513/AnnalsATS.201509-597OC.

137. Cigna, editor. Medical coverage policy: airway clearance devices in the ambulatory setting. 0069 ed2022. p. 1–16.

138. Bidiwala A, Volpe L, Halaby C, Fazzari M, Valsamis C, Pirzada M. A comparison of high frequency chest wall oscillation and intrapulmonary percussive ventilation for airway clearance in pediatric patients with tracheostomy. Postgrad Med. 2017;129(2):276–82. https://doi.org/10.1080/00325481.2017.1264854.

139. Lauwers E, Ides K, Van Hoorenbeeck K, Verhulst S. The effect of intrapulmonary percussive ventilation in pediatric patients: a systematic review. Pediatr Pulmonol. 2018;53(11):1463–74. https://doi.org/10.1002/ppul.24135.

140. Chatwin M, Toussaint M. Will the addition of oscillations in mechanical insufflation-exsufflation ever be beneficial? Respir Care. 2020;65(5):725–8. https://doi.org/10.4187/respcare.07798.

141. Katz S, Selvadurai H, Keilty K, Mitchell M, MacLusky I. Outcome of non-invasive positive pressure ventilation in paediatric neuromuscular disease. Arch Dis Child. 2004;89(2):121–4. https://doi.org/10.1136/adc.2002.018655.

142. Passamano L, Taglia A, Palladino A, Viggiano E, D'Ambrosio P, Scutifero M, et al. Improvement of survival in Duchenne muscular dystrophy: retrospective analysis of 835 patients. Acta Myol. 2012;31(2):121–5.
143. Oskoui M, Levy G, Garland CJ, Gray JM, O'Hagen J, De Vivo DC, et al. The changing natural history of spinal muscular atrophy type 1. Neurology. 2007;69(20):1931–6. https://doi.org/10.1212/01.wnl.0000290830.40544.b9.
144. Fauroux B, Leroux K, Desmarais G, Isabey D, Clement A, Lofaso F, et al. Performance of ventilators for noninvasive positive-pressure ventilation in children. Eur Respir J. 2008;31(6):1300–7. https://doi.org/10.1183/09031936.00144807.
145. Castro-Codesal ML, Olmstead DL, MacLean JE. Mask interfaces for home non-invasive ventilation in infants and children. Paediatr Respir Rev. 2019;32:66–72. https://doi.org/10.1016/j.prrv.2019.03.004.
146. Fauroux B, Lavis JF, Nicot F, Picard A, Boelle PY, Clement A, et al. Facial side effects during noninvasive positive pressure ventilation in children. Intensive Care Med. 2005;31(7):965–9. https://doi.org/10.1007/s00134-005-2669-2.
147. Toussaint M, Chatwin M, Goncalves MR, Gonzalez-Bermejo J, Benditt JO, McKim D, et al. Mouthpiece ventilation in neuromuscular disorders: narrative review of technical issues important for clinical success. Respir Med. 2021;180:106373. https://doi.org/10.1016/j.rmed.2021.106373.
148. De Jesus RW, Samuels CL, Gonzales TR, McBeth KE, Yadav A, Stark JM, et al. Use of nasal non-invasive ventilation with a RAM cannula in the outpatient home setting. Open Respir Med J. 2017;11:41–6. https://doi.org/10.2174/1874306401711010041.
149. Bach JR, Saltstein K, Sinquee D, Weaver B, Komaroff E. Long-term survival in Werdnig-Hoffmann disease. Am J Phys Med Rehabil. 2007;86(5):339–45; quiz 46–8, 79. https://doi.org/10.1097/PHM.0b013e31804a8505.
150. Soudon P, Steens M, Toussaint M. A comparison of invasive versus noninvasive full-time mechanical ventilation in Duchenne muscular dystrophy. Chron Respir Dis. 2008;5(2):87–93. https://doi.org/10.1177/1479972308088715.
151. You P, Strychowsky J, Gandhi K, Chen BA. Anticholinergic treatment for sialorrhea in children: a systematic review. Paediatr Child Health. 2022;27(2):82–7. https://doi.org/10.1093/pch/pxab051.
152. Singh H, Nene Y, Mehta TR, Govindarajan R. Efficacy of botulinum toxin for treating sialorrhea in neuromuscular conditions. Front Neurol. 2020;11:513. https://doi.org/10.3389/fneur.2020.00513.
153. Ture E, Yazar A, Dundar MA, Bakdik S, Akin F, Pekcan S. Treatment of sialorrhea with botulinum toxin A injection in children. Niger J Clin Pract. 2021;24(6):847–52. https://doi.org/10.4103/njcp.njcp_85_20.
154. Shoval HA, Antelis E, Hillman A, Wei X, Tan P, Alejandro R, et al. Onabotulinum toxin A injections into the salivary glands for spinal muscle atrophy type I: a prospective case series of 4 patients. Am J Phys Med Rehabil. 2018;97(12):873–8. https://doi.org/10.1097/phm.0000000000000989.
155. Kim DH, Elsherbini N, Zielinski D, Oskoui M. A case report of systemic intoxication following onabotulinum toxin A injections into the salivary glands in a patient with spinal muscular atrophy type 1. Pediatr Neurol. 2022;129:37–8. https://doi.org/10.1016/j.pediatrneurol.2022.01.005.
156. Hughes A, Lambert EM. Drooling and aspiration of saliva. Otolaryngol Clin North Am. 2022;55(6):1181–94. https://doi.org/10.1016/j.otc.2022.07.007.
157. Piccione JC, McPhail GL, Fenchel MC, Brody AS, Boesch RP. Bronchiectasis in chronic pulmonary aspiration: risk factors and clinical implications. Pediatr Pulmonol. 2012;47(5):447–52. https://doi.org/10.1002/ppul.21587.
158. Chou E, Lindeback R, D'Silva AM, Sampaio H, Neville K, Farrar MA. Growth and nutrition in pediatric neuromuscular disorders. Clin Nutr. 2021;40(6):4341–8. https://doi.org/10.1016/j.clnu.2021.01.013.

159. Toussaint M, Davidson Z, Bouvoie V, Evenepoel N, Haan J, Soudon P. Dysphagia in Duchenne muscular dystrophy: practical recommendations to guide management. Disabil Rehabil. 2016;38(20):2052–62. https://doi.org/10.3109/09638288.2015.1111434.
160. Wadman RI, De Amicis R, Brusa C, Battezzati A, Bertoli S, Davis T, et al. Feeding difficulties in children and adolescents with spinal muscular atrophy type 2. Neuromuscul Disord. 2021;31(2):101–12. https://doi.org/10.1016/j.nmd.2020.12.007.
161. Chatwin M, Bush A, Simonds AK. Outcome of goal-directed non-invasive ventilation and mechanical insufflation/exsufflation in spinal muscular atrophy type I. Arch Dis Child. 2011;96(5):426–32. https://doi.org/10.1136/adc.2009.177832.
162. Inal-Ince D, Savci S, Arikan H, Saglam M, Vardar-Yagli N, Bosnak-Guclu M, et al. Effects of scoliosis on respiratory muscle strength in patients with neuromuscular disorders. Spine J. 2009;9(12):981–6. https://doi.org/10.1016/j.spinee.2009.08.451.
163. LaValva S, Adams A, MacAlpine E, Gupta P, Hammerberg K, Thompson GH, et al. Serial casting in neuromuscular and syndromic early-onset scoliosis (EOS) can delay surgery over 2 years. J Pediatr Orthop. 2020;40(8):e772–9. https://doi.org/10.1097/BPO.0000000000001568.
164. Tangsrud SE, Carlsen KC, Lund-Petersen I, Carlsen KH. Lung function measurements in young children with spinal muscle atrophy; a cross sectional survey on the effect of position and bracing. Arch Dis Child. 2001;84(6):521–4. https://doi.org/10.1136/adc.84.6.521.
165. Swarup I, MacAlpine EM, Mayer OH, Lark RK, Smith JT, Vitale MG, et al. Impact of growth friendly interventions on spine and pulmonary outcomes of patients with spinal muscular atrophy. Eur Spine J. 2021;30(3):768–74. https://doi.org/10.1007/s00586-020-06564-8.
166. Gaume M, Saudeau E, Gomez-Garcia de la Banda M, Azzi-Salameh V, Mbieleu B, Verollet D, et al. Minimally invasive fusionless surgery for scoliosis in spinal muscular atrophy: long-term follow-up results in a series of 59 patients. J Pediatr Orthop. 2021;41(9):549–58. https://doi.org/10.1097/BPO.0000000000001897.
167. Trucco F, Ridout D, Scoto M, Coratti G, Main ML, Muni Lofra R, et al. Respiratory trajectories in type 2 and 3 spinal muscular atrophy in the iSMAC cohort study. Neurology. 2021;96(4):e587–99. https://doi.org/10.1212/WNL.0000000000011051.
168. Chua K, Tan CY, Chen Z, Wong HK, Lee EH, Tay SK, et al. Long-term follow-up of pulmonary function and scoliosis in patients with Duchenne's muscular dystrophy and spinal muscular atrophy. J Pediatr Orthop. 2016;36(1):63–9. https://doi.org/10.1097/BPO.0000000000000396.
169. Kariyawasam D, Carey KA, Jones KJ, Farrar MA. New and developing therapies in spinal muscular atrophy. Paediatr Respir Rev. 2018;28:3–10. https://doi.org/10.1016/j.prrv.2018.03.003.
170. Finkel RS, Mercuri E, Darras BT, Connolly AM, Kuntz NL, Kirschner J, et al. Nusinersen versus sham control in infantile-onset spinal muscular atrophy. N Engl J Med. 2017;377(18):1723–32. https://doi.org/10.1056/NEJMoa1702752.
171. De Vivo DC, Bertini E, Swoboda KJ, Hwu WL, Crawford TO, Finkel RS, et al. Nusinersen initiated in infants during the presymptomatic stage of spinal muscular atrophy: interim efficacy and safety results from the phase 2 NURTURE study. Neuromuscul Disord. 2019;29(11):842–56. https://doi.org/10.1016/j.nmd.2019.09.007.
172. Masson R, Mazurkiewicz-Beldzinska M, Rose K, Servais L, Xiong H, Zanoteli E, et al. Safety and efficacy of risdiplam in patients with type 1 spinal muscular atrophy (FIREFISH part 2): secondary analyses from an open-label trial. Lancet Neurol. 2022;21(12):1110–9. https://doi.org/10.1016/S1474-4422(22)00339-8.
173. Mendell JR, Al-Zaidy SA, Lehman KJ, McColly M, Lowes LP, Alfano LN, et al. Five-year extension results of the phase 1 START trial of onasemnogene abeparvovec in spinal muscular atrophy. JAMA Neurol. 2021;78(7):834–41. https://doi.org/10.1001/jamaneurol.2021.1272.
174. Biggar WD, Skalsky A, McDonald CM. Comparing deflazacort and prednisone in Duchenne muscular dystrophy. J Neuromuscul Dis. 2022;9(4):463–76. https://doi.org/10.3233/JND-210776.

175. Bladen CL, Salgado D, Monges S, Foncuberta ME, Kekou K, Kosma K, et al. The TREAT-NMD DMD Global Database: analysis of more than 7,000 Duchenne muscular dystrophy mutations. Hum Mutat. 2015;36(4):395–402. https://doi.org/10.1002/humu.22758.
176. Patterson G, Conner H, Groneman M, Blavo C, Parmar MS. Duchenne muscular dystrophy: current treatment and emerging exon skipping and gene therapy approach. Eur J Pharmacol. 2023;947:175675. https://doi.org/10.1016/j.ejphar.2023.175675.
177. Khan N, Eliopoulos H, Han L, Kinane TB, Lowes LP, Mendell JR, et al. Eteplirsen treatment attenuates respiratory decline in ambulatory and non-ambulatory patients with Duchenne muscular dystrophy. J Neuromuscul Dis. 2019;6(2):213–25. https://doi.org/10.3233/JND-180351.
178. Mendell JR, Rodino-Klapac L, Sahenk Z, Malik V, Kaspar BK, Walker CM, et al. Gene therapy for muscular dystrophy: lessons learned and path forward. Neurosci Lett. 2012;527(2):90–9. https://doi.org/10.1016/j.neulet.2012.04.078.
179. Elangkovan N, Dickson G. Gene therapy for Duchenne muscular dystrophy. J Neuromuscul Dis. 2021;8(s2):S303–16. https://doi.org/10.3233/jnd-210678.
180. Nicolino M, Byrne B, Wraith JE, Leslie N, Mandel H, Freyer DR, et al. Clinical outcomes after long-term treatment with alglucosidase alfa in infants and children with advanced Pompe disease. Genet Med. 2009;11(3):210–9. https://doi.org/10.1097/GIM.0b013e31819d0996.
181. Shieh PB, Kuntz N, Smith B, Dowling J, Müller-Felber W, Bönnemann CG, et al. ASPIRO gene therapy trial in X-linked myotubular myopathy (XLMTM): update on preliminary safety and efficacy findings up to 72 weeks post-treatment (1053). Neurology. 2020;94(15 Suppl):1053.
182. Rosen DS, Blum RW, Britto M, Sawyer SM, Siegel DM, Society for Adolescent Medicine. Transition to adult health care for adolescents and young adults with chronic conditions: position paper of the Society for Adolescent Medicine. J Adolesc Health. 2003;33(4):309–11. https://doi.org/10.1016/s1054-139x(03)00208-8.
183. Cheng PC, Panitch HB, Hansen-Flaschen J. Transition of patients with neuromuscular disease and chronic ventilator-dependent respiratory failure from pediatric to adult pulmonary care. Paediatr Respir Rev. 2020;33:3–8. https://doi.org/10.1016/j.prrv.2019.03.005.

Chapter 8
The Pediatric to Adult Transition of Patients with Neuromuscular Disease

Jackie Chiang, Kathryn Selby, Jeremy Orr, Aaron Izenberg, and Reshma Amin

Key Concepts in Transition

The concept of "transition of care" first arose in the 1990s and has been defined as a "purposeful, planned, multidisciplinary movement of adolescents and young adults from child-versus-adult-oriented health care systems" [1]. The term "transition" indicates the process of moving from one state to another that involves young people aged 13–25 years and generally involves the families and the professionals associated with the individual [2]. It is important to note that transition is not synonymous with a one-time transfer event [3]. Similarly, the World Health Organization recommends the focus be placed on patients and their needs rather than on clinician-to-clinician "handover" [4]. It requires careful planning and coordination, typically over several years, leading up to the actual transfer of care.

J. Chiang · R. Amin (✉)
Division of Respiratory Medicine, Department of Pediatrics, The Hospital for Sick Children, University of Toronto, Toronto, ON, Canada
e-mail: jackie.chiang@sickkids.ca; reshma.amin@sickkids.ca

K. Selby
Division of Pediatric Neurology, Department of Pediatrics, British Columbia Children's Hospital, University of British Columbia, Vancouver, BC, Canada
e-mail: kselby@cw.bc.ca

J. Orr
Department of Pulmonary and Critical Care Medicine, UC San Diego Health, University of California San Diego, La Jolla, CA, USA
e-mail: j1orr@health.ucsd.edu

A. Izenberg
Division of Neurology, Department of Medicine, Sunnybrook Health Sciences Center, University of Toronto, Toronto, ON, Canada
e-mail: aaron.izenberg@sunnybrook.ca

© The Author(s), under exclusive license to Springer Nature Switzerland AG 2024
N. Lechtzin (ed.), *Pulmonary Complications of Neuromuscular Disease*, Respiratory Medicine, https://doi.org/10.1007/978-3-031-65335-3_8

With the growing awareness of the importance of successful healthcare transitions, the American Academy of Pediatrics, American Academy of Family Physicians, and American College of Physicians-American Society of Internal Medicine published a joint consensus statement on healthcare transitions for young adults with special healthcare needs. This statement indicates that transition in healthcare for young adults with chronic conditions or special healthcare needs is a dynamic, lifelong process that seeks to meet the individual needs of each patient with the goal of maximizing lifelong functioning and potential through the provision of developmentally appropriate, quality care that continues uninterrupted as the patient moves from adolescence to adulthood [5]. Furthermore, the process should be patient-centered, and its cornerstones include (1) flexibility, (2) responsiveness, (3) continuity, (4) comprehensiveness, and (5) coordination [5]. Contributors to *Healthy People 2010*, including the Centers for Disease Control and Prevention, attempted to establish the goal that all individuals with special healthcare needs receive the services needed to make necessary transitions to all aspects of adult life, including healthcare, work, and independent living by 2010 [6]. Unfortunately, despite more than 500,000 youth entering adult healthcare services each year in the United States, only 40% have been found to receive transition support that meets recommended criteria [7].

Complex medical conditions, and especially neuromuscular diseases, pose unique challenges to transition. Firstly, pediatric patients with medical complexity and special healthcare needs are known to have high healthcare utilization. For example, approximately half of all pediatric healthcare expenditure is for children with complexity primarily due to frequent hospitalizations [8] and readmissions. Secondly, there is a wide spectrum of clinical severity in neuromuscular disorders including cognitive and behavioral disability that may influence the patients' own ability to make medical decisions or assume responsibility of care as well as medical comorbidities that will continue to require lifelong care [9]. In one retrospective study of patients with diverse neuromuscular disease transitioned from pediatric to adult neuromuscular care within a tertiary academic center in Canada, over one-third of patients required ongoing adult follow-up for cardiac and respiratory care, nearly a quarter for orthopedic services, and 10–25% required consultation from other subspecialties such as endocrinology, gastroenterology, psychiatry, and speech and language pathology [10]. Thirdly, there is also a high symptom burden in neuromuscular conditions associated with adverse psychosocial outcomes such as reduced quality of life and impairment in adaptive behavior [2]. The development of new therapeutic modalities for neuromuscular conditions that were once fatal in childhood has now allowed these patients to live into adulthood; however, adult healthcare providers may not be as familiar and/or have a lack of experience providing care to these individuals [9]. In addition, reproductive and sexual health and advanced care planning also need to form an integral part of transition education and are often given minimal emphasis, both by pediatric and adult healthcare providers.

Differences Between Pediatric and Adult Models of Care

It is important to recognize that fundamental differences in the model of care occur as patients transition from pediatrics to adult healthcare. In a transitional care scoping review for young people with neurological disorders authored by McGovern et al., pediatric hospitals were deemed to provide more services and resources [11]. In another qualitative interview study of young adults with special healthcare needs, pediatric staff were thought to be more available for questions and support, involving both the patient and the family [12]. In addition, differences were noted in the availability of allied health personnel such as social workers or nurses who understood your illness and had a much more psychosocial approach to your illness [12].

In pediatrics, there is an emphasis on a family-centered approach whereby caregivers often make or significantly contribute to medical decision-making. Families see themselves as having an ongoing role in the care of the young adult and continue to communicate with pediatric providers [12]. In addition, pediatric care often involves multidisciplinary teams [13]. In contrast, adult healthcare places greater autonomy on the patient and has been described to be more "disease centered rather than patient centred" [12]. There is more separation of care across multiple subspecialty clinics and treatment services that often spans more than one institution [11].

In 2012, Oskoui and Wolfson described the current practice and views of neurologists transitioning patients from pediatric to adult care in one province in Canada via a cross-sectional survey of all pediatric and adult neurologists [14]. It was identified that most pediatric neurologists do not have a transition program or policy in place and although an individual health summary document is commonly provided, crucial information was often lacking. Nearly half of all neurologists believed that patients experience a gap in care during the transition process and most agreed that the process was often poorly coordinated. Most surveyed agreed that young adults often did not know their own medical history and that caregivers can remain excessively protective and may not understand the privacy issues of the young adult. Adult practices were described as less paternalistic than pediatric practices, and thus, for example, patients may not be contacted when an appointment was missed. Interestingly, 75% of pediatric neurologists suggested starting the transition process 1–2 years prior to transitioning at 18 years of age, which does not follow current recommendations by the Canadian Pediatric Society or American cademy of Pediatrics, which recommend much earlier initiation [5, 15].

Potential Negative Health Consequences Related to Gaps in Transition

Suboptimal transition can be associated with negative consequences such as poor health outcomes, increased rates of hospitalization, non-adherence, disengagement from healthcare, and missed medical appointments [16, 17]. Young adults who are lost to medical follow-up are more likely to utilize acute care services and experience increasing morbidity and disability [18, 19].

In patients who underwent transplantation, medical outcomes have consistently been shown to deteriorate when patients were transitioned to adult care with non-adherence suspected as a primary reason for this change [20]. In a retrospective study of liver transplant patients who had recently transitioned, the authors found that medication adherence was significantly poorer over time for transitioned patients than for a cohort of adolescent pediatric patients studied over a 3-year period as measured by tacrolimus blood levels [21]. This comparison also suggests that transition itself may be associated with reduced adherence that cannot fully be accounted for by being an adolescent. In addition, the mortality rate was far higher among transitioned patients than patients receiving care exclusively within the pediatric or adult healthcare sector [21].

Data on health consequences after transition are very limited in the neuromuscular population. However, a retrospective comparison of young adults with neuromuscular disease requiring non-invasive ventilation transitioned to adult care in two different respiratory centers, one with a transition program and one without, again highlights the potential care gaps that can occur without a formal transition process. Onofri et al. compared Bambino Gesu Children's Hospital (BGCH) in Rome, Italy, which did not have a formal transition program, to the Royal Brompton Hospital (RBHT) in London, UK, that had an established transition program [22]. Although initiation of non-invasive ventilation is well established to prevent respiratory complications and prolong life in neuromuscular patients, the authors found a significant difference in the starting age for non-invasive support between the two groups. The median age of NIV initiation was 16 years for the BGCH group in contrast to 12 years of age in the RBHT group, although different underlying disease profiles as well as varying diagnostic tools (i.e., polysomnogram versus oximetry-capnography) may have played a role as well. Furthermore, whereas most patients continued to be followed by the pediatric respiratory team at BGCH at 18 years of age, transition was initiated at 15 years of age and completed by 17 years of age at the RBHT.

Patient and Family Perspectives

The definition of transition originally stems from crisis theory, which asserts that people operate in equilibrium with their environment and solve problems by habitual mechanisms. However, when the usual problem-solving strategies do not work, the individual experiences anxiety, fear, and feelings of helplessness [2]. Erik Erikson, a psychologist, theorized that people developmentally progress based on how they adjust to social crises throughout their lives [23]. Transition to adulthood for those with neuromuscular disease not only means navigating the typical social frameworks for all adolescents but also navigating new healthcare domains and practices. It is therefore crucial to take a developmental approach to healthcare transition and incorporate the perspective of the patient (and families) when pursuing transition.

In a qualitative study of young adults with SMA that had transitioned from pediatric to adult care, the experience of transition was described as "challenging and scary" [24]. They reported difficulties associated with learning to navigate a new healthcare system. Participants also described deep sadness associated with declines in functional capacity that occurred in adulthood and many perceived mental healthcare needs to be vital to their well-being after transition.

Family caregivers of patients also identified having a sense of fear of the unknown after many years in the pediatric healthcare environment and that there was insufficient awareness of the vulnerability of young patients in the adult healthcare system [11]. Parents of individuals with Duchenne muscular dystrophy who were interviewed identified strongly as an advocate and medical decision-maker for their sons when they were children but recognized that as they became adults, they needed to support self-determination [25].

Both patients and their caregivers have also reported feeling a sense of abandonment during the transition process as they leave trusted relationships that have inevitably developed over years [11]. Some reasons cited for this include failure to provide a referral to a specific adult service, a long gap between the last pediatric appointment and first adult clinic, and sadness at leaving the pediatric environment. In a cross-sectional study of adolescents with chronic disorders, aged 14–25 years, not yet transitioned to adult care and their parents, approximately 20% reported feeling anxious about the transition process, and 53% of adolescents and 69% of parents preferred a joint transfer meeting with the pediatric and adult specialist. Interestingly, only 24% of adolescents reported being offered this as an option by their healthcare provider.

Barriers and Facilitators to Transition

Patient and Family Factors

The Socioecological Model of Adolescent and Young Adult Readiness for Transition (SMART) has been used to summarize the literature on barriers to transition [26]. SMART is an expert-informed, theory-driven model of transition readiness capturing systems-level barriers and facilitators of transition readiness. The most frequently cited barriers focused on relationships between adolescents, parents, pediatrics, and adult providers (see Table 8.1). Developmental immaturity was cited as a barrier across several chronic conditions, and many adolescents reported that they did not feel ready to take responsibility of their medical condition. Lack of developmental maturity was shown to lead to transition delays, non-adherence, missed appointments, and refusal to manage care independently. In a survey of pediatric and adult healthcare providers' (physicians and nurses) attitudes toward

Table 8.1 Pediatric to adult healthcare transitions for individuals with neuromuscular disease: transition barriers and potential solutions

Transition barrier	Potential solutions
Developmental immaturity or poor self-management	• Early identification of preparedness—Consider the use of Transition Readiness Assessment Questionnaire (TRAQ) • Regular discussions regarding transition planning
Patient/family anxieties and concerns regarding transition	• Early interaction with adult providers • Written materials • Peer connections • Address negative biases
Differences between pediatric and adult care models and financing	• Increased adult provider training in neuromuscular diseases • Identification of community resources including transition coordinators, case managers, and social workers • Attention to potential insurance issues—Obtain authorizations, and change insurance if possible

transition in young adults with chronic illnesses in Sweden, age, maturity, and family situations were considered the most important initiators for transition [27].

Adolescents also feared the loss of relationships with pediatric providers, forming new relationships with adult providers, and perceptions of poorer quality of care in adult settings attributed to less time spent with patients, lack of "caring" or experience, or not prioritizing patient needs in emergency situations. In addition, both patient and caregiver lack of knowledge pertaining to the underlying disease, medications, therapies, and the transition process were highlighted as other barriers to transition. Finally, lack of self-management skills related to poor adherence, lack of independence, low health literacy, unfamiliarity with scheduling medical appointments, and navigating the adult healthcare system are also important barriers.

To foster relationships with adult care providers, earlier interaction with adult providers and the creation of joint clinic visits attended by both pediatric and adult health care providers have been recommended [26]. In addition, a structured transition plan, written educational materials to address common concerns, and connecting patients with peers who have already transitioned have been suggested as other strategies to overcome misinformed beliefs [26, 28]. To foster development of skills and self-efficacy, the following recommendations were highlighted: begin transition preparation early in adolescence by embedding transition discussions into regular clinic flow to normalize the discussion, provide education on transition responsibility potentially in the form of group classes, encourage independent visits as adolescents, and use technology to target disease knowledge and other self-management strategies [26].

It is also essential that pediatric practitioners be mindful of avoiding negative bias during discussions of transition and adult care. The transition process should be normalized, and the difference in culture between pediatric and adult care should be discussed in a neutral manner (e.g., greater focus on patient autonomy). Furthermore, the development of new relationships with adult providers should be highlighted while acknowledging that transition also means the loss of pediatric care provider relationships [28].

Healthcare Systems

As described earlier, there are marked differences in general practices between pediatric and adult care. The largest difference likely being the relative ease of availability to numerous subspecialties, including neurology, respiratory medicine, cardiology, gastroenterology, orthopedics, and physiatrists, all within the same pediatric institution [29]. In addition, pediatric care often takes place within multidisciplinary teams with access to social work, dietician, speech, physical therapy, and occupation therapy. In contrast, this is not the norm in adult healthcare, which can prove to be a greater challenge to navigate.

Individually, the pediatric care provider may lack the time or knowledge to coordinate a transition process and/or may be unfamiliar with the existing community resources [30]. At times, the patient and family may consider the pediatric subspecialist to be their primary physician and have had limited contact with their primary care provider, which has been identified to be a significant barrier to transition. Adult healthcare providers may have had little training or exposure to certain neuromuscular conditions previously considered pediatric diseases. In a survey of adult physicians regarding their perspective on caring for those with chronic disorders of childhood onset, 40% indicated they did not feel comfortable caring for such patients and were influenced by lack of training in adolescent development and care of complex disorders as well as deficient knowledge of the literature [31]. The level of comfort of adult neurologists in providing care for neuromuscular patients was reported to be much lower in comparison to youth with headaches or epilepsy [32]. They may also be concerned with the increased healthcare demands of these patients [30]. Even if adult practitioners are willing to assume care, there may be a lack of program funding and physician compensation needed to support continuous shared and integrated care during the transition process to adult healthcare providers and adult specialty clinics for neuromuscular patients [30].

Proposed solutions to some of these barriers include early identification of and relationship building with community resources (such as primary care physicians), ensuring access to a social worker or psychologist for pediatric and adult transition clinics and preparing families for the change in models of care [28]. With respect to lack of funding or resources, it has been suggested that healthcare providers identify sources of grant funding for transition clinics that include local, national, and non-traditional sources and seek sustainable funding and institutional buy-in with demonstration of program value [28]. Funding for maintenance shared by pediatric and adult programs could be considered. While cost-effectiveness may be challenging to demonstrate, other outcome measures such as clinical outcomes or patient satisfaction may be used. Finally, it was highlighted that advocacy for transition and dissemination of results is needed at institutional, local and national levels [28].

Health Insurance

For countries where access to medical care is tied to health insurance, adolescents transitioning to adulthood may face problems when they are no longer covered by their parents' insurance plans. Insurance provisions with respect to preexisting medical conditions may limit or even preclude eligibility for obtaining their own insurance [13]. Young adults with chronic conditions often require insurance coverage for multiple subspecialty services, diagnostic tests, medical equipment, and medication prescriptions. And yet, sufficiently comprehensive insurance plans are often not available to individuals with disabilities. In addition, psychological, communication, or mobility supports are often not covered or may be limited to a certain number of hours per year [13].

In the United States, adult Medicaid plans are not as comprehensive as those for children [29]. Social Security Insurance also reassesses eligibility when an individual turns 18 years of age using adult disability standards, which may mean that some patients may lose their benefits creating additional financial strain on families [29]. Furthermore, pediatric and adult hospitals may not participate in the same insurance plans, thus forcing patients to switch insurance policies in order to receive the subspecialty expert care they require [29]. For other patients, this barrier may result in patients seeking medical care in centers that do not have neuromuscular expertise. One solution highlighted by the Children's Hospital of Philadelphia (CHOP) was to obtain prior authorization approving patients to receive specialized care by specific neuromuscular experts at the adult partnering hospital, Hospital of the University of Pennsylvania (HUP), when insurance was incompatible [29]. Another suggestion to facilitate access to adult care and to aid in insurance issues was to employ a transition coordinator or a transition navigator to help prepare young adult patients with the transition process [26].

Criteria for Successful Transition

As a result of the AAP,, and ACP guidelines [33] and the call for established transition practices from pediatric to adult healthcare, the *Got Transition*, a federally funded American national resource center and program on healthcare transition, was developed with the aim of using evidence-driven strategies for clinicians, patients, and caregivers to improve the transition process. Now in its third iteration, the Got Transition 3.0 program has been widely adopted and describes six core elements that outline the necessary basic components of a structured transition process (see Fig. 8.1). These are as follows: (1) transition policy, (2) tracking and monitoring, (3) transition readiness and/or orientation to adult practice, (4) transition planning, (5) transfer of care, and (6) transition completion and ongoing care with the adult healthcare team.

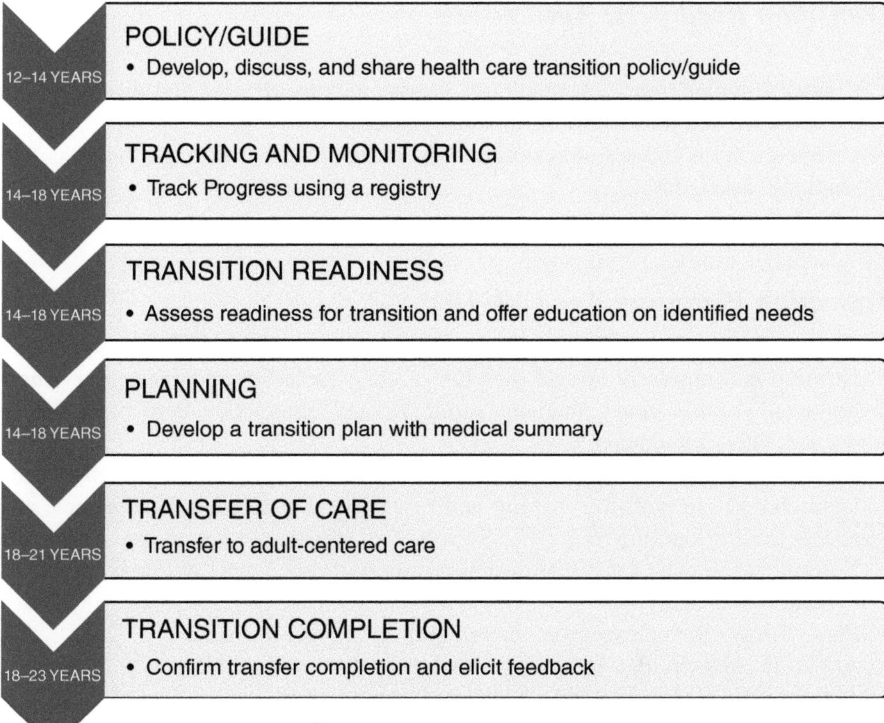

Fig. 8.1 Got Transition 3.0 six core elements of healthcare transition

Transition Policy Co-Development

- Develop a transition policy/statement with input from youth and caregivers that describes the practice's approach to transition as well as an adult approach to care in terms of privacy and consent.
- Educate staff about the approach to transition and roles of the patient, caregiver, and pediatric and adult healthcare team in the transition process, taking into account cultural values.
- Display transition policy/statement in an accessible place, discuss and share with patient and caregiver, and regularly review as part of ongoing care.

Tracking and Monitoring: Aged 14–18

- Establish criteria and process for identifying transition-aged young adults.
- Develop process to track receipt of the six core elements of transition, integrating with the electronic medical record when possible.

Transition Readiness: Aged 14–18

- Conduct regular transition readiness assessments to identify and discuss needs for self-care and how to use healthcare services.
- Offer education and resources on needed skills identified through the transition readiness assessment.

Transition Planning: Aged 14–18

- Develop and regularly update the plan of care, including readiness assessment findings, youth's goals, medical summary and emergency care plan, and if needed, legal documents.
- Prepare young adults and caregivers for an adult approach to care, including legal changes in decision-making and privacy and consent, self-advocacy, and access to information.
- Determine the need for decision-making supports for youth, and make referrals to legal resources.
- Plan with youth and caregiver the optimal timing of transition.
- Assist in identifying an adult clinician and provide linkages to insurance resources (if applicable) and community support services.
- Obtain consent for release of medical information.

Transfer of Care: Aged 18–21

- Complete transfer package including the final transition readiness assessment, plan of care, medical summary and emergency care plan, and, if needed, legal documents.
- Confirm date of the first adult clinical appointment.
- Prepare letter with transfer package, send to adult clinician, and confirm receipt of package.
- Communicate with adult clinician about pending transition.
- Confirm the pediatric clinicians' responsibility for care until youth seen by adult clinician.
- Transition patient when their condition is as stable as possible.

Transition Completion: Aged 18–23

- Contact patient and caregiver 3–6 months after the last pediatric visit to confirm attendance at the first adult appointment.
- Elicit anonymous feedback from patient and caregiver on their transition experience.
- Communicate with adult clinician confirming completion of transition, and offer consultative assistance as needed.
- Build ongoing and collaborative partnerships with adult primary and specialty care clinicians.

A number of questionnaires have been developed to assess transition readiness. Among them, the Transition Readiness Assessment Questionnaire (TRAQ), which was developed in 2011, has overall shown high internal reliability and construct validity [34]. In addition, it has been translated into many different languages lending support to cross-cultural validity [35–39]. A higher TRAQ score translates to greater knowledge of disease, skill, self-efficacy, positive outlook toward the future, and health-related quality of life [40–43]. Conversely, a lower TRAQ score has been related to medication non-adherence [44]. In a review of randomized controlled trials utilizing the TRAQ to evaluate transition program interventions, Takeuchi et al. identified 261 reports and 3 randomized control studies where TRAQ was the outcome measure [45]. In two of the three randomized control studies, a web-based and nurse directed program, interventions were shown to improve transition readiness. It was confirmed that increasing the score between the intervention and control group allows for assessment of the quality of transition readiness and that therefore employing efficacious interventions can improve health-related outcomes.

Future Considerations

Despite the clear mandate to provide quality medical services to youth transitioning to adult care from pediatric care, there is unfortunately a paucity of literature evaluating the transition process in individuals with neuromuscular disease. Although there are broader healthcare transition guidelines that exist, there are no guidelines established for neuromuscular patients who have unique challenges and considerations to consider. As a result, there are gaps in knowledge and comfort with transitioning and caring for these medically complex individuals in adult health systems.

It has yet to be clear whether transitional care interventions established for one condition can be applied effectively to service other conditions [46]. Transition programs guided by well-established overarching transition principles likely need to be tailored to specific disease considerations. All relevant stakeholders, including patients and family caregivers, need to be included in the process. Thereafter, longitudinal evaluation of post-transition outcomes, such as health-related outcomes, treatment adherence, healthcare costs, and perceptions of care received by neuromuscular patients, is essential. In addition, understanding the neuromuscular adult lifestyle, including education, career, and psychosocial well-being, can provide insights on how to optimize health self-management [47], autonomy, and timing of transition. Certain facilitators and barriers to transition will likely be unique to individuals with neuromuscular disease and may be different between different conditions given the wide spectrum of disease severity, comorbidities, and cognitive profile that can be found.

Healthcare providers will need to utilize a more holistic, developmental perspective when approaching the transition process, which should include not only disease management awareness but also understanding the adolescent learning style, what they know about their disease, level of self-management, and satisfaction with care [47]. Advanced planning, preparation, collaboration, and communication are all important to ensuring a successful transition [3]. Development of training programs for clinicians and establishment of standard neuromuscular practice guidelines for transition should be prioritized to advance the care of individuals with neuromuscular disease.

References

1. Blum RW, Garell D, Hodgman CH, et al. Transition from child-centered to adult health-care systems for adolescents with chronic conditions. A position paper of the Society for Adolescent Medicine. J Adolesc Health. 1993;14(7):570–6. https://doi.org/10.1016/1054-139x(93)90143-d.
2. Baldanzi S, Ricci G, Simoncini C, Cosci ODCM, Siciliano G. Hard ways towards adulthood: the transition phase in young people with myotonic dystrophy. Acta Myol. 2016;35(3):145–9. https://www.ncbi.nlm.nih.gov/pubmed/28484315, https://www.ncbi.nlm.nih.gov/pmc/articles/PMC5416743/pdf/1128-2460-35-145.pdf.
3. Willis LD. Transition from pediatric to adult care for young adults with chronic respiratory disease. Respir Care. 2020;65(12):1916–22. (In eng). https://doi.org/10.4187/respcare.08260.
4. World Health Organization. Transitions of care. Geneva: World Health Organization; 2016.
5. American Academy of Pediatrics, American Academy of Family Physicians, American College of Physicians-American Society of Internal Medicine. A consensus statement on health care transitions for young adults with special health care needs. Pediatrics. 2002;110(6 Pt 2):1304–6. https://www.ncbi.nlm.nih.gov/pubmed/12456949.
6. Prevention CfDCa, National Institute on Disability and Rehabilitation Research aUDoE. Disability and secondary conditions. Healthy People 2010. Washington, DC: Public Health Service US Department of Health and Human Services; 2000.
7. McManus MA, Pollack LR, Cooley WC, et al. Current status of transition preparation among youth with special needs in the United States. Pediatrics. 2013;131(6):1090–7. https://doi.org/10.1542/peds.2012-3050.
8. Davis AM, Brown RF, Taylor JL, Epstein RA, McPheeters ML. Transition care for children with special health care needs. Pediatrics. 2014;134(5):900–8. https://doi.org/10.1542/peds.2014-1909.
9. Tilton AH. Transition of children with neurological disorders. Curr Neurol Neurosci Rep. 2018;18(4):14. https://doi.org/10.1007/s11910-018-0822-x.

10. Menon D, Gonorazky HD, Dowling JJ, et al. Clinical profile and multidisciplinary needs of patients with neuromuscular disorders transitioning from paediatric to adult care. Neuromuscul Disord. 2022;32(3):206–12. https://doi.org/10.1016/j.nmd.2021.12.002.

11. McGovern E, Pringsheim T, Medina A, et al. Transitional care for young people with neurological disorders: a scoping review with a focus on patients with movement disorders. Mov Disord. 2021;36(6):1316–24. https://doi.org/10.1002/mds.28381.

12. Reiss JG, Gibson RW, Walker LR. Health care transition: youth, family, and provider perspectives. Pediatrics. 2005;115(1):112–20. https://doi.org/10.1542/peds.2004-1321.

13. Transition of care provided for adolescents with special health care needs. American Academy of Pediatrics Committee on Children with Disabilities and Committee on Adolescence. Pediatrics. 1996;98(6 Pt 1):1203–6. https://www.ncbi.nlm.nih.gov/pubmed/8951283.

14. Oskoui M, Wolfson C. Current practice and views of neurologists on the transition from pediatric to adult care. J Child Neurol. 2012;27(12):1553–8. https://doi.org/10.1177/0883073812439249.

15. Transition to adult care for youth with special health care needs. Paediatr Child Health. 2007;12(9):785–93. https://doi.org/10.1093/pch/12.9.785.

16. Pai ALH, Ostendorf HM. Treatment adherence in adolescents and young adults affected by chronic illness during the health care transition from pediatric to adult health care: a literature review. Child Health Care. 2011;40(1):16–33. https://doi.org/10.1080/02739615.2011.537934.

17. Cole R, Ashok D, Razack A, Azaz A, Sebastian S. Evaluation of outcomes in adolescent inflammatory bowel disease patients following transfer from pediatric to adult health care services: case for transition. J Adolesc Health. 2015;57(2):212–7. https://doi.org/10.1016/j.jadohealth.2015.04.012.

18. White PH. Access to health care: health insurance considerations for young adults with special health care needs/disabilities. Pediatrics. 2002;110(6 Pt 2):1328–35. (In eng).

19. Williams RG. Fumbling the handoff: managing the transition to adult care for adolescents with chronic conditions. J Adolesc Health. 2009;44(4):307–8. (In eng). https://doi.org/10.1016/j.jadohealth.2009.01.001.

20. Watson AR. Non-compliance and transfer from paediatric to adult transplant unit. Pediatr Nephrol. 2000;14(6):469–72. https://doi.org/10.1007/s004670050794.

21. Annunziato RA, Emre S, Shneider B, Barton C, Dugan CA, Shemesh E. Adherence and medical outcomes in pediatric liver transplant recipients who transition to adult services. Pediatr Transplant. 2007;11(6):608–14. (In eng). https://doi.org/10.1111/j.1399-3046.2007.00689.x.

22. Onofri A, Tan H-L, Cherchi C, et al. Transition to adult care in young people with neuromuscular disease on non-invasive ventilation. Ital J Pediatr. 2019;45(1):90. https://doi.org/10.1186/s13052-019-0677-z.

23. Erikson EH (1968). Identity: youth and crisis. Norton & Co.

24. Wan HWY, Carey KA, D'Silva A, Kasparian NA, Farrar MA. "Getting ready for the adult world": how adults with spinal muscular atrophy perceive and experience healthcare, transition and well-being. Orphanet J Rare Dis. 2019;14(1):74. https://doi.org/10.1186/s13023-019-1052-2.

25. Yamaguchi M, Suzuki M. Becoming a back-up carer: parenting sons with Duchenne muscular dystrophy transitioning into adulthood. Neuromuscul Disord. 2015;25(1):85–93. https://doi.org/10.1016/j.nmd.2014.09.001.

26. Gray WN, Schaefer MR, Resmini-Rawlinson A, Wagoner ST. Barriers to transition from pediatric to adult care: a systematic review. J Pediatr Psychol. 2018;43(5):488–502. https://doi.org/10.1093/jpepsy/jsx142.

27. Sparud-Lundin C, Berghammer M, Moons P, Bratt EL. Health care providers' attitudes towards transfer and transition in young persons with long term illness—a web-based survey. BMC Health Serv Res. 2017;17(1):260. https://doi.org/10.1186/s12913-017-2192-5.

28. Nurre E, Smith AW, Jenkins A, Horewitz D, Modi AC. Barriers and facilitators to developing transition clinics for adolescents and young adults with chronic conditions. Clin Pediatr (Phila). 2019;58(13):1444–8. https://doi.org/10.1177/0009922819875533.

29. Cheng PC, Panitch HB, Hansen-Flaschen J. Transition of patients with neuromuscular disease and chronic ventilator-dependent respiratory failure from pediatric to adult pulmonary care. Paediatr Respir Rev. 2020;33:3–8. https://doi.org/10.1016/j.prrv.2019.03.005.
30. American Academy of Pediatrics Committee on Children With Disabilities. The role of the pediatrician in transitioning children and adolescents with developmental disabilities and chronic illnesses from school to work or college. American Academy of Pediatrics. Committee on Children With Disabilities. Pediatrics. 2000;106(4):854–6. https://doi.org/10.1542/peds.106.4.854.
31. Hunt S, Sharma N. Pediatric to adult-care transitions in childhood-onset chronic disease: hospitalist perspectives. J Hosp Med. 2013;8(11):627–30. https://doi.org/10.1002/jhm.2091.
32. Oskoui M, Wolfson C. Treatment comfort of adult neurologists in childhood onset conditions. Can J Neurol Sci. 2012;39(2):202–5. https://doi.org/10.1017/s0317167100013238.
33. Transition G. Six core elements of health care transition. https://www.gottransition.org/six-core-elements/.
34. Sawicki GS, Lukens-Bull K, Yin X, et al. Measuring the transition readiness of youth with special healthcare needs: validation of the TRAQ—Transition Readiness Assessment Questionnaire. J Pediatr Psychol. 2011;36(2):160–71. (In eng). https://doi.org/10.1093/jpepsy/jsp128.
35. De Cunto CL, Eymann A, Britos ML, et al. Cross-cultural adaptation of the Transition Readiness Assessment Questionnaire to Argentinian Spanish. Arch Argent Pediatr. 2017;115(2):181–7. https://doi.org/10.5546/aap.2017.eng.181.
36. Kiziler E, Yildiz D, Eren Fidanci B. Validation of Transition Readiness Assessment Questionnaire in Turkish adolescents with diabetes. Balkan Med J. 2018;35(1):93–100. https://doi.org/10.4274/balkanmedj.2016.1415.
37. Perica MS, Mayer M, Bukovac LT. Readiness for transition–Croatian version and pilot evaluation of the Transition Readiness Assessment Questionnaire (TRAQ) in rheumatologic patients. Ann Rheum Dis. 2019;2019(78):1349–50.
38. Culen C, Herle M, König M, et al. Be on TRAQ—cross-cultural adaptation of the Transition Readiness Assessment Questionnaire (TRAQ 5.0) and pilot testing of the German Version (TRAQ-GV-15). J Transit Med. 2019;1. https://doi.org/10.1515/jtm-2018-0005.
39. Chapados P, Aramideh J, Lamore K, et al. Getting ready for transition to adult care: tool validation and multi-informant strategy using the Transition Readiness Assessment Questionnaire in pediatrics. Child Care Health Dev. 2021;47(5):645–53. https://doi.org/10.1111/cch.12872.
40. Carlsen K, Haddad N, Gordon J, et al. Self-efficacy and resilience are useful predictors of transition readiness scores in adolescents with inflammatory bowel diseases. Inflamm Bowel Dis. 2017;23(3):341–6. (In eng). https://doi.org/10.1097/mib.0000000000001038.
41. Stewart KT, Chahal N, Kovacs AH, et al. Readiness for transition to adult health care for young adolescents with congenital heart disease. Pediatr Cardiol. 2017;38(4):778–86. (In eng). https://doi.org/10.1007/s00246-017-1580-2.
42. Pereira Júnior ADC, Castilho ECD, Borges TL, Santos PLD, Carvalho AMP, Miasso AI. An integrative review of non-pharmacological therapeutic interventions in children with mental health problems. Compr Child Adolesc Nurs. 2020;43(4):245–59. (In eng). https://doi.org/10.1080/24694193.2019.1621961.
43. Corsello A, Pugliese D, Bracci F, et al. Transition of inflammatory bowel disease patients from pediatric to adult care: an observational study on a joint-visits approach. Ital J Pediatr. 2021;47(1):18. (In eng). https://doi.org/10.1186/s13052-021-00977-x.
44. Rosen D, Annunziato R, Colombel JF, Dubinsky M, Benkov K. Transition of inflammatory bowel disease care: assessment of transition readiness factors and disease outcomes in a young adult population. Inflamm Bowel Dis. 2016;22(3):702–8. (In eng). https://doi.org/10.1097/mib.0000000000000633.
45. Takeuchi J, Yanagimoto Y, Sato Y, et al. Efficacious interventions for improving the transition readiness of adolescents and young adult patients with chronic illness: a narrative review

of randomized control trials assessed with the transition readiness assessment questionnaire. Front Pediatr. 2022;10:983367. (In eng). https://doi.org/10.3389/fped.2022.983367.

46. Crowley R, Wolfe I, Lock K, McKee M. Improving the transition between paediatric and adult healthcare: a systematic review. Arch Dis Child. 2011;96(6):548–53. (In eng). https://doi.org/10.1136/adc.2010.202473.

47. Haarbauer-Krupa J, Alexander NM, Mee L, et al. Readiness for transition and health-care satisfaction in adolescents with complex medical conditions. Child Care Health Dev. 2019;45(3):463–71. (In eng). https://doi.org/10.1111/cch.12656.

Chapter 9
Respiratory Care of the Individual with Muscular Dystrophy

Sherri Lynne Katz and Marielena Linda DiBartolo

Disease Presentation and Progression in Muscular Dystrophy

Muscular dystrophy (MD) refers to a group of inherited diseases resulting in progressive muscular weakness. They are caused by defects intrinsic to the muscle structure and result in muscle breakdown [1]. These diseases vary in their inheritance, prevalence, presentation, and course (see Table 9.1). In general, the muscular dystrophies are considered in two groups: those that are congenital (presenting in the newborn period) and those that present later. This chapter will discuss respiratory management for those diseases which involve the respiratory musculature, with Duchenne muscular dystrophy (DMD), the most common and best studied, presented as the primary model.

S. L. Katz (✉)
Children's Hospital of Eastern Ontario, Ottawa, ON, Canada

Children's Hospital of Eastern Ontario Research Institute, Ottawa, ON, Canada

University of Ottawa, Ottawa, ON, Canada
e-mail: skatz@cheo.on.ca

M. L. DiBartolo
Children's Hospital of Eastern Ontario, Ottawa, ON, Canada

University of Ottawa, Ottawa, ON, Canada
e-mail: mdibartolo@cheo.on.ca

© The Author(s), under exclusive license to Springer Nature Switzerland AG 2024
N. Lechtzin (ed.), *Pulmonary Complications of Neuromuscular Disease*, Respiratory Medicine, https://doi.org/10.1007/978-3-031-65335-3_9

Table 9.1 Summary of muscular dystrophies

Name	Gene/protein	Inheritance	Prevalence	Extraskeletal systems involved			
				Respiratory	Cardiac	Bulbar	CNS (cognition, seizures)
DMD	Dystrophin	X-linked	1/3500–5000 males	X	X	X	X
Becker MD	Dystrophin	X-linked	1/7250 males	X	X	X	X
Myotonic dystrophy	Tri-nucleotide repeat on chromosome 19 or 3	AD	14/100,000 worldwide (189/100,000 in Saguenay region of Quebec)	X	X	X	X
Fascioscapular-humeral MD	Contraction of D4Z4/ SMCHD1/DNMT3B	AD/de novo Incomplete penetrance	1/8–20,000	Uncommon	Uncommon	X	X
Limb-girdle MD	20 subtypes	AR	1/14,500– 123,000	X	X		
Oculopharyngeal MD		AD	1/1000 in QC, 1/100,000 worldwide			X	Uncommon
Congenital MDs							
Ulrich/Bethlem MD	Collagen VI	AD and AR		X			
Merosin- deficient	Merosin	AR		X			X
Fukuyama/muscle-eye-brain/Walker-Warburg	Dystroglycans	AR		X	X		X

References for table [1–6]. *AD* autosomal dominant, *AR* autosomal recessive, *CNS* central nervous system, *DMD* Duchenne muscular dystrophy, *MD* muscular dystrophy

Presentation

By definition, the congenital MD presents with muscle weakness at birth or in early infancy, though with a wide range of phenotypes [7]. DMD typically presents in early childhood, with delay in gross motor milestones including independent sitting, rising, and standing [1]. The Gowers sign, whereby an individual pushes themselves from prone to A-frame position and then uses their hands to "walk up" their legs to raise themselves to a standing position, is classically described in DMD (see Fig. 9.1) [8]. This sign can, however, present in any condition associated with weakness of the pelvic girdle or proximal lower limbs, including other MD, neuromuscular disorders, and rheumatologic disorders [8]. A further classic physical examination finding is pseudohypertrophy of the calf muscles (relative to the atrophy of the proximal lower limb muscles), seen in Duchenne and Becker MD [9].

Given the X-linked inheritance, both Duchenne and Becker MD predominantly affect males, though female carriers may show mild symptoms based on the pattern of X-inactivation [10, 11]. Boys with DMD are more severely affected and generally diagnosed by age 4 years [10]. Boys with Becker MD present later, around age 8 years, with much less rapid and more variable presentation and progression [10].

Progression

Generally, boys with DMD lose ambulation in early adolescence (30% by 10 years, 90% by 15 years) [12, 13] and often require ventilatory support for nocturnal hypoventilation in later adolescence (20–40% by 20 years) [14, 15].

DMD generally has a predictable progression. Respiratory progression generally tracks with changes in ambulation. Development of cardiac problems, however, is less predictable, with little genotypic-phenotypic correlation.

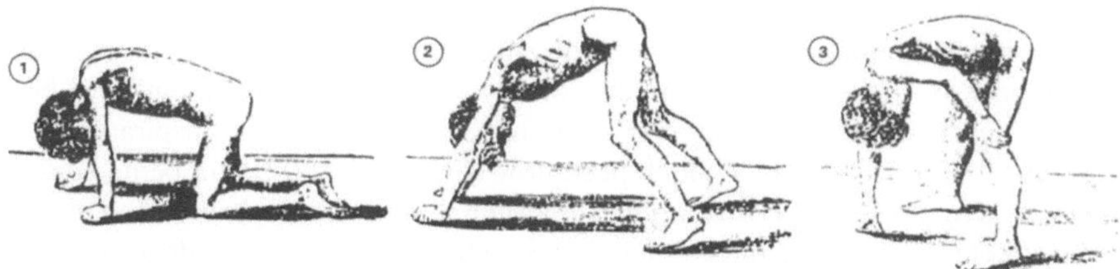

Fig. 9.1 Depiction of Gowers sign. (By William Richard Gowers (1845–1915)—Gowers W. R. Clinical lecture on pseudohypertrophic muscular paralysis. Lancet 1879; ii, 73–5. Public Domain, https://commons.wikimedia.org/w/index.php?curid=6072589 accessed June 6, 2023)

Morbidity and Mortality

While both respiratory failure and cardiomyopathy are leading causes of death in DMD, with more intensive management of respiratory complications, cardiac dysfunction has become the major limitation to survival, accounting for 30–50% of deaths [16]. Non-cardiopulmonary causes account for up to 20% of deaths and include injury-related pulmonary embolism, gastrointestinal complications, and stroke [17].

Median life expectancy remains in the third decade, though is increasing over time with greater use of steroid therapy, management of respiratory failure, and introduction of emerging treatments. Median life expectancy without ventilatory support is reported to be 19 years and 30 years with ventilatory support. Presented differently, mortality by age 20 years is reported in up to 16% of individuals with DMD, and among those surviving to adulthood, mortality was as high as 60% by age 30 years [18–20].

Pathophysiology of Respiratory Problems in MD

Weak Cough/Atelectasis/Pneumonia

As weakness of the respiratory muscles progresses, cough becomes inefficient and ineffective. In DMD, weakness of the expiratory muscles, as demonstrated by reduction in the gastric pressure during cough (Pgas) develops first. Weakness of the inspiratory muscles, particularly the diaphragm, occurs later [21]. The result is reduced cough force, because of both decreased expiratory muscle strength and reduced total lung capacity due to inadequate inspiratory muscle strength. Contractures of the chest wall, respiratory muscle fibrosis, and kyphoscoliosis all reduce chest wall compliance, and these mechanical disadvantages increase the load on respiratory muscles [22]. Finally, atelectasis contributes to lower lung volumes and cough strength by reducing compliance of the lung [22].

These factors all result in decreased ability to clear airway secretions and put children with MD at risk of pneumonia and acute respiratory failure. Respiratory illnesses are the most common cause of hospitalization and death in congenital MD and remain an important cause of morbidity and mortality in DMD [23]. Frequency of episodes of pneumonia and number of days of antibiotic treatment have been found to correlate with measures of pulmonary function, with an inspiratory vital capacity (IVC) <1.1 L and a cough peak flow (CPF) of <160 L/min being specific and sensitive thresholds to discriminate between those individuals who had already been affected by a severe infection and those who had not [24]. Incidence of pneumonia is reported to be 0.8 episodes/year in DMD and mixed neuromuscular populations [24, 25]. It is important to recognize that due to respiratory muscle weakness, individuals may not present with typical signs of increased work of breathing as one would typically expect for severe illness and impending respiratory failure [7]. Thus, a low threshold for further investigation (chest X-ray, blood gas) is important.

Sleep Disordered Breathing/Diurnal Respiratory Failure

As upper airway and respiratory muscles weaken, maintenance of airway patency and ventilation become more challenging, especially during sleep. With the loss of tone in pharyngeal and intercostal muscles during sleep, particularly in REM, obstructive sleep apnea (OSA) may develop before hypoventilation. This risk increases with the presence of obesity which often can result from steroid treatment. Adenotonsillar hypertrophy can also contribute to the risk of OSA, particularly in young children. OSA may present with typical symptoms of snoring and parent-witnessed obstruction. However, clinical symptoms are not a reliable predictor of OSA in this population, and so a high degree of suspicion should be maintained. The presence of OSA can also contribute to hypoventilation.

The constellation of deficits that contribute to weak cough (diaphragmatic weakness, poor chest wall compliance due to muscle fibrosis and kyphoscoliosis) also results in hypoventilation. The supine position, in the setting of diaphragmatic weakness, further impairs ventilation due to reduced vital capacity [26]. In DMD, development of nocturnal hypoventilation typically follows loss of ambulation. In the congenital MDs, respiratory failure may occur early (by age 10 years), while individuals are still ambulatory, particularly in those conditions where early diaphragmatic weakness is a key feature (e.g., Ulrich MD) [7]. There is emerging evidence that suggests that variations in B-adrenergic genotype may influence the age at which boys with DMD develop nocturnal hypoventilation [27]. Morning headaches can be a sign of nocturnal hypoventilation, though again individuals may be relatively asymptomatic [28]. Once forced vital capacity (FVC) drops below 50–60% predicted, assessment for hypoventilation becomes especially important [7, 29, 30]. As pulmonary function worsens, hypoventilation then progresses to impact waking hours.

Multi-disciplinary Aspects of Care That Impact the Respiratory System

As MD is a progressive condition that affects many organ systems, its management should therefore address the multi-system problems that arise, as each has a significant impact on health. Ideally, this should be provided in the context of a multi-disciplinary clinic, where there is access to a range of specialists in each aspect of the disease, who communicate with each other to provide coordinated, multi-faceted, patient-centered care.

Cardiac

Cardiac problems, including heart failure secondary to cardiomyopathy and resultant arrhythmia, are major sources of morbidity and mortality for individuals with DMD, particularly since respiratory supports help manage respiratory failure [31]. A recent systematic review reported, based on registry data, that 70% of individuals with DMD have cardiomyopathy by 15 years of age and almost all do by age 20 years [20]. Thirty to fifty percent of DMD-related mortality is estimated to be attributable to cardiac disease [16].

Early diagnosis and management are critical for improving quality of life and longevity, but signs and symptoms of cardiac disease may be subtle and insidious [32]. Proactive screening is recommended, beginning in the ambulatory and early non-ambulatory stage. Baseline cardiac assessment should include an electrocardiogram and echocardiogram to evaluate function and identify any anatomical abnormalities that could affect long-term health [32]. An annual cardiac assessment and echocardiogram is recommended for asymptomatic individuals, particularly after age 10, when the risk of left ventricular dysfunction increases [32]. Cardiac MRI is recommended as the gold standard non-invasive test for assessing cardiac function in individuals who can cooperate for the procedure without the need for sedation. An electrocardiogram and a cardiac imaging are also recommended prior to any major surgical procedures [33].

Since progressive myocardial fibrosis leads to ventricular dysfunction, with progression to the late ambulatory stage, more frequent cardiac monitoring is recommended. Surveillance at this stage should also include periodic 24-h Holter monitoring given the increased risk of arrhythmia [32]. For individuals with heart failure and ejection fraction below 35%, placement of an implantable defibrillator should be considered [32].

Angiotensin-converting enzyme (ACE) inhibitors, angiotensin receptor blockers (ARB), beta-blockers, and/or aldosterone agonists may be used to treat cardiac dysfunction. In many cases, ACE and ARB may be considered for prophylactic therapy in asymptomatic individuals without evidence of cardiomyopathy to improve long-term cardiovascular outcomes, including longer survival and lower rates of hospitalization for heart failure [16, 34]. Beta-blockers and/or aldosterone agonists are often started when systolic dysfunction develops [16]. The use of implantable cardioverter defibrillators and ventricular assist devices may also be considered in individuals with advanced cardiac disease [16]. Although there is variability in the implementation of cardiac therapies in this population, it is clear that attention to cardiac complications and possible treatments are critical to survival of individuals with DMD.

Musculoskeletal Care

Maintenance of ambulation and motor function and avoidance of development of scoliosis, bone loss, and joint contractures are the main goals of musculoskeletal care [32]. The care team for this aspect of DMD may include physiotherapists, occupational therapists, physiatrists, neurologists, endocrinologists, and/or orthopedic surgeons [35]. In the ambulatory individual, foot surgery to improve varus positioning and/or surgery on the Achilles tendon to improve the range of dorsiflexion may assist in improving gait; clinical evaluation for scoliosis should be done annually, with X-rays if there are any concerns noted [32]. In non-ambulatory individuals, inspection of the spine should be performed with each clinical encounter, and a spine radiograph should be obtained when the individual first becomes non-ambulant and/or if clinical evaluation is challenging because of obesity. Spine X-rays are recommended every 6 months for individuals who are not yet skeletally mature and then annually after skeletal maturity in the late non-ambulatory stage because of the higher likelihood of progression of scoliosis [35].

In the current era, where many individuals with DMD are treated with corticosteroids, progression of scoliosis to the point of needing surgical intervention is less common. Steroid treatment prolongs the time that individuals are ambulant and may slow progression of scoliosis. Nonetheless, posterior spinal fusion is recommended for individuals who are non-ambulatory and who have a spinal curve in the sitting position greater than 20–30°, who have not reached puberty and who have not been treated with corticosteroids [32]. In this select population, surgical intervention benefits function, sitting balance and tolerance, and quality of life, while reducing pain and preventing further progression of scoliosis.

Maintenance of bone health is also critical to avoid osteoporosis and fractures, particularly in individuals treated with corticosteroids [36]. Progressive myopathy also predisposes to osteoporosis which increases fracture risk. Vertebral fractures may be asymptomatic but can result in chronic back pain and spine deformity if they are not treated. Low-trauma long bone fractures can result in loss of ambulation, and in rare instances have been associated with fat embolism syndrome, which can be fatal.

Bone mineral density measurement is recommended annually to monitor the overall trajectory of bone health and fragility in individuals with DMD and can be used to guide the frequency of spinal imaging, as well as the onset of treatment [36]. Monitoring of 25-hydroxyvitamin D levels and assessment of calcium intake annually can also be helpful for bone health assessment.

Intravenous bisphosphonate treatment should be initiated for those with symptomatic and asymptomatic fractures and/or evidence of bone loss [37]. Intravenous zoledronic acid has been shown to improve bone mineral density compared to placebo in boys with DMD [37]. Treatment should be guided by an expert in the management of osteoporosis.

Swallowing and Nutrition

Nutrition should be optimized in individuals with DMD to meet metabolic demands and avoid catabolism. Obesity, however, should be avoided as this can increase strain on the respiratory system and predisposition to sleep disordered breathing.

The delivery of nutrition must be achieved safely, with attention to oromotor skills so that aspiration is prevented [1]. In the presence of coughing or choking with feeds, a videofluoroscopic feeding study may be useful to determine safety of feeding of different textures. In instances where oral feeding is not safe, or insufficient to meet nutritional needs, supplementary tube feeding may be considered. The use of a gastrostomy tube is preferred over nasogastric feeds where possible, both for individual comfort and reduced risk of tube dislodgement causing aspiration. A gastrostomy tube, however, requires sedation or anesthetic for insertion, and the risks inherent in undertaking such a procedure must also be weighed against benefit.

Transition to Adult Care

The process of transition from pediatric to adult care is best described as a continuum rather than an event [38, 39]. Preparation is key to success and needs to begin early. Establishment of the individual's understanding of their disease and autonomy in medical care as well as participation in medical appointments are early steps in the transition process. This should start in early adolescence, depending on maturity and the developmental stage [39]. It is also important for adolescents and their families to understand the infrastructure for care at adult institutions, which may differ substantially from pediatric clinics in the multi-disciplinary care environment, psychosocial supports, decision-making and consent processes, and degree of family involvement [38, 40]. Parents may also find it difficult to relinquish decision-making to the young adult and allow the adolescent their independence. A contingency plan for a substitute decision-maker should, however, be put in place. Goals and any desired limitations of care should be discussed and documented prior to transition to adult care. Discussion of issues relevant to adolescents and young adults including sexuality, fertility, career, and employment counseling should begin with the pediatric team and be continued in adult care [40].

There are several models for transition of care from other chronic diseases that have been shown to be successful and can be emulated in neuromuscular disease. These include (1) patient education to ensure a full understanding of their medical condition, (2) combined or "overlap" clinics with the presence of both pediatric and adult care providers, and (3) a transition coordinator who ensures transfer of the necessary health information and serves as a liaison between pediatric and adult care teams [40].

Clinical Respiratory Assessment of the Individual with MD

Clinical evaluation of respiratory health for individuals with neuromuscular conditions relies on a combination of symptom assessment and physical examination findings, along with daytime and nocturnal laboratory tests. Decline in health may be gradual and difficult to discern without objective health measures evaluated for change over time.

History

Medical history should focus on symptoms that may indicate weak cough and predilection to poor tolerance of respiratory infections, as well as those that help identify the presence of sleep disordered breathing. A thorough medical history may also identify changes in the function of other systems that impact on the respiratory system.

Symptoms of Weak Cough

As cough becomes weaker, clearance of airway secretions becomes a greater challenge. This may first manifest at times of increased secretion burden, as occurs with intercurrent respiratory infections [30]. Information on how upper respiratory tract infections are handled may therefore be very telling. The duration of symptoms and interventions required are important markers of severity and ability to handle respiratory stressors. Episodes that are more severe may result in physician visits, the need for antibiotics, and/or hospitalization.

With disease progression, poor handling of secretions may become a constant problem. Individuals with neuromuscular disease may describe a rattling in the back of their throat and/or a feeling that secretions feel stuck in their chest and difficult to clear after coughing.

Symptoms of Sleep Disordered Breathing

Detection of nocturnal hypoventilation, the most common type of sleep disordered breathing which manifests in neuromuscular disease, can be difficult [41]. Symptoms develop insidiously and are not specific. In many cases, individuals with slower disease progression may be asymptomatic, and symptoms may only be appreciated retrospectively once sleep disordered breathing is treated [41]. Some symptoms, including daytime fatigue and poor growth may be attributed to disease progression rather than being identified as being related to nocturnal hypoventilation. A "fear of going to sleep" may be erroneously ascribed to anxiety. Morning headaches are a more specific flag for nocturnal hypoventilation and can be attributed to the presence of hypercapnia.

Obstructive sleep apnea may occur in neuromuscular conditions that result in hypotonia of the upper airway [42]. This may be identifiable by the presence of snoring and/or apneas followed by a gasp. It may also come to attention due to identification of daytime fatigue and/or morning headaches.

Physical Examination

Physical examination begins with assessment of vital signs. Individuals who have weak respiratory muscles may not be able to take deep breaths, resulting in a rapid shallow breathing pattern with tachypnea [43]. Evaluation of oxygen saturation becomes very important to identify changes in respiratory status in such individuals [32]. End-tidal or transcutaneous carbon dioxide measurements are also useful clinical measurements that can be part of a physical examination and may identify developing respiratory failure [32].

The use of accessory muscles of respiration such as tracheal tug and intercostal or subcostal indrawing may indicate increased work of breathing, although with advanced disease this may not be visible, as weak muscles may not be able to effect the increased muscle effort required. A paradoxical respiratory pattern may indicate a relative imbalance of weakness of different respiratory muscle groups [43].

Inspection of the chest wall provides information on fixed restriction of the ribcage, such as with kyphoscoliosis. Assessment of chest wall excursion is also useful to assess motion of the chest wall. Auscultation of the lung fields may identify areas of atelectasis or consolidation with decreased air entry or crackles.

A qualitative evaluation of cough strength may supplement objective measures and may be the sole indicator in individuals who are unable to perform pulmonary function tests [44]. Asking the individual to cough as hard as they can will identify those who are unable to produce a cough of sufficient strength to clear airway secretions.

Finally, examination of other organ systems may uncover other health issues that impact the respiratory system. Growth failure in children can indicate a negative energy balance due to either inadequate intake or increased energy expenditure which may be due to cardiorespiratory difficulties [1]. Obesity may predispose to obstructive sleep apnea [42]. The presence of nasal mucosal edema and/or adenotonsillar hypertrophy may also contribute to upper airway obstruction resulting in obstructive sleep apnea [42]. The presence of heart murmurs, hepatomegaly, and/or pedal edema may indicate the presence of cardiomyopathy [32]. Finally, increasing kyphoscoliosis may cause strain on the respiratory system by limiting expansion of the chest wall with respiration [32].

Pulmonary Function Testing

Individuals with neuromuscular disease develop a restrictive pattern on pulmonary function testing whereby lung volumes are decreased in proportion to airflow [45]. Forced vital capacity (FVC) is the lung function parameter most closely associated with morbidity and mortality [45–47]. Longitudinal assessment of FVC percent predicted allows identification of more rapid decline that can be a harbinger of disease progression. FVC below 1 L has been associated with substantially increased mortality [45, 46, 48]. Total lung capacity declines over time, and residual volume-to-total lung capacity ratio increases as expiratory muscle weakness develops with inability to empty the lungs during expiration [47]. A decrease of greater than 20% in supine as compared to sitting FVC is consistent with diaphragmatic weakness and may be an indicator of the need to screen for sleep disordered breathing [7].

Cough strength is most commonly assessed with cough peak flow (CPF), in L/min of expiratory flow [45]. In children 12 years and older, as well as in adults, a CPF below 270 L/min is indicative of an individual at risk of impaired airway clearance during respiratory infections and below 160 L/min is indicative of poor airway clearance [30, 49]. These thresholds are often utilized to determine the need to initiate airway clearance therapies. In younger children, percent-predicted CPF are available by age and sex, which can be useful to identify reduced cough strength [50].

Respiratory muscle strength can be assessed with surrogate measures, including maximal inspiratory and expiratory pressures (MIP, MEP). These measures, however, depend on sustained effort by the participant, which can be challenging for individuals with muscle weakness [45]. Decline in MIP and MEP may be a sensitive measure of respiratory muscle weakness as these values may be low even if CPF and FVC are still in the normal range [45]. Sniff nasal pressure is an alternate measure of respiratory muscle strength which can be used for longitudinal assessment [45]. Together with FVC percent predicted, sniff nasal pressure has been proposed to best predict the overall decline in respiratory function [21].

Finally, chest wall distensibility can be assessed by maximal inspiratory capacity (MIC), a measure of the amount of air that can fill the lungs at end inspiration after an assisted breath-stacking or lung volume recruitment maneuver [51]. The difference between the MIC and vital capacity is indicative of distensibility of the chest wall with a lung volume recruitment maneuver [52].

Nocturnal Gas Exchange Assessment

Polysomnography is the gold standard test for sleep disordered breathing assessment in neuromuscular disease, which provides the most comprehensive evaluation of gas exchange, sleep architecture, and respiratory pattern [53]. It is used to determine whether obstructive or central sleep apnea and nocturnal hypoventilation are present. Nocturnal hypoventilation on polysomnography in adults has been defined by the American Academy of Sleep Medicine (AASM) as an arterial pCO_2 (or surrogate) during sleep greater than 55 mmHg for at least 10 min and/or an increase in 10 mmHg of pCO_2 from baseline awake supine value to a value exceeding 50 mmHg for at least 10 min [54]. In children, nocturnal hypoventilation is defined by a carbon dioxide measurement above 50 mmHg for at least 25% of total sleep time, according to the AASM [54]. Recently, there has been an interest in applying a less stringent definition of hypoventilation in individuals with neuromuscular disease who may benefit from intervention sooner [32]. Nonetheless, the identification of nocturnal hypoventilation is an indication for initiation of nocturnal respiratory support with non-invasive ventilation.

In resource-limited settings, polysomnography may not be readily available. In such instances, at-home polygraphy or dual monitoring of oxygen saturation and carbon dioxide may be used to assess for impairments in nocturnal gas exchange [30, 32, 55]. Overnight oximetry may also be used as a screening tool to assess for nocturnal hypoventilation, although it is not very sensitive as periods of hypercapnia may occur without desaturation [30, 56, 57].

Frequency of Clinical Evaluation

Respiratory

Clinical evaluations provide opportunities to develop relationships with children and families, give anticipatory guidance, and perform clinical evaluations that inform treatment plans. The frequency of assessment will increase with advancing disease, as the need for respiratory interventions increases [32].

While ambulatory, children and caregivers should be educated about respiratory complications that are associated with MD [38]. Immunizations should be provided to prevent infection whenever possible. These may include pneumococcal, inactive influenza and SARS-CoV2 vaccines, as well as immunization with respiratory syncytial virus monoclonal antibody [32]. Pulmonary function testing can be performed beginning at age 6 years and should be monitored annually for ambulatory individuals [32]. Assessment of gas exchange during sleep may also be considered if there are symptoms of sleep disordered breathing and/or in the presence of obesity [30, 32].

In non-ambulatory individuals, it is recommended that pulmonary function testing is performed every 6 months [32]. This can include measurement of forced vital capacity, maximal inspiratory and expiratory pressures, and peak cough flow [32]. Oxygen saturation and carbon dioxide (end-tidal or transcutaneous) can also be evaluated at each clinic visit. Polysomnography can be considered if clinically indicated and may be helpful as a preoperative evaluation if a surgical procedure is planned and pulmonary function testing cannot be performed [32]. Although it is difficult to predict the presence of sleep disordered breathing and the need for nocturnal respiratory support based on daytime clinical parameters, evaluation of nocturnal gas exchange is recommended at a minimum when FVC is <50% predicted and/or the absolute value of MIP is <60 mmHg, in the presence of daytime hypercapnia (CO_2 >45 mmHg) and/or if oxygen saturation is <95% in room air [32]. A high index of suspicion for sleep disordered breathing is prudent, and nocturnal gas exchange evaluation should be considered with less obvious markers of the presence of nocturnal hypoventilation and/or in a child who has shown clinical deterioration [30, 40, 41].

For non-ambulatory individuals with declining pulmonary function, attention should be paid to the presence of daytime fatigue, dyspnea, difficulty concentrating, and/or presence of morning headaches [32, 41]. These symptoms may indicate the need for daytime-assisted ventilation. Individuals with very low FVC (<680 mL) are at particularly high risk of diurnal respiratory failure [32].

Cardiac

Cardiovascular morbidity, in particular cardiomyopathy, is a significant cause of morbidity and mortality in boys with MD. Proactive evaluation by a cardiologist is recommended, especially since signs and symptoms of cardiac dysfunction may be subtle in the non-ambulatory individual [32]. It is recommended that individuals with MD undergo baseline electrocardiogram and non-invasive imaging to screen for underlying anatomical abnormalities that could contribute to health problems [32]. Echocardiography is the primary tool of cardiac evaluation in young children. Cardiac MRI can also be used to assess cardiac function [16]. Until the age of 10, annual evaluation with electrocardiogram and non-invasive imaging is recommended. Cardiac evaluation after the age of 10 should occur at least annually due to the increased risk of left ventricular dysfunction, and frequency should increase if there are any symptoms of heart failure or evidence of cardiac dysfunction on testing [32]. Prior to any surgical procedure, cardiac function assessment is also recommended [32].

As there is an increased risk of cardiac rhythm abnormalities, individuals with DMD should be screened with periodic 24-h Holter monitoring. The optimal frequency of monitoring is unclear but may be reasonable to perform annually in the presence of left ventricular dysfunction or development of myocardial fibrosis [16, 32].

Respiratory Management of MD

General

In general, treatments are supportive and aimed at health maintenance with optimized nutrition, improvement of airway clearance, and management of hypoventilation. A multi-disciplinary approach is essential as outlined above. There are currently no specific, disease-modifying therapies available as standard of care for most of the MDs, except for DMD.

Vaccinations/Anticipatory Guidance

Children with MD should receive routine childhood immunizations—there is no contraindication to receiving live vaccines. In addition, children should be treated with annual influenza vaccine, as well as 23-valent pneumococcal polysaccharide vaccine (PPSV23) [7, 32]. Treatment with RSV prophylaxis should be considered for children under 2 years of age. Early initiation of antibiotics can also help prevent severe respiratory infections [7].

Corticosteroids

Steroid (prednisone, deflazacort) use for >1 year has been found to improve/delay progression of muscle weakness with a delay in loss of ambulation as well as upper limb milestones in DMD [15, 58]. On average, males with DMD not treated with steroids become non-ambulatory at age 10, whereas males treated with at least 5 years of steroids become non-ambulatory at age 13. There is evidence from observational studies that suggest that deflazacort may be associated with later age of loss of ambulation than prednisone [12]. Treatment with steroids can improve and prevent decline of pulmonary function, with higher peak forced vital capacity and peak expiratory flow values, later onset of decline, and slower rate of decline [48, 59]. Given that risk of death is fourfold greater when forced vital capacity is less than 1 L (5-year survival drops to 8%) [46], and steroids delay progressive loss of lung function to this threshold, there is improvement in survival with steroid therapy [15]. Steroids may also slow the development of scoliosis and reduce the need for scoliosis surgery by age 18 [58]. In addition, individuals treated with steroids were less likely to need ventilatory support [60]. Unfortunately, the use of steroids is associated with significant potential side effects, including obesity, hypertension, hyperglycemia, osteopenia, and adrenal suppression [31]. Work is underway to identify alternatives (e.g., Vamolarone, a synthetic steroid) that minimize these complications. The use of systemic steroids is not currently indicated for other MD [31].

Secretion Management

An impaired ability to cough and clear secretions increases the risk of atelectasis and pneumonia. Therapies that enhance airway clearance can improve cough efficacy, thereby assisting with secretion removal, maintenance of compliance, and distensibility of the chest wall and may slow the decline in pulmonary function. Proximal airway clearance therapies are recommended in clinical care guidelines to be used regularly when cough peak flow is reduced (<270 L/min in individuals 12 years or older), when forced vital capacity falls below 40–60% and if there is subjective evidence of a weak cough [30, 32, 40, 61, 62]. Introduction of airway clearance therapies is recommended early, so that individuals are comfortable with performing these treatments at times of exacerbation. Airway clearance therapies can also be increased at times of respiratory infection or exacerbation to assist with removal of respiratory secretions. Distal airway clearance therapies are recommended as adjuncts to proximal airway clearance therapies [63].

Proximal Airway Clearance

Proximal airway clearance therapies assist lung inflation, followed by coughing which may be spontaneous or assisted with an abdominal thrust or negative pressure. These techniques help augment cough force to remove secretions from the large airways and pharynx. Studies comparing the outcome of lung volume recruitment (LVR) and mechanical in-exsufflation (MI-E) during acute exacerbations suggest that MI-E may result in greater efficacy of secretion clearance and improvement in gas exchange, although no differences in efficacy between cough augmentation techniques were found in a recent systematic review [63–66]. Proximal airway clearance therapies have been used for many years with few complications, although pneumothorax, bradycardia, tachycardia, and transient hypotension have been reported with treatment [63, 67–69].

Lung Volume Recruitment

This therapy consists of assisting inspiration by application of positive pressure, which may be delivered via mask/mouthpiece interface with a self-inflating bag with one-way valve or with a ventilator. Breaths may be stacked, with the cooperation of the individual to hold their breath with a closed glottis between positive pressure breaths. These techniques fill the lungs to maximal inspiratory capacity and then utilize the elastic recoil of the lungs to assist with cough [63, 70]. Small studies of the acute effects of LVR have shown that it increases respiratory system compliance, decreases respiratory rate and rapid shallow breathing index, improves lung volumes and cough peak flow, and may raise voice volume and ability to speak longer phrases [71–77]. Longer-term retrospective cohort studies of LVR used twice daily in young men with DMD and advanced lung disease have demonstrated an 89% reduction in rate of decline in forced vital capacity and that the peak of maximal vital capacity decline was delayed by 5 years [78, 79]. In addition, cough peak flow achieved following a lung volume recruitment maneuver can be maintained for up to 8 years in a range that produces a cough effective for airway clearance [52]. A systematic review showed acute improvements in cough peak flow with LVR, most significant in those with lower baseline CPF, but less clear long-term benefits of therapy [80]. Two randomized controlled trials of LVR in children with neuromuscular disease have not shown sustained long-term improvements in lung function with LVR but included individuals with fairly mild baseline lung function impairments [81, 82].

Manually Assisted Cough

While some individuals may be able to generate sufficient expiratory airflow to cough spontaneously, the expiratory phase of cough may be enhanced with the application of an abdominal or thoracic thrust to produce a manually assisted cough [83]. An abdominal or thoracic thrust may be self-delivered or applied by a caregiver [63]. The addition of manually assisted expiration increases cough peak flow beyond that achieved with an inspiratory maneuver alone, particularly in those with lower lung function [63, 75, 84–86]. This is not always routinely applied in children.

Mechanical In-exsufflation

Mechanical in-exsufflation delivers positive pressure to achieve lung inflation, followed by negative pressure to simulate a cough and remove secretions from the large airways. This therapy is recommended specifically in clinical care guidelines to be used in individuals who are very weak, have impaired bulbar function, and/or are not able to cooperate with manual techniques [30, 40]. Immediate effects of MI-E include increased cough peak flow, vital capacity, inspiratory capacity, expiratory reserve volume, and mucus clearance [73, 87–92]. Prospective studies and systematic review, however, have not shown sustained improvements in lung function with MI-E, although one study showed that forced vital capacity stabilized in the first 2 years of regular MI-E use compared to the 2 years prior to onset of therapy [87, 93, 94]. Nonetheless, studies in which MI-E was integrated into a plan of care have shown that it can reduce frequency of hospitalizations, pneumonia, episodes of respiratory failure, and need for tracheostomy [95–98]. Furthermore, regular MI-E has been shown to be associated with an increase in maximal insufflation capacity over time despite a decreasing vital capacity, suggesting that chest wall distensibility is maintained [99].

Settings for mechanical insufflation vary from ±20 to 40 cm water, typically. The use of greater expiratory flows than inspiratory flows, longer inspiratory time, and a pause between inspiration and expiration may enhance secretion movement and may also reduce laryngeal closure as well as aspiration of oral secretions [100, 101].

Respiratory Muscle Training

While respiratory muscle training has been explored to improve strength, there is conflicting data in DMD. Studies are limited by sample size and differences in techniques. A recent Cochrane review found no clear improvement in either DMD or Becker MD [102]. No data exist on whether respiratory muscle training is useful in congenital MD [7].

Distal Airway Clearance Therapies

These therapies assist in the mobilization of respiratory secretions from the peripheral to central airways but need to be followed by an effective cough to clear them from the respiratory tract. There are several techniques which may be used to provide this treatment. Manually performed chest percussion is followed by vibration of the chest wall which generates a rapid extra-thoracic force at the beginning of expiration, followed by oscillatory compressions during the rest of the expiratory phase [63]. High-frequency chest wall oscillation uses an air pulse generator to deliver intermittent positive airflow into a jacket [63]. Intra-pulmonary percussive ventilation delivers high-frequency bursts of air via a pneumatic device which both mobilizes secretions proximally and inflates areas of the lung distal to secretions [63].

Distal airway clearance therapies do not depend upon the cooperation of the individual, nor on the presence of intact bulbar function [63]. They are recommended as adjuncts to proximal airway clearance techniques and may be particularly useful in ventilator-assisted individuals and others with very impaired cough efficacy. Evidence-based guidelines for the use of such therapies are lacking.

Medications and Other Adjuncts

Medications that affect viscosity and volume of secretions are of unclear benefit in individuals with neuromuscular disease and have not been well studied. Caution should be exercised with the use of drying medications such as glycopyrrolate (Robinul, Baxter Pharmaceutical, Deerfield, IL) which may be used to reduce oral secretions, as thickening of lower airway secretions may make expectoration more difficult and may increase mucus plugging [103, 104]. Anticholinergics such as scopolamine and atropine drops may provide more local action and fewer systemic effects but still have risks of drying or thickening lower airway secretions. Botulinum toxin (Botox, Allergan Inc., Irvine, CA) may be useful as more targeted therapy for upper airway and oral secretions, although they also have not been well-studied and there are reports of worsening bulbar function after their use in individuals with neuromuscular conditions [103–108].

Nebulized mucolytics such as dornase (Pulmozyme, Genentech Inc. South San Francisco, CA), *N*-acetylcysteine (Mucomyst, Apothecon Inc. Princeton, NJ), and hypertonic saline may be beneficial in specific instances of mucus plugging, in conjunction with other airway clearance techniques [103, 109]. The British Thoracic Society guidelines suggest the use of nebulized normal saline in children with tenacious secretions [30].

Humidification and suctioning are additional adjunctive therapies that may be used. They may be particularly useful for individuals with a tracheostomy, in whom humidification may avoid mucus plugging and suctioning to the distal end of the tracheostomy tube is frequently used to clear the large airways of mucus [40, 44].

Management of Sleep Disordered Breathing and Respiratory Failure

Sleep Disordered Breathing

Sleep disordered breathing is usually treated with non-invasive respiratory support. In individuals without neuromuscular disease, obstructive sleep apnea is usually treated with continuous positive airway pressure (CPAP). The continuous pressure provided by CPAP serves to stent open the oropharynx, thereby reducing the obstruction to inspiratory airflow. However, when higher pressures are required to overcome obstruction, this can be an impediment to expiration in the setting of neuromuscular weakness. High CPAP pressures may also inflate the lungs to a point of further decreased compliance, at which point the respiratory muscle strength may be insufficient to generate adequate tidal volumes. Given this, and the fact that development of nocturnal hypoventilation is inevitable, while CPAP may be used if no hypoventilation is yet present, bilevel positive airway pressure (BPAP)/non-invasive ventilation is often the initial treatment of choice for obstructive sleep apnea in the context of MD. BPAP provides an expiratory positive airway pressure (EPAP) analogous to CPAP but then also a higher inspiratory positive airway pressure (IPAP). This second pressure is delivered either in response to the individual initiating a breath, thereby triggering the device or at a set rate ("backup rate"). The EPAP serves to stent the upper airway and maintain lung inflation to prevent atelectasis, while the delivery of the IPAP improves the tidal volume, thereby improving ventilation. Generally, the goal in management of hypoventilation in MD is to allow respiratory muscle rest by setting a backup rate similar to the individual's natural rate, such that a minority of breaths are triggered by the individual. Non-invasive ventilation should also be initiated once there is clear evidence of nocturnal hypoventilation, as well as when the FVC is <50% predicted or MIP is <60 cm H_2O [32]. More stringent definitions of hypoventilation have been advocated, including CO_2 >50 mmHg for >2% of sleep time, an increase in CO_2 of 10 mmHg above awake baseline for >2% of sleep time, or an oxygen saturation of <88% for >2% of sleep time of at least 5 min [32].

The use of non-invasive ventilation in populations of children with a variety of neuromuscular diseases, including children with MD, has been shown to improve symptoms of daytime sleepiness and headache and improve sleep quality and gas exchange during sleep. Retrospective data show that when compared to the year prior to initiation of NIV, individuals made one-third of the number of visits to their primary care provider and experienced half the number of respiratory infections requiring antibiotics in the year following initiation of NIV [110]. This same study found that hospitalization rates decreased by more than half once NIV was started [110]. In another group of children with neuromuscular disorders, initiation of NIV resulted in a 85% drop in hospital days and almost 70% fewer days in the intensive care unit [111]. Treatment with NIV has been shown to improve survival, as noted above [19, 112, 113]. Overall, adherence with NIV is good, with hours of usage increasing with age and as pulmonary function declines [114].

While NIV is well-tolerated by individuals with neuromuscular disease, potential complications include skin breakdown from the interface and risk of aspiration of gastric contents if the individual vomits and is unable to remove the mask interface [115]. For this reason, nasal interfaces for NIV are preferred over oronasal interfaces. If an oronasal interface is used, an awake caregiver may need to be present to attend to individuals if they cannot remove the mask themselves.

Diurnal Respiratory Failure

Daytime ventilation is indicated when resting oxygen saturation is less than 95%, CO_2 is >45 mmHg or if symptoms of dyspnea are present [32]. This can be delivered via mask interface, mouthpiece (also known as "sip" ventilation), or tracheostomy. Improvement in survival with management of daytime hypoventilation is similar regardless of method [116].

Non-invasive Ventilation

Daytime ventilation via mask interface can be safe, effective, and well-tolerated [117]. Practice is variable, however, as this may interfere with social interaction, and therefore it is important that a shared decision-making approach is employed. A nasal mask interface is preferred to keep the mouth free for speech and nutritional intake as well as for safety. However, if weakness is so significant that the mouth cannot be held closed, this may result in insufficient ventilation due to air leak. At times this may be mitigated with the use of a chin strap. Ventilation via an oronasal mask is also an option. However, safety concerns arise with both chin strap and oronasal mask, due to the risk of aspiration should the individual vomit and be unable to remove the mask or open their mouth adequately. In addition, with the prolonged use of NIV, the risk of skin breakdown increases, and attention must be paid to careful skin care and assessment to prevent and treat pressure ulcers. Finally, with many hours of continuous use, there is a risk of development of midface hypoplasia, which must be monitored [115].

Mouthpiece Ventilation

Mouthpiece ventilation (MPV) involves the use of a portable home mechanical ventilator, typically with a single-limb open circuit, with mouthpiece assembly [118]. The entire assembly can be mounted on a wheelchair, with the mouthpiece mounted on an adjustable support arm to facilitate independent access. Breaths are delivered by the ventilator in response to negative pressure generated by a "sip" on the mouthpiece [118]. It thus provides on-demand ventilation with freedom from the interference of a mask on the face, while providing skin rest and normalized verbal communication [117]. The use of MPV requires the ability to sufficiently seal lips around the mouthpiece [7]. Use also necessitates adequate cognitive/developmental status and ability to communicate (Video of mouthpiece ventilation, Canadian Alternatives in Noninvasive Ventilation, https://canventottawa.ca/EducationModules/Phase/4, https://youtu.be/qtc0kj7fIMs).

MPV provides a safe alternative to tracheostomy when mask-interface ventilation during the day fails or is unacceptable to the individual [117, 119]. Even a short (2 h) period of MPV use during the afternoon has been shown to relieve daytime respiratory muscle loading and dyspnea [120]. MPV has been shown to stabilize vital capacity, adequately manage hypoventilation, and improve long-term survival in individuals with DMD [117, 121]. It has also been shown to improve quality of life [122]. One study showed that when provided with a choice, all individuals with DMD and their families chose 24-h NIV including MPV [117]. MPV can also be used to perform independent lung volume recruitment maneuvers [117]. It may also improve dysphagia, though the mechanism for this is unclear [123]. Challenges of MPV include air leak from the nose or mouth [124], and some individuals may experience increased salivation and vomiting [125]. Attention must be paid to the choice of ventilator when prescribing MPV, as not all ventilators have software designed for this purpose, resulting in frequent nuisance alarms due to the open circuit [126].

Tracheostomy

Tracheostomy provides a more secure airway and more direct airway access for clearance, though with additional risks. Tracheostomy is controversial in the management of DMD and other MD. Some groups strongly recommend ongoing use of NIV when 24-h ventilation is required [32, 62]. Indications for tracheostomy include individual preference, worsening bulbar function, frequent aspiration, inability of the individual to use NIV, or failure of NIV, for instance, due to inability to appropriately fit a mask [7, 32, 62]. Tracheostomy is associated with higher risks of tracheal injury, chronic hypersecretion, and more frequent lower respiratory infections than NIV [116]. Individuals with tracheostomy are also less likely to live at home, given the additional care requirements associated with tracheostomy care [116]. Significant risks associated with tracheostomy include occlusion and accidental decannulation, either of which may be fatal. For children, or any individual not able to manage tracheostomy care independently, constant presence of a trained, awake caregiver may be necessary [127].

Emerging Therapies

Several disease-modifying therapies are on the horizon for individuals with DMD. They may induce exon skipping or target molecular pathways downstream of the absence of functional dystrophin [31, 128]. Trials are ongoing to evaluate their efficacy, including their effects on the respiratory system. It is possible that these treatments may significantly alter disease progression. Similar strategies are under investigation for treatment of the congenital MDs [129]. Optimization of health of the respiratory and other systems is therefore critical so that individuals can take the best advantage of new therapies that emerge for these disorders.

References

1. Birnkrant DJ, Bushby K, Bann CM, Apkon SD, Blackwell A, Brumbaugh D, et al. Diagnosis and management of Duchenne muscular dystrophy, part 1: diagnosis, and neuromuscular, rehabilitation, endocrine, and gastrointestinal and nutritional management. Lancet Neurol. 2018;17(3):251–67. https://doi.org/10.1016/s1474-4422(18)30024-3.
2. Guien C, Blandin G, Lahaut P, Sanson B, Nehal K, Rabarimeriarijaona S, et al. The French National Registry of patients with facioscapulohumeral muscular dystrophy. Orphanet J Rare Dis. 2018;13(1):218. https://doi.org/10.1186/s13023-018-0960-x.
3. Deenen JC, Arnts H, van der Maarel SM, Padberg GW, Verschuuren JJ, Bakker E, et al. Population-based incidence and prevalence of facioscapulohumeral dystrophy. Neurology. 2014;83(12):1056–9. https://doi.org/10.1212/WNL.0000000000000797.
4. Flanigan KM, Coffeen CM, Sexton L, Stauffer D, Brunner S, Leppert MF. Genetic characterization of a large, historically significant Utah kindred with facioscapulohumeral dystrophy. Neuromuscul Disord. 2001;11(6–7):525–9. https://doi.org/10.1016/s0960-8966(01)00201-2.
5. Brais B. Oculopharyngeal muscular dystrophy: a polyalanine myopathy. Curr Neurol Neurosci Rep. 2009;9(1):76–82. https://doi.org/10.1007/s11910-009-0012-y.
6. Kang PB, Morrison L, Iannaccone ST, Graham RJ, Bönnemann CG, Rutkowski A, et al. Evidence-based guideline summary: evaluation, diagnosis, and management of congenital muscular dystrophy: report of the guideline development subcommittee of the American Academy of Neurology and the practice issues review panel of the American Association of Neuromuscular & Electrodiagnostic Medicine. Neurology. 2015;84(13):1369–78. https://doi.org/10.1212/wnl.0000000000001416.

7. Wang CH, Bonnemann CG, Rutkowski A, Sejersen T, Bellini J, Battista V, et al. Consensus statement on standard of care for congenital muscular dystrophies. J Child Neurol. 2010;25(12):1559–81. https://doi.org/10.1177/0883073810381924.

8. Chang RF, Mubarak SJ. Pathomechanics of Gowers' sign: a video analysis of a spectrum of Gowers' maneuvers. Clin Orthop Relat Res. 2012;470(7):1987–91. https://doi.org/10.1007/s11999-011-2210-6.

9. Cros D, Harnden P, Pellissier JF, Serratrice G. Muscle hypertrophy in Duchenne muscular dystrophy. A pathological and morphometric study. J Neurol. 1989;236(1):43–7. https://doi.org/10.1007/bf00314217.

10. Lovering RM, Porter NC, Bloch RJ. The muscular dystrophies: from genes to therapies. Phys Ther. 2005;85(12):1372–88.

11. Mathews KD. Muscular dystrophy overview: genetics and diagnosis. Neurol Clin. 2003;21(4):795–816. https://doi.org/10.1016/s0733-8619(03)00065-3.

12. Bello L, Gordish-Dressman H, Morgenroth LP, Henricson EK, Duong T, Hoffman EP, et al. Prednisone/prednisolone and deflazacort regimens in the CINRG Duchenne Natural History Study. Neurology. 2015;85(12):1048–55. https://doi.org/10.1212/wnl.0000000000001950.

13. Kim S, Zhu Y, Romitti PA, Fox DJ, Sheehan DW, Valdez R, et al. Associations between timing of corticosteroid treatment initiation and clinical outcomes in Duchenne muscular dystrophy. Neuromuscul Disord. 2017;27(8):730–7. https://doi.org/10.1016/j.nmd.2017.05.019.

14. Pandya S, James KA, Westfield C, Thomas S, Fox DJ, Ciafaloni E, et al. Health profile of a cohort of adults with Duchenne muscular dystrophy. Muscle Nerve. 2018;58(2):219–23. https://doi.org/10.1002/mus.26129.

15. McDonald CM, Henricson EK, Abresch RT, Duong T, Joyce NC, Hu F, et al. Long-term effects of glucocorticoids on function, quality of life, and survival in patients with Duchenne muscular dystrophy: a prospective cohort study. Lancet. 2018;391(10119):451–61. https://doi.org/10.1016/s0140-6736(17)32160-8.

16. Villa C, Auerbach SR, Bansal N, Birnbaum BF, Conway J, Esteso P, et al. Current practices in treating cardiomyopathy and heart failure in Duchenne muscular dystrophy (DMD): understanding care practices in order to optimize DMD heart failure through ACTION. Pediatr Cardiol. 2022;43(5):977–85. https://doi.org/10.1007/s00246-021-02807-7.

17. Wahlgren L, Kroksmark AK, Tulinius M, Sofou K. One in five patients with Duchenne muscular dystrophy dies from other causes than cardiac or respiratory failure. Eur J Epidemiol. 2022;37(2):147–56. https://doi.org/10.1007/s10654-021-00819-4.

18. Broomfield J, Hill M, Guglieri M, Crowther M, Abrams K. Life expectancy in Duchenne muscular dystrophy: reproduced individual patient data meta-analysis. Neurology. 2021;97(23):e2304–14. https://doi.org/10.1212/wnl.0000000000012910.

19. Landfeldt E, Thompson R, Sejersen T, McMillan HJ, Kirschner J, Lochmüller H. Life expectancy at birth in Duchenne muscular dystrophy: a systematic review and meta-analysis. Eur J Epidemiol. 2020;35(7):643–53. https://doi.org/10.1007/s10654-020-00613-8.

20. Szabo SM, Salhany RM, Deighton A, Harwood M, Mah J, Gooch KL. The clinical course of Duchenne muscular dystrophy in the corticosteroid treatment era: a systematic literature review. Orphanet J Rare Dis. 2021;16(1):237. https://doi.org/10.1186/s13023-021-01862-w.

21. Khirani S, Ramirez A, Aubertin G, Boulé M, Chemouny C, Forin V, et al. Respiratory muscle decline in Duchenne muscular dystrophy. Pediatr Pulmonol. 2014;49(5):473–81. https://doi.org/10.1002/ppul.22847.

22. Panitch HB. The pathophysiology of respiratory impairment in pediatric neuromuscular diseases. Pediatrics. 2009;123(Suppl 8):S215.

23. Panitch HB. Respiratory issues in the management of children with neuromuscular disease. Respir Care. 2006;51(8):885–93.

24. Dohna-Schwake C, Ragette R, Teschler H, Voit T, Mellies U. Predictors of severe chest infections in pediatric neuromuscular disorders. Neuromuscul Disord. 2006;16(5):325–8.

25. Bach JR, Rajaraman R, Ballanger F, Tzeng AC, Ishikawa Y, Kulessa R, et al. Neuromuscular ventilatory insufficiency: effect of home mechanical ventilator use v oxygen therapy on pneumonia and hospitalization rates. Am J Phys Med Rehabil. 1998;77(1):8–19.

26. Fromageot C, Lofaso F, Annane D, Falaize L, Lejaille M, Clair B, et al. Supine fall in lung volumes in the assessment of diaphragmatic weakness in neuromuscular disorders. Arch Phys Med Rehabil. 2001;82(1):123–8. https://doi.org/10.1053/apmr.2001.18053.

27. Kelley EF, Cross TJ, Snyder EM, McDonald CM, Hoffman EP, Bello L. Influence of β(2) adrenergic receptor genotype on risk of nocturnal ventilation in patients with Duchenne muscular dystrophy. Respir Res. 2019;20(1):221. https://doi.org/10.1186/s12931-019-1200-1.

28. Sawnani H, Thampratankul L, Szczesniak RD, Fenchel MC, Simakajornboon N. Sleep disordered breathing in young boys with Duchenne muscular dystrophy. J Pediatr. 2015;166(3):640–5.e1. https://doi.org/10.1016/j.jpeds.2014.12.006.

29. Khan A, Frazer-Green L, Amin R, Wolfe L, Faulkner G, Casey K, et al. Respiratory management of patients with neuromuscular weakness: an American College of Chest Physicians clinical practice guideline and expert panel report. Chest. 2023;164:394. https://doi.org/10.1016/j.chest.2023.03.011.

30. Hull J, Aniapravan R, Chan E, Chatwin M, Forton J, Gallagher J, et al. British Thoracic Society guideline for respiratory management of children with neuromuscular weakness. Thorax. 2012;67:i1–40.

31. Birnkrant DJ, Bello L, Butterfield RJ, Carter JC, Cripe LH, Cripe TP, et al. Cardiorespiratory management of Duchenne muscular dystrophy: emerging therapies, neuromuscular genetics, and new clinical challenges. Lancet Respir Med. 2022;10(4):403–20. https://doi.org/10.1016/s2213-2600(21)00581-6.

32. Birnkrant DJ, Bushby K, Bann CM, Alman BA, Apkon SD, Blackwell A, et al. Diagnosis and management of Duchenne muscular dystrophy, part 2: respiratory, cardiac, bone health, and orthopaedic management. Lancet Neurol. 2018;17(4):347–61. https://doi.org/10.1016/s1474-4422(18)30025-5.

33. Andrews JG, Soim A, Pandya S, Westfield CP, Ciafaloni E, Fox DJ, et al. Respiratory care received by individuals with Duchenne muscular dystrophy from 2000 to 2011. Respir Care. 2016;61(10):1349–59. https://doi.org/10.4187/respcare.04676.

34. El-Aloul B, Altamirano-Diaz L, Zapata-Aldana E, Rodrigues R, Malvankar-Mehta MS, Nguyen CT, et al. Pharmacological therapy for the prevention and management of cardiomyopathy in Duchenne muscular dystrophy: a systematic review. Neuromuscul Disord. 2017;27(1):4–14. https://doi.org/10.1016/j.nmd.2016.09.019.

35. Apkon SD, Alman B, Birnkrant DJ, Fitch R, Lark R, Mackenzie W, et al. Orthopedic and surgical management of the patient with Duchenne muscular dystrophy. Pediatrics. 2018;142(Suppl 2):S82–9. https://doi.org/10.1542/peds.2018-0333J.

36. Ward LM, Hadjiyannakis S, McMillan HJ, Noritz G, Weber DR. Bone health and osteoporosis management of the patient with Duchenne muscular dystrophy. Pediatrics. 2018;142(Suppl 2):S34–42. https://doi.org/10.1542/peds.2018-0333E.

37. Ward LM, Choudhury A, Alos N, Cabral DA, Rodd C, Sbrocchi AM, et al. Zoledronic acid vs placebo in pediatric glucocorticoid-induced osteoporosis: a randomized, double-blind, phase 3 trial. J Clin Endocrinol Metab. 2021;106(12):e5222–35. https://doi.org/10.1210/clinem/dgab458.

38. Cheng PC, Panitch HB, Hansen-Flaschen J. Transition of patients with neuromuscular disease and chronic ventilator-dependent respiratory failure from pediatric to adult pulmonary care. Paediatr Respir Rev. 2020;33:3–8. https://doi.org/10.1016/j.prrv.2019.03.005.

39. Accogli G, Ferrante C, Fanizza I, Oliva MC, Gallo I, De Rinaldis M, et al. Neuromuscular disorders and transition from pediatric to adult care in a multidisciplinary perspective: a narrative review of the scientific evidence and current debate. Acta Myol. 2022;41(4):188–200. https://doi.org/10.36185/2532-1900-083.

40. Amin R, MacLusky I, Zielinski D, Adderley R, Carnevale F, Chiang J, et al. Pediatric home mechanical ventilation: a Canadian Thoracic Society clinical practice guideline executive summary. Can J Respir Crit Care Sleep Med. 2017;1(1):7–36.

41. Katz SL. Assessment of sleep-disordered breathing in pediatric neuromuscular diseases. Pediatrics. 2009;123(Suppl 4):S222–5.

42. Aboussouan LS. Sleep-disordered breathing in neuromuscular disease. AmJ Respir Crit Care Med. 2015;191(9):979–89.

43. Bourke SC. Respiratory involvement in neuromuscular disease. Clin Med (Lond). 2014;14(1):72–5. https://doi.org/10.7861/clinmedicine.14-1-72.

44. Katz SL. Section 5: airway clearance. Can J Respir Crit Care Sleep Med. 2018;2(sup1):32–40. https://doi.org/10.1080/24745332.2018.1494979.

45. Miller K, Mayer OH. Pulmonary function testing in patients with neuromuscular disease. Pediatr Pulmonol. 2021;56(4):693–9. https://doi.org/10.1002/ppul.25182.

46. Phillips MF, Quinlivan RC, Edwards RH, Calverley PM. Changes in spirometry over time as a prognostic marker in patients with Duchenne muscular dystrophy. Am J Respir Crit Care Med. 2001;164(12):2191–4.

47. Leon-Astudillo C, Okorie CUA, McCown MY, Dy FJ, Puranik S, Prero M, et al. ATS Core Curriculum 2022. Pediatric pulmonary medicine: updates in pediatric neuromuscular disease. Pediatr Pulmonol. 2023;58(7):1866–74. https://doi.org/10.1002/ppul.26448.

48. McDonald CM, Gordish-Dressman H, Henricson EK, Duong T, Joyce NC, Jhawar S, et al. Longitudinal pulmonary function testing outcome measures in Duchenne muscular dystrophy: long-term natural history with and without glucocorticoids. Neuromuscul Disord. 2018;28(11):897–909. https://doi.org/10.1016/j.nmd.2018.07.004.

49. Bushby K, Finkel R, Birnkrant DJ, Case LE, Clemens PR, Cripe L, et al. Diagnosis and management of Duchenne muscular dystrophy, part 2: implementation of multidisciplinary care [Erratum appears in Lancet Neurol. 2010 Mar;9(3):237]. Lancet Neurol. 2010;9(2):177–89.

50. Bianchi C, Baiardi P, Bianchi C, Baiardi P. Cough peak flows: standard values for children and adolescents. Am J Phys Med Rehabil. 2008;87(6):461–7.

51. Kang SW, Bach JR. Maximum insufflation capacity. Chest. 2000;118(1):61–5.

52. Katz SL, Barrowman N, Monsour A, Su S, Hoey L, McKim D. Long-term effects of lung volume recruitment on maximal inspiratory capacity and vital capacity in Duchenne muscular dystrophy. Ann Am Thorac Soc. 2016;13(2):217–22.

53. Aurora RN, Zak RS, Karippot A, Lamm CI, Morgenthaler TI, Auerbach SH, et al. Practice parameters for the respiratory indications for polysomnography in children. Sleep. 2011;34(3):379–88.

54. Berry RB, Budhiraja R, Gottlieb DJ, Gozal D, Iber C, Kapur VK, et al. Rules for scoring respiratory events in sleep: update of the 2007 AASM manual for the scoring of sleep and associated events. Deliberations of the sleep apnea definitions task force of the American Academy of Sleep Medicine. J Clin Sleep Med. 2012;8(5):597–619. https://doi.org/10.5664/jcsm.2172.

55. Kotterba S, Patzold T, Malin JP, Orth M, Rasche K. Respiratory monitoring in neuromuscular disease—capnography as an additional tool? Clin Neurol Neurosurg. 2001;103(2):87–91.

56. Paiva R, Krivec U, Aubertin G, Cohen E, Clement A, Fauroux B. Carbon dioxide monitoring during long-term noninvasive respiratory support in children 1. Intensive Care Med. 2009;35(6):1068–74.

57. Trucco F, Pedemonte M, Fiorillo C, Tan H-L, Carlucci A, Brisca G, et al. Detection of early nocturnal hypoventilation in neuromuscular disorders. J Int Med Res. 2018;46(3):1153–61. https://doi.org/10.1177/0300060517728857.

58. Gloss D, Moxley RT III, Ashwal S, Oskoui M. Practice guideline update summary: corticosteroid treatment of Duchenne muscular dystrophy: report of the guideline development subcommittee of the American Academy of Neurology. Neurology. 2016;86(5):465–72. https://doi.org/10.1212/wnl.0000000000002337.

59. Henricson EK, Abresch RT, Cnaan A, Hu F, Duong T, Arrieta A, et al. The cooperative international neuromuscular research group Duchenne natural history study: glucocorticoid treatment preserves clinically meaningful functional milestones and reduces rate of disease progression as measured by manual muscle testing and other commonly used clinical trial outcome measures. Muscle Nerve. 2013;48(1):55–67. https://doi.org/10.1002/mus.23808.

60. Koeks Z, Bladen CL, Salgado D, van Zwet E, Pogoryelova O, McMacken G, et al. Clinical outcomes in Duchenne muscular dystrophy: a study of 5345 patients from the TREAT-NMD DMD global database. J Neuromuscul Dis. 2017;4(4):293–306. https://doi.org/10.3233/jnd-170280.
61. Finder JD, Birnkrant D, Carl J, Farber HJ, Gozal D, Iannaccone ST, et al. Respiratory care of the patient with Duchenne muscular dystrophy: ATS consensus statement. Am J Respir Crit Care Med. 2004;170(4):456–65.
62. Sheehan DW, Birnkrant DJ, Benditt JO, Eagle M, Finder JD, Kissel J, et al. Respiratory management of the patient with Duchenne muscular dystrophy. Pediatrics. 2018;142(Suppl 2):S62–s71. https://doi.org/10.1542/peds.2018-0333H.
63. Chatwin M, Toussaint M, Gonçalves MR, Sheers N, Mellies U, Gonzales-Bermejo J, et al. Airway clearance techniques in neuromuscular disorders: a state of the art review. Respir Med. 2018;136:98–110. https://doi.org/10.1016/j.rmed.2018.01.012.
64. Rafiq MK, Bradburn M, Proctor AR, Billings CG, Bianchi S, McDermott CJ, et al. A preliminary randomized trial of the mechanical insufflator-exsufflator versus breath-stacking technique in patients with amyotrophic lateral sclerosis. Amyotroph Lateral Scler Frontotemporal Degener. 2015;16(7–8):448–55. https://doi.org/10.3109/21678421.2015.1051992.
65. Siriwat R, Deerojanawong J, Sritippayawan S, Hantragool S, Cheanprapai P. Mechanical insufflation-exsufflation versus conventional chest physiotherapy in children with cerebral palsy. Respir Care. 2018;63(2):187–93. https://doi.org/10.4187/respcare.05663.
66. Morrow B, Argent A, Zampoli M, Human A, Corten L, Toussaint M. Cough augmentation techniques for people with chronic neuromuscular disorders. Cochrane Database Syst Rev. 2021;4(4):Cd013170. https://doi.org/10.1002/14651858.CD013170.pub2.
67. McDonald LA, Berlowitz DJ, Howard ME, Rautela L, Chao C, Sheers N. Pneumothorax in neuromuscular disease associated with lung volume recruitment and mechanical insufflation-exsufflation. Respirol Case Rep. 2019;7(6):e00447. https://doi.org/10.1002/rcr2.447.
68. Suri P, Burns SP, Bach JR. Pneumothorax associated with mechanical insufflation-exsufflation and related factors. Am J Phys Med Rehabil. 2008;87(11):951–5.
69. Westermann EJ, Jans M, Gaytant MA, Bach JR, Kampelmacher MJ. Pneumothorax as a complication of lung volume recruitment. J Bras Pneumol. 2013;39(3):382–6. https://doi.org/10.1590/s1806-37132013000300017.
70. Sheers N, Howard ME, Berlowitz DJ. Respiratory adjuncts to NIV in neuromuscular disease. Respirology. 2019;24(6):512–20. https://doi.org/10.1111/resp.13431.
71. Molgat-Seon Y, Hannan LM, Dominelli PB, Peters CM, Fougere RJ, McKim DA, et al. Lung volume recruitment acutely increases respiratory system compliance in individuals with severe respiratory muscle weakness. ERJ Open Res. 2017;3(1):00135. https://doi.org/10.1183/23120541.00135-2016.
72. Cesareo A, LoMauro A, Santi M, Biffi E, D'Angelo MG, Aliverti A. Acute effects of mechanical insufflation-exsufflation on the breathing pattern in stable subjects with Duchenne muscular dystrophy. Respir Care. 2018;63(8):955–65. https://doi.org/10.4187/respcare.05895.
73. Bach JR. Mechanical insufflation-exsufflation. Comparison of peak expiratory flows with manually assisted and unassisted coughing techniques. Chest. 1993;104(5):1553–62.
74. Dohna-Schwake C, Ragette R, Teschler H, Voit T, Mellies U. IPPB-assisted coughing in neuromuscular disorders 2. Pediatr Pulmonol. 2006;41(6):551–7.
75. Trebbia G, Lacombe M, Fermanian C, Falaize L, Lejaille M, Louis A, et al. Cough determinants in patients with neuromuscular disease. Respir Physiol Neurobiol. 2005;146(2–3):291–300.
76. Mellies U, Goebel C. Optimum insufflation capacity and peak cough flow in neuromuscular disorders. Ann Am Thorac Soc. 2014;11(10):1560–8. https://doi.org/10.1513/AnnalsATS.201406-264OC.
77. De Troyer A, Deisser P. The effects of intermittent positive pressure breathing on patients with respiratory muscle weakness. Am Rev Respir Dis. 1981;124(2):132–7. https://doi.org/10.1164/arrd.1981.124.2.132.

78. McKim DA, Katz SL, Barrowman N, Ni A, Leblanc C. Lung volume recruitment slows pulmonary function decline in Duchenne muscular dystrophy. Arch Phys Med Rehabil. 2012;93(7):1117–22.

79. Chiou M, Bach JR, Jethani L, Gallagher MF. Active lung volume recruitment to preserve vital capacity in Duchenne muscular dystrophy. J Rehabil Med. 2017;49(1):49–53. https://doi.org/10.2340/16501977-2144.

80. O'Sullivan R, Carrier J, Cranney H, Hemming R. Effect of lung volume recruitment on pulmonary function in progressive childhood-onset neuromuscular disease: a systematic review. Arch Phys Med Rehabil. 2021;102(5):976–83. https://doi.org/10.1016/j.apmr.2020.07.014.

81. Sawnani H, Mayer OH, Modi AC, Pascoe JE, McConnell K, McDonough JM, et al. Randomized trial of lung hyperinflation therapy in children with congenital muscular dystrophy. Pediatr Pulmonol. 2020;55(9):2471–8. https://doi.org/10.1002/ppul.24954.

82. Katz SL, Mah JK, McMillan HJ, Campbell C, Bijelić V, Barrowman N, et al. Routine lung volume recruitment in boys with Duchenne muscular dystrophy: a randomised clinical trial. Thorax. 2022;77(8):805–11. https://doi.org/10.1136/thoraxjnl-2021-218196.

83. Camela F, Gallucci M, Ricci G. Cough and airway clearance in Duchenne muscular dystrophy. Paediatr Respir Rev. 2019;31:35–9. https://doi.org/10.1016/j.prrv.2018.11.001.

84. Bianchi C, Carrara R, Khirani S, Tuccio MC. Independent cough flow augmentation by glossopharyngeal breathing plus table thrust in muscular dystrophy. Am J Phys Med Rehabil. 2014;93(1):43–8. https://doi.org/10.1097/PHM.0b013e3182975bfa.

85. Ishikawa Y, Bach JR, Komaroff E, Miura T, Jackson-Parekh R. Cough augmentation in Duchenne muscular dystrophy. Am J Phys Med Rehabil. 2008;87(9):726–30.

86. Brito MF, Moreira GA, Pradella-Hallinan M, Tufik S. Air stacking and chest compression increase peak cough flow in patients with Duchenne muscular dystrophy. J Bras Pneumol. 2009;35(10):973–9. https://doi.org/10.1590/s1806-37132009001000005.

87. Chatwin M, Ross E, Hart N, Nickol AH, Polkey MI, Simonds AK. Cough augmentation with mechanical insufflation/exsufflation in patients with neuromuscular weakness. Eur Respir J. 2003;21(3):502–8.

88. Sivasothy P, Brown L, Smith IE, Shneerson JM. Effect of manually assisted cough and mechanical insufflation on cough flow of normal subjects, patients with chronic obstructive pulmonary disease (COPD), and patients with respiratory muscle weakness. Thorax. 2001;56(6):438–44.

89. Mustfa N, Aiello M, Lyall RA, Nikoletou D, Olivieri D, Leigh PN, et al. Cough augmentation in amyotrophic lateral sclerosis. Neurology. 2003;61(9):1285–7.

90. Santos DB, Boré A, Castrillo LDA, Lacombe M, Falaize L, Orlikowski D, et al. Assisted vital capacity to assess recruitment level in neuromuscular diseases. Respir Physiol Neurobiol. 2017;243:32–8. https://doi.org/10.1016/j.resp.2017.05.001.

91. Jung JH, Oh HJ, Lee JW, Suh MR, Park J, Choi WA, et al. Improvement of peak cough flow after the application of a mechanical in-exsufflator in patients with neuromuscular disease and pneumonia: a pilot study. Ann Rehabil Med. 2018;42(6):833–7. https://doi.org/10.5535/arm.2018.42.6.833.

92. Fauroux B, Guillemot N, Aubertin G, Nathan N, Labit A, Clement A, et al. Physiologic benefits of mechanical insufflation-exsufflation in children with neuromuscular diseases. Chest. 2008;133(1):161–8.

93. Chatwin M, Simonds AK, Chatwin M, Simonds AK. The addition of mechanical insufflation/exsufflation shortens airway-clearance sessions in neuromuscular patients with chest infection. Respir Care. 2009;54(11):1473–9.

94. Auger C, Hernando V, Galmiche H. Use of mechanical insufflation-exsufflation devices for airway clearance in subjects with neuromuscular disease. Respir Care. 2017;62(2):236–45.

95. Gomez-Merino E, Bach JR. Duchenne muscular dystrophy: prolongation of life by noninvasive ventilation and mechanically assisted coughing. Am J Phys Med Rehabil. 2002;81(6):411–5.

96. Bach JR, Goncalves M. Ventilator weaning by lung expansion and decannulation. Am J Phys Med Rehabil. 2004;83(7):560–8.

97. Miske LJ, Hickey EM, Kolb SM, Weiner DJ, Panitch HB. Use of the mechanical in-exsufflator in pediatric patients with neuromuscular disease and impaired cough. Chest. 2004;125(4):1406–12.

98. Veldhoen ES, Verweij-van den Oudenrijn LP, Ros LA, Hulzebos EH, Papazova DA, van der Ent CK, et al. Effect of mechanical insufflation-exsufflation in children with neuromuscular weakness. Pediatr Pulmonol. 2020;55(2):510–3. https://doi.org/10.1002/ppul.24614.

99. Bach JR, Mahajan K, Lipa B, Saporito L, Goncalves M, Komaroff E. Lung insufflation capacity in neuromuscular disease. Am J Phys Med Rehabil. 2008;87(9):720–5.

100. Andersen TM, Hov B, Halvorsen T, Røksund OD, Vollsæter M. Upper airway assessment and responses during mechanically assisted cough. Respir Care. 2021;66(7):1196–213. https://doi.org/10.4187/respcare.08960.

101. Winck JC, Gonçalves MR, Lourenço C, Viana P, Almeida J, Bach JR. Effects of mechanical insufflation-exsufflation on respiratory parameters for patients with chronic airway secretion encumbrance. Chest. 2004;126(3):774–80. https://doi.org/10.1378/chest.126.3.774.

102. Silva IS, Pedrosa R, Azevedo IG, Forbes AM, Fregonezi GA, Dourado Junior ME, et al. Respiratory muscle training in children and adults with neuromuscular disease. Cochrane Database Syst Rev. 2019;9(9):Cd011711. https://doi.org/10.1002/14651858.CD011711.pub2.

103. Kravitz RM. Airway clearance in Duchenne muscular dystrophy. Pediatrics. 2009;123(Suppl 5):S231.

104. Finkel RS, Mercuri E, Meyer OH, Simonds AK, Schroth MK, Graham RJ, et al. Diagnosis and management of spinal muscular atrophy: part 2: pulmonary and acute care; medications, supplements and immunizations; other organ systems; and ethics. Neuromuscul Disord. 2018;28(3):197–207. https://doi.org/10.1016/j.nmd.2017.11.004.

105. Meijer JW, van Kuijk AA, Geurts AC, Schelhaas HJ, Zwarts MJ. Acute deterioration of bulbar function after botulinum toxin treatment for sialorrhoea in amyotrophic lateral sclerosis. Am J Phys Med Rehabil. 2008;87(4):321–4. https://doi.org/10.1097/PHM.0b013e318164a931.

106. Reid SM, Johnstone BR, Westbury C, Rawicki B, Reddihough DS. Randomized trial of botulinum toxin injections into the salivary glands to reduce drooling in children with neurological disorders. Dev Med Child Neurol. 2008;50(2):123–8. https://doi.org/10.1111/j.1469-8749.2007.02010.x.

107. Shehee L, O'Rourke A, Garand KL. The role of radiation therapy and botulinum toxin injections in the management of sialorrhea in patients with amyotrophic lateral sclerosis: a systematic review. J Clin Neuromuscul Dis. 2020;21(4):205–21. https://doi.org/10.1097/cnd.0000000000000273.

108. van Hulst K, Kouwenberg CV, Jongerius PH, Feuth T, van den Hoogen FJ, Geurts AC, et al. Negative effects of submandibular botulinum neurotoxin A injections on oral motor function in children with drooling due to central nervous system disorders. Dev Med Child Neurol. 2017;59(5):531–7. https://doi.org/10.1111/dmcn.13333.

109. Crescimanno G, Marrone O. Successful treatment of atelectasis with Dornase alpha in a patient with congenital muscular dystrophy. Rev Port Pneumol. 2014;20(1):42–5. https://doi.org/10.1016/j.rppneu.2012.12.002.

110. Dohna-Schwake C, Podlewski P, Voit T, Mellies U. Non-invasive ventilation reduces respiratory tract infections in children with neuromuscular disorders. Pediatr Pulmonol. 2008;43(1):67–71. https://doi.org/10.1002/ppul.20740.

111. Katz S, Selvadurai H, Keilty K, Mitchell M, Maclusky I. Outcome of non-invasive positive pressure ventilation in paediatric neuromuscular disease 1. Arch Dis Child. 2004;89(2):121–4.

112. Simonds AK, Muntoni F, Heather S, Fielding S. Impact of nasal ventilation on survival in hypercapnic Duchenne muscular dystrophy. Thorax. 1998;2002(53):949–52.

113. Bach JR, Martinez D. Duchenne muscular dystrophy: continuous noninvasive ventilatory support prolongs survival. Respir Care. 2011;56(6):744–50. https://doi.org/10.4187/respcare.00831.

114. Hurvitz MS, Bhattacharjee R, Lesser DJ, Skalsky AJ, Orr JE. Determinants of usage and non-adherence to noninvasive ventilation in children and adults with Duchenne muscular dystrophy. J Clin Sleep Med. 2021;17(10):1973–80. https://doi.org/10.5664/jcsm.9400.
115. Castro-Codesal ML, Olmstead DL, MacLean JE. Mask interfaces for home non-invasive ventilation in infants and children. Paediatr Respir Rev. 2019;32:66–72. https://doi.org/10.1016/j.prrv.2019.03.004.
116. Soudon P, Steens M, Toussaint M. A comparison of invasive versus noninvasive full-time mechanical ventilation in Duchenne muscular dystrophy. Chron Respir Dis. 2008;5(2):87–93. https://doi.org/10.1177/1479972308088715.
117. McKim DA, Griller N, LeBlanc C, Woolnough A, King J. Twenty-four hour noninvasive ventilation in Duchenne muscular dystrophy: a safe alternative to tracheostomy. Can Respir J. 2013;20(1):e5–9. https://doi.org/10.1155/2013/406163.
118. Pinto T, Chatwin M, Banfi P, Winck JC, Nicolini A. Mouthpiece ventilation and complementary techniques in patients with neuromuscular disease: a brief clinical review and update. Chron Respir Dis. 2017;14(2):187–93. https://doi.org/10.1177/1479972316674411.
119. Bach JR, Alba AS, Saporito LR. Intermittent positive pressure ventilation via the mouth as an alternative to tracheostomy for 257 ventilator users. Chest. 1993;103(1):174–82.
120. Toussaint M, Chatwin M, Gonçalves MR, Gonzalez-Bermejo J, Benditt JO, McKim D, et al. Mouthpiece ventilation in neuromuscular disorders: narrative review of technical issues important for clinical success. Respir Med. 2021;180:106373. https://doi.org/10.1016/j.rmed.2021.106373.
121. Bach JR, Gonçalves MR, Hon A, Ishikawa Y, De Vito EL, Prado F, et al. Changing trends in the management of end-stage neuromuscular respiratory muscle failure: recommendations of an international consensus. Am J Phys Med Rehabil. 2013;92(3):267–77. https://doi.org/10.1097/PHM.0b013e31826edcf1.
122. Bach JR. A comparison of long-term ventilatory support alternatives from the perspective of the patient and care giver. Chest. 1993;104(6):1702–6. https://doi.org/10.1378/chest.104.6.1702.
123. Toussaint M, Steens M, Wasteels G, Soudon P. Diurnal ventilation via mouthpiece: survival in end-stage Duchenne patients. Eur Respir J. 2006;28(3):549–55. https://doi.org/10.1183/09031936.06.00004906.
124. Hess DR. The growing role of noninvasive ventilation in patients requiring prolonged mechanical ventilation. Respir Care. 2012;57(6):900–18; discussion 18–20. https://doi.org/10.4187/respcare.01692.
125. Nava S, Navalesi P, Gregoretti C. Interfaces and humidification for noninvasive mechanical ventilation. Respir Care. 2009;54(1):71–84.
126. Khirani S, Ramirez A, Delord V, Leroux K, Lofaso F, Hautot S, et al. Evaluation of ventilators for mouthpiece ventilation in neuromuscular disease. Respir Care. 2014;59(9):1329–37. https://doi.org/10.4187/respcare.03031.
127. St-Laurent A, Zielinski D, Qazi A, AlAwadi A, Almajed A, Adamko DJ, et al. Chronic tracheostomy care of ventilator-dependent and -independent children: clinical practice patterns of pediatric respirologists in a publicly funded (Canadian) healthcare system. Pediatr Pulmonol. 2023;58(1):140–51. https://doi.org/10.1002/ppul.26171.
128. Markati T, Oskoui M, Farrar MA, Duong T, Goemans N, Servais L. Emerging therapies for Duchenne muscular dystrophy. Lancet Neurol. 2022;21(9):814–29. https://doi.org/10.1016/s1474-4422(22)00125-9.
129. Zambon AA, Muntoni F. Congenital muscular dystrophies: what is new? Neuromuscul Disord. 2021;31(10):931–42. https://doi.org/10.1016/j.nmd.2021.07.009.

Chapter 10
Respiratory Care of the ALS Patient

Matthew Berlinger and Noah Lechtzin

Introduction

Amyotrophic lateral sclerosis is a progressive multisystem neurodegenerative disease characterized by involvement of upper motor and lower motor neurons of the central nervous system. ALS often presents with focal weakness which then progresses to involve weakness in the limbs as well as bulbar and respiratory muscles; however, given the heterogeneity of the syndrome, clinical presentations vary. Typically, death occurs due to respiratory failure and occurs in 3–5 years from the time of diagnosis [1].

Epidemiology

The global incidence of ALS is approximately 1.75–3 per 100,000 persons per year; however, there are geographical differences in the incidence of ALS throughout the world, for example, Northern Europe vs. Asia [2]. This may be explained by a lower prevalence of ALS genes in the Asian populations [3, 4]. Recent population studies demonstrate a prevalence of 4.1–8.4 per 100,000 person years [2]. Incidence and prevalence in ALS are expected to increase due to an ageing population as well as improved management [5, 6]. Sporadic ALS comprises about 90% of the cases,

M. Berlinger
LSU Health School of Medicine, Pulmonary and Critical Care Medicine, Baton Rouge, LA, USA

N. Lechtzin (✉)
Pulmonary and Critical Care Medicine, Johns Hopkins Medicine, Baltimore, MD, USA
e-mail: nlechtz@jhmi.edu

N. Lechtzin (ed.), *Pulmonary Complications of Neuromuscular Disease*, Respiratory Medicine, https://doi.org/10.1007/978-3-031-65335-3_10

while familial ALS makes up approximately 10% [7]. Median age at onset is between 51 and 66 years; however, familial ALS tends to have an earlier age of onset compared with sporadic ALS. The male-to-female ratio of ALS in sporadic cases approaches 2:1; however, in the familial cases, it is closer to 1:1 [2].

Risk Factors

Genes

Familial ALS refers to those cases that occur in the setting of a family history of ALS and accounts for 10% of all cases of ALS [7]. The remaining 90% of cases occur in individuals without family histories of ALS and are considered sporadic. Seventy percent of familial cases have mutations within established ALS genes; however, only 15% of sporadic cases are associated with established mutations within ALS-associated genes [8]. Inheritance patterns of familial ALS occur in an autosomal dominant pattern and in genes with high penetrance. In 1993, the first ALS-related gene was discovered: SOD1 [9]. Since the initial discovery of SOD1, more than 120 genetic variants have been discovered to be associated with the risk of developing ALS [10]. In general, the genes associated with the risk of developing ALS can be divided into three loose categories: protein quality control and degradation, RNA metabolism, and cytoskeletal and axonal transport. The most common penetrant mutations are *C9orf72, TARDBP, SOD1,* and *FUS* [11]. *Genetic variants that increase the risk of developing ALS are of growing interest.* For example, in patients with ALS with genetic mutations in the genes that code for enzyme ephrin A4 (EPHA4), lower levels of expression of EPHA4 tend to live longer [12]. Accelerated progression of disease can be seen in certain mutations of the SOD1 gene or even fulminant, childhood-onset disease in certain FUS/TLS mutations [13, 14].

Sex, Aging, and Environmental Exposures

In addition to the genetic risk factors previously discussed, other factors contribute to a higher risk of developing disease. For example, males are at increased risk of developing ALS than females [15]. Furthermore, ALS is a disease of aging and occurs in older patients [16]. There are environmental risk factors that increase the risk of developing ALS and include smoking, lower BMI, and strenuous and repetitive exercise [17–21]. Certain occupational exposures such as heavy metals, pesticides, and beta-methylamino-l-alanine (BMAA) have been associated with an increased risk of developing ALS [15]. Even certain viral infections such as HIV and other ssRNA viruses may increase the risk of developing ALS [22–24].

Pathophysiology (See Fig. 10.1)

The neuropathological hallmark of ALS is characterized by cell death of upper and lower motor neurons in the motor cortex and spinal cord. As previously mentioned, mutations in genes that influence protein homeostasis, RNA metabolism, and cytoskeletal pathways disrupt normal cellular functions and result in protein aggregation, mitochondrial dysfunction, cytoplasmic and axonal transport defects, disturbed RNA metabolism and DNA repair, oligodendrocyte dysfunction and neuroinflammation, ubiquitinated protein inclusions, and cellular death. [1, 10] In over 95% of all cases of ALS, these inclusions are composed of TAR DNA-binding protein 43 (TDP-43) [25]. Degeneration of motor neurons in the lateral aspects of the spinal cord will result in thinning and sclerosis. As further motor neuron death occurs, there is thinning of the ventral roots resulting in denervation and atrophy of the muscles of the tongue, oropharynx, and limbs. In ALS with frontotemporal dementia, neuronal degeneration can occur throughout the frontal and temporal lobes [26].

Clinical Features

The initial symptoms of ALS vary with the degree of upper and lower motor neuron involvement and regional distribution of involvement. The two most common subtypes fall under the category of classic ALS and include spinal ALS and bulbar ALS. Patients with spinal ALS will often present with focal unilateral weakness in distal extremities. Further symptoms may include muscle cramping in the early mornings, twitching, or even fasciculations. Weakness caused by denervation will be associated with muscle wasting and atrophy. Patients with bulbar ALS will report issues with chewing, swallowing, and movements of the face and tongue. While

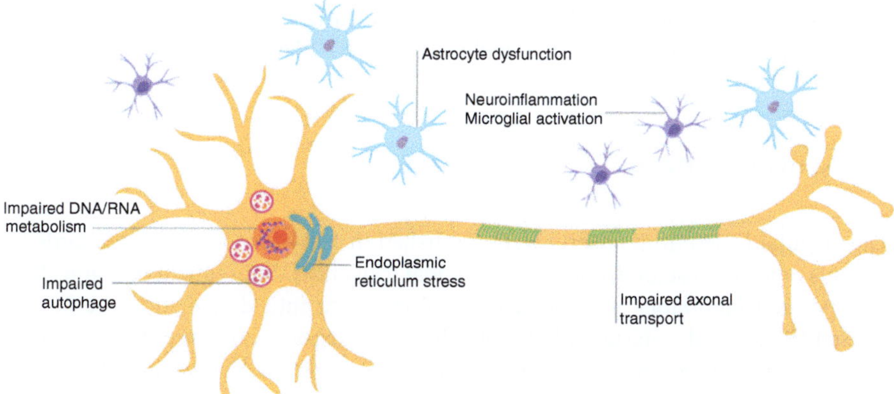

Fig. 10.1 Disease mechanisms contributing to neurodegeneration in ALS. (Adapted from Llieva et al. [134])

most patients will be labeled as having classic ALS, it is increasingly recognized that there is heterogeneity within the clinical syndrome resulting in different presenting symptoms as well as clinical trajectories. For example, a small subset of patients may present with diaphragm weakness as the presenting problem, will complain of dyspnea at rest and upon exertion as well as orthopnea, and are described as having respiratory ALS. Patients with respiratory onset disease have a worse prognosis than those with classic ALS [27]. Primary lateral sclerosis and progressive muscular atrophy are other clinical entities that represent the clinical heterogeneity of the ALS syndrome.

There are a combination of signs associated with upper motor neuron (UMN) and lower motor neuron (LMN) involvement. LMN findings include muscle weakness, reduced muscle tone, atrophy, and fasciculations. UMN signs include hyperreflexia, increased muscle tone, and slowed movements. In addition to findings of motor dysfunction, it has become increasingly recognized that patients with ALS may experience cognitive and behavioral changes that may even be present early in the course of the disease. These include loss of normal language and executive function. There are often behavioral changes such as increased apathy or irritability. Patients may exhibit signs of depression or even sleep disturbance. Finally, some patients will experience signs of dementia or will meet diagnostic criteria for frontotemporal dementia.

Diagnosis

ALS is diagnosed clinically and relies on clinical history and exam findings for diagnosis with electromyography to confirm the extent of denervation. Serologic testing is warranted to rule out potentially reversible entities resembling ALS. Given the clinical heterogeneity of ALS, there are often delays in diagnosis and referrals to appropriate specialists. The median time from the onset of symptoms of ALS to diagnosis is 10–16 months [1]. In efforts to aid in earlier diagnosis and referral, different scoring systems have been developed (Table 10.1).

El Escorial Criteria

The original El Escorial criteria were published in 1994 for inclusion standards for patients entering research studies and clinical trials [28]. Subsequent revisions have incorporated laboratory and electrophysiologic data into diagnostic criteria. The revised El Escorial criteria include four distinct categories: definite ALS; probable ALS; probable ALS, laboratory supported; and possible ALS. Based on these criteria, a definitive diagnosis of ALS requires upper and lower motor neuron involvement in at least three of four anatomic regions (cranial, cervical, thoracic, and lumbar regions) [29]. It is important to note that laboratory, electrophysiological,

Table 10.1 Diagnostic criteria for ALS

Revised El Escorial criteria	
Possible ALS	Presence of upper motor neuron and lower motor neuron signs in one region or upper motor neuron signs in two or three regions, such as monomelic ALS, progressive bulbar palsy, and primary lateral sclerosis
Probable ALS, laboratory supported	Presence of upper motor neuron and lower motor neuron signs in one region with evidence by EMG of lower motor neuron involvement in another region
Probable ALS	Presence of upper motor neuron and lower motor neuron signs in at least two regions with upper motor neuron sign rostral to lower motor neuron signs
Definite ALS	Presence of upper motor neuron and lower motor neuron signs in three anatomical regions
Gold Coast criteria	
Progressive motor impairment documented by history or repeated clinical assessment, preceded by normal motor function	
AND	
The presence of upper and lower motor neuron dysfunction in at least one body region, with	
Upper and lower motor neuron dysfunction noted in the same body region if only one region is involved or lower motor neuron dysfunction in at least TWO body regions	
AND	
Investigations excluding other disease processes	

Refs. [29, 31]

and neuroimaging results should not show evidence of other pathological processes to suggest an alternative diagnosis. One of the criticisms of the El Escorial criteria is that labeling patients with "possible ALS" is often confusing for patients, families, and physicians and would suggest an alternative diagnosis; however, almost all patients initially diagnosed with possible ALS will have disease progression and die from complications of ALS [30].

Gold Coast Criteria

The Gold Coast criteria were developed to identify patients earlier in their disease course and capture the broad features of the disease [31]. The Gold Coast criteria define ALS by the following:

- Progressive motor impairment, documented by history or repeated clinical assessment, preceded by normal motor function.
- Upper and lower motor neuron dysfunction in at least one body region or lower motor neuron dysfunction in at least two body regions.
- Investigative findings that exclude alternative diseases.

Multiple studies have demonstrated improved sensitivity for diagnosis of ALS when compared to the El Escorial criteria with comparable specificity [32, 33].

Staging and Prognosis

Staging systems have been developed to better identify where an individual is in their disease course. These systems are useful tools that help counsel patients, allocate resources, and design clinical trials. The King's staging system defines four stages based on regional body involvement as well as respiratory and nutritional failure [34]. Another scoring system, the ALS Milano-Torino Staging (ALS-MiToS), is based on a functional rating scale based on four functional domains (movement, swallowing, communication, and breathing) [35]. As patients progress along stages, there is decreased median survival. Early in the disease course, the King's staging system outperforms the ALS-MiToS system, while in the later stage, the ALS-MiToS system is better [36]. Currently, these staging systems are predominantly used in research settings [37].

Clinicians largely utilize the Amyotrophic Lateral Sclerosis Functional Rating Score-Revised (ALSFRS-R) to monitor disease progression [38]. Within this scoring system, respiratory involvement carries prognostic information. One limitation with the ALSFRS-R is that subscores can improve based on symptoms management despite ongoing functional decline and disease progression [39]. New scoring systems and prognostic scores are being developed to overcome limitations from ALSFRS-R and provide meaningful prognostic data based on age and clinical features including respiratory involvement and genetic factors; however, these models require further validation [40, 41].

Treatment

ALS is a progressive and incurable disease with treatment focused on disease-modifying agents and symptomatic management. Two medications that have been shown to slow the progression of disease are riluzole and edaravone [42–44]. Riluzole works by blocking the release of glutamate, which is thought to promote neuronal injury in ALS. The most common adverse effects of riluzole are elevated liver enzymes and decreased energy. There are reports of fatal hepatic failure and pancreatitis; however, these are rare. Edaravone is an antioxidant thought to relieve motor nerve death caused by oxidative stress. Edaravone seems to have limited efficacy in patients with early ALS [45].

Recognition of the clinical heterogeneity as well as genetic features that contribute to the development of ALS has led to emerging treatment paradigms. Gene therapy is an avenue that holds promise in treatment of patients with ALS [46]. Antisense oligonucleotides can be used to target mRNA and pre-RNA in patients with gain-of-function mutations such as *SOD1*, *C9orf72*, *FUS*, and *ATAXN2* [47]. Monoclonal antibodies targeting abnormal protein aggregates are under investigation [48]. Therapies aimed at altering the immune system are being evaluated for use in patients with ALS. Increasing T regulatory cells may slow disease progression [49]. Masitinib is a tyrosine kinase inhibitor that may decrease microglial activation and showed promise in early clinical trials [50, 51]. Stem cells are yet another avenue that is being explored and seems to be well tolerated with early promise; however, trials have not shown long-lasting efficacy [52].

Complications of ALS and Respiratory Manifestations

Respiratory Dysfunction

Respiratory compromise can be an early- or late-stage manifestation of ALS and is associated with worsening morbidity and mortality once it occurs. In ALS, the respiratory system can be affected at several anatomic levels and can manifest due to inspiratory muscle weakness and subsequent hypoventilatory failure, expiratory muscle weakness and decreased airway clearance, and bulbar muscle dysfunction causing issues with airway protection, speech, or swallowing (see Fig. 10.2).

Respiratory failure due to respiratory muscle weakness can often develop insidiously. Early on, manifestations may only occur during sleep, resulting in symptoms of sleep disordered breathing. These include morning headaches and daytime fatigue, though the symptoms may be subtle and attributed to other causes. As further muscle weakness occurs, patients may begin to report additional symptoms including dyspnea and orthopnea. When expiratory muscle weakness occurs, patients will report issues with weak or ineffective cough and increased secretions. This can increase the risk of respiratory infections and subsequent morbidity and mortality.

Bulbar Symptoms

When bulbar involvement occurs in ALS, patients will present with symptoms of dysphagia and dysarthria. When upper motor neuron involvement occurs in bulbar ALS, patients will report slow, labored, and distorted speech. This pattern of speech disturbance is defined as spastic dysarthria. When LMN involvement occurs and results in dysarthria, this is known as flaccid dysarthria. Patients will have tongue wasting and fasciculations. Regardless of initial manifesting symptoms, 80–95% of patients with ALS will have trouble with communication at some point in their disease course [53]. With bulbar involvement, patients will also develop dysphagia. These patients will experience malnutrition, weight loss, dehydration, and

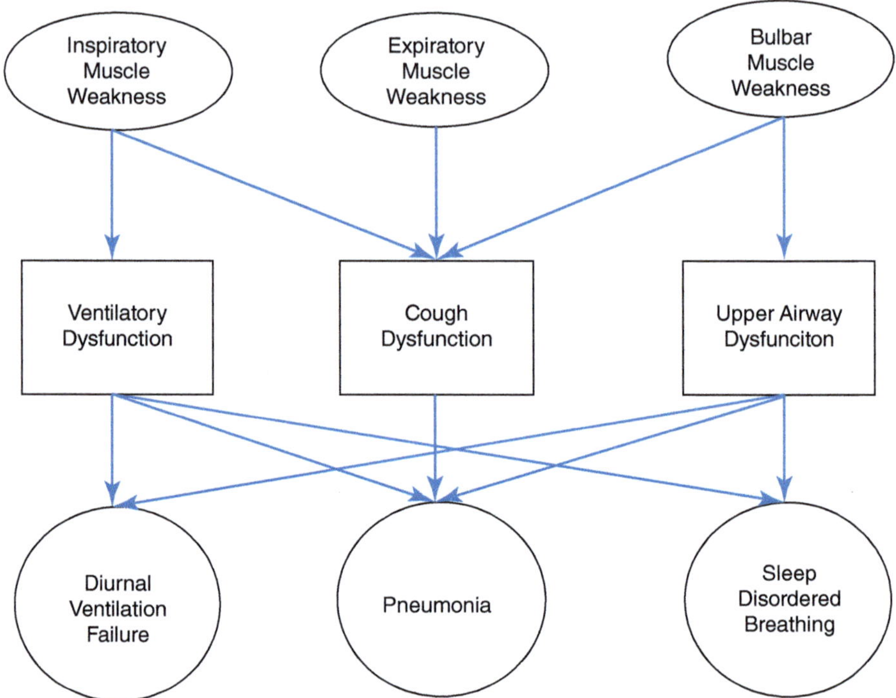

Fig. 10.2 Pathogenesis of respiratory dysfunction in ALS. (Reprinted with permission of the American Thoracic Society. Copyright © 2024 American Thoracic Society. All rights reserved. Benditt and Boitano [135])

aspiration events, which may worsen respiratory compromise. Weight loss and malnourishment are predictors of mortality in ALS and should be monitored closely [54, 55].

Cognitive Impairment

Cognitive impairment is becoming an increasingly recognized entity in ALS [56–58]. Degenerative changes can be seen in the frontotemporal lobes in patients with ALS and may manifest as behavioral complications or executive and language dysfunction [59–61]. Behavioral changes may include apathy, disinhibition, and delusions. Depression is frequently encountered; however, it is unclear if this can be attributed to the pathogenesis of ALS or a consequence of the symptoms of the disease. Mild behavioral and language dysfunction can be some of the earliest manifestations of the disease; however, they may go unnoticed until motor manifestations develop. Frontotemporal dysfunction is diagnosed retrospectively once motor manifestations become apparent. It is also becoming increasingly recognized that ALS and frontotemporal dementia (FTD) exist on a clinical spectrum with pure motor ALS representing one end of the spectrum, while pure FTD represents the other end of the spectrum. Approximately 15% of patients will meet all criteria for frontotemporal dementia [58, 62].

Sleep Disorders

Disorders of sleep and wakefulness may also manifest in patients with ALS. As previously discussed, some of the earliest manifestations of weakness involving the muscles of respiration leading to hypoventilation will occur when patients are supine and when sleeping; however, sleep disturbances have also been observed in patients with preserved diaphragmatic and respiratory muscle functions. These patients will commonly report increased sleep latency, have reduced slow-wave sleep, reduced sleep efficiency, and disturbance in the duration of REM and non-REM sleep [63–67]. Neuroimaging and pathologic studies have suggested that the pathophysiology of ALS extends beyond the motor cortex and may involve areas in the brain stem involved in REM sleep [68]. These anatomic and radiographic findings may explain the disturbances that some patients with ALS will experience. Restless leg syndrome (RLS) is the unpleasant sensation of "creeping" or aching in the lower extremities that is relieved with movement. There are studies demonstrating an association with RLS and patients with ALS [69–71]. Regardless of the mechanism of sleep disturbance in ALS, it is important for physicians to inquire about sleep and wake disorders in ALS as these can lead to decreased quality of life for these patients and may be a sign of respiratory complications that should be addressed [67, 72–75].

Evaluation of Pulmonary Status in ALS

Symptom Assessment and Physical Exam

Complications of respiratory failure are the most common causes of death in patients with ALS; therefore, early and periodic assessments for signs and symptoms of respiratory deterioration are necessary [1, 76, 77]. The initial assessment should occur at the time of diagnosis. Providers should ask patients about symptoms of dyspnea, orthopnea, sleep disturbances, daytime somnolence, morning headaches, weak cough, dysphagia, or dysarthria.

Patients may speak in a softer voice which may be an early sign of respiratory muscle weakness. Upon further examination, there may be decreased chest wall movement, use of accessory muscles of respiration, and paradoxical abdominal movement. Tachypnea may be present or even dyspnea with minimal activities such as assisted transfer or speaking.

Pulmonary Function Testing

Formal assessment of respiratory function should occur at the time of diagnosis and every 3–6 months thereafter [77]. Spirometry is the primary respiratory test in patients with ALS with upright forced vital capacity (FVC) being used to assess disease progression, overall prognosis, and timing of initiation of non-invasive ventilation (NIV) [78]. Supine FVC has also been shown to correlate with diaphragmatic strength and is a more sensitive test for the assessment of diaphragmatic muscle weakness in patients with ALS [79].

Despite widespread use in ALS centers, FVC has several limitations in tracking respiratory function in ALS. One such limitation is that diaphragmatic weakness can be present despite a normal FVC. Studies have shown that lung volumes can remain stable despite progression of diaphragmatic muscle weakness, and FVC has been shown to remain stable until late in the disease course [80]. Furthermore, FVC is non-specific for diaphragmatic weakness and can be reduced in other restrictive lung diseases and in conditions such as obesity. Finally, measurement of vital capacity requires strength of facial muscles to form a seal around the mouthpiece which may be limited in some patients with ALS [81]. These limitations have prompted some clinicians and researchers to consider specific tests looking at respiratory muscle strength in addition to FVC when evaluating patients with ALS.

Maximal inspiratory pressure (MIP) and maximal expiratory pressure (MEP) are alternative tests that can be used in assessing respiratory muscle weakness. Using a non-invasive mask or mouth piece, patients are encouraged to maximally inhale or exhale against an occluded valve, and the resultant pressure is recorded. Normal values almost always exclude respiratory muscle weakness; however, in patients with facial muscle weakness or cognitive impairment, these tests may underestimate inspiratory and expiratory respiratory muscle strength and may be difficult to interpret [82, 83]. In these circumstances sniff nasal pressure (SNp) may be used.

In the SNp maneuver, patients have one nostril occluded with a probe connected to a pressure transducer and inhale through their noses. Studies have shown that SNp is an accurate measure of inspiratory muscle strength and is easier for patients with facial muscle weakness to perform reliably [84]. Finally, SNp has be shown to have the greatest decline leading to the need for non-invasive ventilation (NIV) [85].

Cough peak flow (CPF) and peak expiratory flow (PEF) are two additional non-invasive tools that can be used to assess expiratory muscles strength [82]. These tests can be used when the MEP is difficult to interpret. CPF uses a peak flow meter adapted to an anesthesia face mask and can be used to assess the ability for ALS patients to cough. PEF measures the maximal flow generated from full inspiration.

Transdiaphragmatic pressure (Pdi) and cough gastric pressure (Pga) are invasive measures that can accurately and reproducibly assess inspiratory and expiratory muscle weakness. Pdi is assessed by placing balloon catheters in the stomach and mid-esophagus and recording the pressure differences while the patient inspires. Cough Pga utilizes a similar technique where a balloon catheter is passed into the stomach and patients are asked to cough maximally until no further increase in cough Pga is observed. While accurate and reliable, these tests are invasive, may not be tolerated in many patients, and are therefore largely research tools.

Nocturnal Oximetry, Polysomnography, and Arterial Blood Gas (ABG)

As previously discussed, patients with ALS often report sleep disturbances that are correlated with the severity of their ALS [74]. In rapid eye movement (REM) sleep, skeletal muscle tone is reduced, and sleep disordered breathing and oxygen desaturation events in the setting of muscle weakness are more likely to occur. Obstructive apneas occur more often in patients with bulbar involvement [63, 86]. Nocturnal oximetry and polysomnography can be useful tools to assess for nocturnal desaturation events and sleep disordered breathing in patients with ALS. Nocturnal pulse oximetry has a prognostic value, and nocturnal desaturations correlate with respiratory muscle weakness [87]. Initiation of NIV based on nocturnal desaturations rather than evidence of daytime respiratory compromise has been associated with increased survival [88, 89].

Arterial blood gas assessment can be used to assess for nocturnal and daytime hypoventilation and be utilized for initiation for NIV. While abnormalities in gas exchange represent an indication for initiation of NIV, early in the disease course, arterial blood gas assessment will have a limited value as hypoventilation and subsequent desaturation events generally occur later in the disease course [90]. Non-invasive assessment of hypercarbia using transcutaneous CO_2 monitors is becoming increasingly common [91].

Management of Hypoventilation

Figure 10.3 provides an overview of respiratory care interventions. While our understanding of the cause and pathophysiology of ALS has grown tremendously, leading to an expanding number of medical therapies for ALS [92], respiratory failure remains the most common cause of death in ALS, and ventilatory support remains the most effective, life-prolonging therapy. Furthermore, there is strong evidence showing that ventilatory support can improve health-related quality of life, sleep quality, dyspnea, and cognitive function [93]. Both the European Federation of Neurological Societies and American Academy of Neurology recommend the use of non-invasive ventilation for people with ALS (pALS) [77, 94].

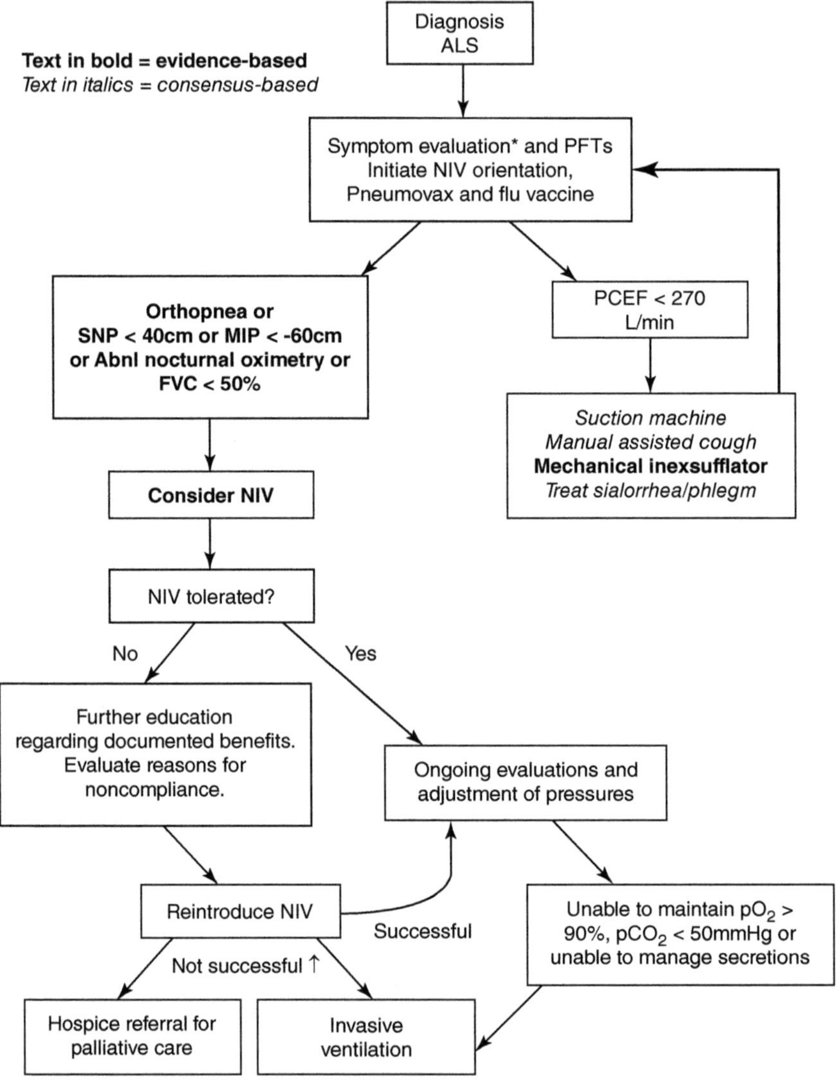

PFT = pulmonary function tests; PCEF = peak cough expiratory flow; NIV = noninvasive ventilation; SNP = sniff nasal pressure; MIP = maximal inspiratory pressure; FVC = forced vital capacity (supine or erect); Abnl nocturnal oximetry = pO_2 <4% from baseline. *Symptoms suggestive of nocturnal hypoventilation: frequent arousals morning headaches excessive day time sleep-iness, vivid dreams. *If NIV is not tolerated or accepted in the setting of advancing respiratory compromise, consider invasive ventilation or referral to hospice.

Fig. 10.3 A proposed respiratory management algorithm. (From Miller et al. [94])

Respiratory muscle weakness leads to hypoventilation, hypercarbia, hypoxia, and dyspnea in pALS [95]. The goal of ventilatory support therefore is to treat hypoventilation leading to improvements in gas exchange, dyspnea, poor sleep, and survival. In virtually all cases, the initial ventilatory strategy should be with non-invasive ventilation (NIV). NIV has many advantages over tracheostomy and invasive ventilation. It can be started and stopped easily, does not require surgery, has fewer complications, has fewer burdens on caregivers, and is less costly [96]. While NIV is generally considered the standard of care for ALS, the actual use of NIV is likely sub-optimal. Published studies may underestimate NIV use, but recent data suggests that only 20–50% of patients are prescribed NIV [97–99].

The criteria for initiating NIV vary in different parts of the world. In the United States, decisions are often based on pulmonary function testing, particularly FVC or maximal inspiratory pressure, and are largely dictated by medical insurance reimbursement criteria. European providers place more emphasis on respiratory symptoms such as orthopnea and dyspnea for initiating NIV and also use overnight oximetry more than US providers [100]. In general NIV should be considered when patients develop dyspnea and orthopnea and have evidence of a decline in respiratory muscle strength. While Medicare reimbursement guidelines use FVC <50% as one criteria for bilevel positive pressure ventilation, there is evidence that starting NIV earlier may be more beneficial. Also, the use of MIP or nocturnal desaturation has been shown to detect respiratory abnormalities earlier than spirometry. Other parameters that can be considered for initiating NIV include transcutaneous CO_2 monitoring [91], sniff nasal pressure [101], and diaphragm ultrasound [102].

NIV can be initiated quickly in many different settings ranging from home to outpatient clinic, in patient hospitalization, or sleep lab. There is little evidence to support one approach over another, and how NIV is started is often determined by provider preference and resources. Most people with ALS initially hypoventilate during sleep, and the majority of patients start using NIV overnight and progress to more usage as their disease progresses, with many eventually using NIV essentially 24 h/day. There are several NIV interfaces to consider including nasal masks, nasal pillows, full-face masks, and mouthpieces [103]. In contrast to other neuromuscular diseases in which bulbar weakness may not occur, all patients with ALS will have bulbar involvement, which can limit the ability of patients to use nasal masks or mouthpiece ventilation. Nevertheless, it is beneficial for patients to be given the option of using a variety of interfaces, and being able to switch between different interfaces can help avoid facial skin breakdown.

There are no adequate studies to guide selection of devices for NIV, nor mode of ventilation [103]. In the United States, device selection may be limited by insurance coverage and contracts with durable medical equipment providers. The options include bilevel positive pressure devices, bilevel positive pressure devices with auto-titrating volume targeted modes, and volume-cycled devices. Regardless of the mode, a device that provides a backup respiratory rate is needed, as pALS may have an unstable respiratory drive [81]. Given the progressive course of ALS, there also needs to be frequent monitoring of ventilatory parameters with the expectation that more ventilatory support will be needed as respiratory muscle weakness progresses. There is also evidence that PEEP should be avoided or minimized, as it has been shown to worsen sleep parameters [104].

There is only one randomized trial of NIV, comparing ventilatory support to no support. This was conducted at a time when the use of NIV was uncommon in the United Kingdom and was not considered the standard of care. In this trial of people with advanced disease, NIV improved quality of life and prolonged survival by 205 days in those with better bulbar function [64]. There are multiple observational studies demonstrating improvements in survival with NIV, as well as improvements in sleep quality, cognitive function, and overall quality of life [105–107]. While it is difficult to accurately estimate the duration of survival benefit afforded by NIV from observational studies, recent estimates are over 1.5 years [98]. As disease advances, people with ALS typically require ventilatory support for longer periods of time and often progress to using it continuously. It is at this point that decisions regarding tracheostomy and invasive ventilation arise. Because all people with ALS have progressive bulbar involvement, they generally reach a point at which secretion clearance and tolerance of NIV are difficult and generally decide between hospice and palliative management vs. tracheostomy.

It is imperative to have discussions about tracheostomy and other end of life decisions early in the course of ALS. This allows patients and families time to learn about various options and make decisions that are consistent with their goals and beliefs. In the United States, only 2% of people with ALS opt for tracheostomy and long-term ventilation; this is similar to rates in Germany, though in Japan rates are much higher at approximately 27% [108]. There are many factors that impact the use of tracheostomy and ventilation including insurance coverage, provider attitude, and cultural beliefs. The Japanese government covers the cost of long-term ventilation, whereas in the United States, there can be substantial out-of-pocket costs for families. In the United States, it is well accepted that patients have autonomy to refuse life-sustaining measures, whereas in Japan, there has traditionally been an expectation for patients to follow treatment recommendations from their physicians.

There are many reasons that people with ALS frequently decline tracheostomy and long-term ventilation in addition to expected medical costs. ALS is usually very advanced by the time a tracheostomy would be required, with loss of limb function, anarthria, and severe dysphagia. In this setting, long-term ventilation may be seen as a burdensome, invasive approach that will prolong survival, but not add to quality of life. Additionally, the hospital stay following tracheostomy is generally long, with an average of 52 days in one study [109]. There is also a heavy burden on family members who provide care for a pALS on long-term mechanical ventilation that needs to be considered. While health insurance will often cover some nursing assistance in the home, family members are expected to contribute substantially in daily care.

While tracheostomy and long-term ventilation are utilized by a small percentage of pALS, there are older studies suggesting that people with ALS who undergo tracheostomy and long-term ventilation are often happy with the decision and have an acceptable quality of life [110]. The life expectancy on long-term ventilation varies widely. A study in Italy reported median survival of 253 days [109], whereas a study in Japan found median survival of 2220 days [111], and there are pALS who live for more than 10 years on continuous ventilatory support after tracheostomy.

Another intervention that has been tried to improve diaphragmatic strength and treat hypoventilation is phrenic nerve stimulation or implantation of a phrenic nerve pacemaker. Phrenic nerve stimulation is not a new concept, and phrenic nerve electrodes that are implanted in the chest have been successfully used to treat congenital central hypoventilation syndrome [112]. However, the surgery is extensive enough that this has not been entertained for pALS. In the late 1990s, a group at Case Western Reserve University developed a laparoscopic technique for implanting electrodes on the underside of the diaphragm at the site of the phrenic nerve insertion [113]. This was used successfully for patients with spinal cord injuries and was then tested in pALS [114]. Initial case series and observational studies showed that the procedure was safe, improved sleep, and raised the possibility that survival improved [115, 116]. This led to two randomized trials, which were both stopped early due to increased mortality in the participants assigned to phrenic nerve stimulation [88, 117]. These results essentially ended further investigation in this area.

Ineffective Cough and Secretion Management

Airway Clearance Techniques

In addition to inadequate ventilation due to respiratory muscle weakness, patients with ALS also develop ineffective cough and difficulty with secretion management. An effective cough requires a coordinated inspiratory muscle effort, glottic closure, and forced expiration. Weakened cough may result in recurrent pneumonia, mucous plugging, atelectasis, and worsened gas exchange [118, 119]. One tool that can be used to assess the adequacy of patients to generate an effective cough is the peak cough flow (PCF) [120]. Normal values are greater than 270 L/min, and values less than 270 L/min are an indication to initiate airway clearance techniques (ACTs). ACTs can be divided into two categories: proximal and peripheral.

Proximal ACTs include breath stacking, manually assisted cough, and mechanical and insufflation-exsufflation (MIE) device. In stacked breath-assisted inspiration, patients will have repeated inspirations to increase intrathoracic pressure prior to exhalation. This can be achieved via various techniques. Glossopharyngeal breathing (GPB) is a technique in which patients can auto-air stack using the mouth, tongue, pharynx, and larynx to pump air into the lungs and overcome inspiratory muscle weakness. Once patients feel full of air, they then are instructed to cough. If patients are unable to perform GPB, they can also perform breath stacking in a passive manner. This can be done in several ways including lung volume recruitment, which uses a one-way valve connected to a manual resuscitation bag. If patients are on a home ventilator, they can be taught to breath stack in volume control modes. If patients are unable to tolerate the breath stacking technique, a single breath-assisted inspiration can be used.

One technique that can be used to assist both inspiration and expiration involves utilizing a single or stacked breath with a manually assisted cough (MAC). In a manually assisted cough, patients will experience inflation of the respiratory system to a desired volume followed by compression of the abdomen or chest to increase expiratory flow from an assistant. While MAC requires an assistant to help perform the maneuver, it is a low-cost option that does not require specialized equipment.

Mechanical insufflation-exsufflation (MIE) devices are another tool that can be utilized to assist with coughing in patients with neuromuscular weakness [119, 121, 122]. These devices apply positive and negative pressure swings sequentially via a mouthpiece or mask in an effort to mimic airflow changes that would be seen in a normal cough. Initial settings on the device include adjustments to the positive and negative pressures; the inspiratory, expiratory, and pause times; and the inspiratory flow. These settings can be adjusted to patient comfort and needs. The use of MIE devices can be done both in the setting of acute illness and part of a multimodal secretion management strategy. Airflow obstruction with exsufflation has been shown to occur in patients with ALS; however, this finding was demonstrated in patients with bulbar symptoms in ALS [123, 124]. Severe airflow obstruction in this setting can limit the efficacy of the MIE devices; however, this may be managed by decreasing the inspiratory flows and pressures while increasing the insufflation time [125]. Its worth noting that MIE devices can improve PCF; however, this improvement is not superior to alternative airway clearance techniques mentioned [126]. Complications of MIE devices are rare but may include abdominal bloating, distension, pneumothorax, nausea, bradycardia, or tachycardia [127, 128]. A limitation to MIE devices may also include cost and size of the device. Some of the newer devices have internal and external batteries, making transportation easier.

Peripheral airway clearance techniques are aimed at loosening secretions and enhancing transport of mucus from the peripheral to central airways and may have a role in the setting of treating patients with ALS. Peripheral airway techniques can include manual or instrumental techniques. Manual techniques are simple and include chest percussion, vibrations, or shaking. These techniques are thought to aid in secretion clearance by increasing peak expiratory flow to move secretions to the central airways for clearance via cough or suction. There is limited data on the efficacy of this technique; however, it is a well-tolerated low-cost option for patients to help mobilize secretions.

High-frequency chest wall oscillation (HFCWO) is a technique that utilizes a device to provide compression of the chest wall at frequencies that are similar to the resonant frequency of the lung. Using transient oscillatory increases in airflow, secretions are vibrated from the peripheral to central airways. HFCWO has been shown to improve respiratory symptoms in patients with ALS, and in a subgroup, some patients showed a decrease rate of FVC decline [129]. HFCWO has also been shown to decrease medical costs, inpatient admissions, and pneumonia costs in patients with neuromuscular disease [76]. It is important to note that while HCFWO can move secretions from the peripheral to central airways, proximal airway clearance techniques are still needed to clear the central airways.

Oral Secretion Management

Many patients with ALS will also struggle with excessive oral secretions. Secretions are either thin and watery or thick and copious, and there are treatment strategies that may help with each type. Patients with thin watery secretions often have tongue weakness that limits their ability to redistribute secretions throughout the mouth. Modalities for secretion management in these patients includes anticholinergic agents, botulinum toxin injection, and radiation therapy. Initial therapy is patient and provider dependent; however, the least invasive choice should be considered first. Anticholinergic agents include scopolamine, glycopyrrolate, sublingual atropine, and amitriptyline. Doses should be increased to a treatment effect, and if the response is minimal, a different agent may be used. Some providers may choose a multi-agent approach; however, this results in limited symptomatic improvement and increases the risk of adverse effects, which include drowsiness, urinary retention, constipation, and confusion. Botulinum toxin injection is an alternative treatment option for pALS who achieve limited benefit with anticholinergic agents or are intolerant of medication side effects. Submandibular and/or parotid glands can be injected every 2–3 months. Treatments are usually well tolerated; however, there is a risk that in some patients this may result in paralysis of the surrounding musculature and potential for worsening bulbar function. Finally surgical ligation or radiation of the salivary glands may provide more definitive treatment in some patients. Patients opting to receive high beam radiation will undergo treatment over 5 days. Patients must be able to lie flat to receive treatment.

Thick secretions may occur in patients with bulbar disease and those with dehydration or receiving anticholinergic medications. Providers should pay close attention to patients' hydration status and may need to increase overall free water intake. Saline nebulizers and home humidifiers can help patients thin out tenacious secretions.

Dysphagia, Aspiration, and Nutrition Management

As bulbar function worsens in pALS, dysphagia, aspiration, weight loss, and malnutrition can occur. ALS patients who are malnourished have an increased risk for death, and early assessment for dysphagia and malnutrition are included in guideline recommendations [54, 55, 77]. Complaints of dysphagia should prompt evaluation by a speech therapist with bedside and video fluoroscopic assessments. Speech therapists can be helpful in recommending behavioral adaptations including modification of food consistency as well as various techniques to minimize risk of aspiration [130]. Nutritionists can monitor body weight and make recommendations regarding additional dietary supplements. Percutaneous endoscopic gastrostomy (PEG) tube placement should be discussed as soon as symptoms of dysphagia occur or in the setting of rapid weight loss (>10% premorbid bodyweight). Enteral nutrition may slow disease progression and improve survival [94]. An assessment of respiratory function is necessary before placement, and current guidelines recommend PEG tube placement be considered before the FVC ≤50% [77, 94]. If the FVC is ≤50%, PEG tube placement may still be done; however, close anesthesia monitoring is essential, and patients may need to use NIV during the procedure.

Palliative Care and End of Life Care in ALS

ALS is a progressive and incurable neurodegenerative disease that causes limb paralysis, loss of speech and swallowing, inability to clear oral and respiratory secretions, shortness of breath, and ultimately respiratory failure. Common symptoms include cramps, pain, depression, fear, anxiety, emotional lability, sialorrhea, constipation, cognitive impairment, and laryngospasm. Palliative care aims to reduce symptoms without expectation of a cure and is one of the most important aspects of care for pALS. ALS care is best provided by a multidisciplinary team in order to address the various complications that arise, which compromise quality of life with ALS. Teams generally include a neurologist, nurse, physical therapist, occupational therapist, speech pathologist, social worker, research coordinator, mental health coordinator, gastroenterologist, orthotist, and respiratory care provider. A study in the Netherlands found that patients receiving care in a multidisciplinary clinic were more likely to receive appropriate supportive devices and had better scores for social functioning and mental health [131].

The median survival from diagnosis is approximately 3 years, though there is a great deal of variability. It is important to be proactive in discussing potential supportive interventions such as wheelchair use, feeding tubes, ventilatory support, and hospice. The timing of these discussions needs to be tailored to the individual patient and inevitably needs to be addressed sequentially over the course of the disease. Additionally, discussions about the end of life care should be initiated by providers and should occur throughout the course of the illness.

The majority of patients present with limb weakness, and maintaining mobility with ankle foot orthoses, manual wheelchairs, and ultimately power chairs is a straightforward progression. The decision to pursue gastrostomy tubes is less straightforward, though most patients who have a gastrostomy placed are happy with the decision. The American Academy of Neurology Practice Guideline recommends gastrostomy for those with weight loss and dysphagia, and they are safer to place when the forced vital capacity is above 50% predicted [94].

Sialorrhea is quite common and can greatly interfere with a patient's daily functioning. Techniques to address excessive saliva include suctioning, anticholinergic medications, and botulinum toxin injection for particularly refractory cases [132].

Respiratory symptoms such as dyspnea and congestion are common in ALS and can be treated effectively using ventilatory support and secretion clearance techniques as described above. Supplemental oxygen is rarely needed unless a patient has an underlying lung disease not related to ALS; however, at times oxygen will be given in hospice. Laryngospasm is a relatively uncommon occurrence, <4% of patients, but can present with the sudden inability to breathe. This is very distressing and often prompts calls to 911. Fortunately laryngospasm usually only lasts a few minutes and ends spontaneously before serious consequences occur. Management can be difficult, but education and reassurance can do a lot to help patients manage this troubling symptom. If laryngospasm is frequent or particularly difficult to manage, low-dose, sublingual benzodiazepines can help [133]. For patients who pursue tracheostomy and long-term ventilation, it is important to discuss circumstances that would prompt them to discontinue ventilatory support. Termination of ventilatory support, which will hasten death, is a legal and accepted decision for people with ALS.

Most people with ALS do not opt for long-term invasive ventilation and frequently pursue hospice care when the disease becomes advanced. Home hospice programs are often the most appropriate service for pALS with advanced disease. However, eligibility criteria for hospice are strict, and hospice programs may not have much familiarity with ALS. Therefore it is helpful for ALS providers to have relationships with local hospice programs and provide them with education about the disease and the needs of pALS. Education of patients and their families and friends, coupled with proactive use of supportive equipment and medications, can do a great deal to improve the quality of life for those with ALS. Multidisciplinary care teams are in the best position to provide care for these complex patients and foster ongoing research which will ultimately benefit future patients.

Conclusion

ALS is considered a rare condition, but it affects over 30,000 people in the United States and is a devastating illness for patients, families, and friends. It is rapidly progressive and ultimately leads to functional quadriplegia, inability to speak and swallow, and respiratory failure. Though intense research efforts have been underway to develop curative therapies for ALS, and new medical therapies have been approved, respiratory support for pALS currently has the biggest impact on the quality of life and survival. Pulmonary providers are crucial for evaluating pALS, discussing goals of care, and initiating therapies. Non-invasive ventilation has been shown to improve respiratory symptoms, sleep quality, cognitive function, and survival. While relatively few pALS choose tracheostomy and long-term ventilation, it is important for patients to be taught about the pros and cons of this modality and allowed to make informed decisions about their care. Bulbar weakness coupled with weakness of the inspiratory and expiratory muscle weakness places patients at high risk for aspiration, mucus plugging, and respiratory failure. Assisted cough techniques and other methods to improve secretion clearance are necessary for pALS and can allow the successful use of non-invasive ventilation for a relatively long time.

References

1. Brown RH, Al-Chalabi A. Amyotrophic lateral sclerosis. N Engl J Med. 2017;377(2):162–72. https://doi.org/10.1056/NEJMra1603471.
2. Longinetti E, Fang F. Epidemiology of amyotrophic lateral sclerosis: an update of recent literature. Curr Opin Neurol. 2019;32(5):771–6. https://doi.org/10.1097/WCO.0000000000000730.
3. Kim HJ, Oh KW, Kwon MJ, et al. Identification of mutations in Korean patients with amyotrophic lateral sclerosis using multigene panel testing. Neurobiol Aging. 2016;37:209.e9–209.e16. https://doi.org/10.1016/j.neurobiolaging.2015.09.012.
4. Kwon MJ, Baek W, Ki CS, et al. Screening of the SOD1, FUS, TARDBP, ANG, and OPTN mutations in Korean patients with familial and sporadic ALS. Neurobiol Aging. 2012;33(5):1017.e17–23. https://doi.org/10.1016/j.neurobiolaging.2011.12.003.
5. Arthur KC, Calvo A, Price TR, Geiger JT, Chiò A, Traynor BJ. Projected increase in amyotrophic lateral sclerosis from 2015 to 2040. Nat Commun. 2016;7(1):12408. https://doi.org/10.1038/ncomms12408.
6. Gowland A, Opie-Martin S, Scott KM, et al. Predicting the future of ALS: the impact of demographic change and potential new treatments on the prevalence of ALS in the United Kingdom, 2020–2116. Amyotroph Lateral Scler Front Degener. 2019;20(3–4):264–74. https://doi.org/10.1080/21678421.2019.1587629.
7. Mulder DW, Kurland LT, Offord KP, Beard CM. Familial adult motor neuron disease: amyotrophic lateral sclerosis. Neurology. 1986;36(4):511–7. https://doi.org/10.1212/wnl.36.4.511.
8. Ranganathan R, Haque S, Coley K, Shepheard S, Cooper-Knock J, Kirby J. Multifaceted genes in amyotrophic lateral sclerosis-frontotemporal dementia. Front Neurosci. 2020;14:684. https://doi.org/10.3389/fnins.2020.00684.
9. Rosen DR, Siddique T, Patterson D, et al. Mutations in Cu/Zn superoxide dismutase gene are associated with familial amyotrophic lateral sclerosis. Nature. 1993;362(6415):59–62. https://doi.org/10.1038/362059a0.
10. Taylor JP, Brown RH, Cleveland DW. Decoding ALS: from genes to mechanism. Nature. 2016;539(7628):197–206. https://doi.org/10.1038/nature20413.
11. Brown RH Jr. Amyotrophic lateral sclerosis and other motor neuron diseases. In: Loscalzo J, Fauci A, Kasper D, Hauser S, Longo D, Jameson JL, editors. Harrison's principles of internal medicine. 21th ed. McGraw-Hill Education; 2022. accessmedicine.mhmedical.com/content.aspx?aid=1201640039. Accessed 11 Dec 2023.
12. Van Hoecke A, Schoonaert L, Lemmens R, et al. EPHA4 is a disease modifier of amyotrophic lateral sclerosis in animal models and in humans. Nat Med. 2012;18(9):1418–22. https://doi.org/10.1038/nm.2901.
13. Berdyński M, Miszta P, Safranow K, et al. SOD1 mutations associated with amyotrophic lateral sclerosis analysis of variant severity. Sci Rep. 2022;12(1):103. https://doi.org/10.1038/s41598-021-03891-8.
14. Goldstein O, Inbar T, Kedmi M, et al. FUS-P525L juvenile amyotrophic lateral sclerosis and intellectual disability: evidence for association and oligogenic inheritance. Neurol Genet. 2022;8(4):e200009. https://doi.org/10.1212/NXG.0000000000200009.
15. Ingre C, Roos PM, Piehl F, Kamel F, Fang F. Risk factors for amyotrophic lateral sclerosis. Clin Epidemiol. 2015;7:181–93. https://doi.org/10.2147/CLEP.S37505.
16. Marin B, Fontana A, Arcuti S, et al. Age-specific ALS incidence: a dose-response meta-analysis. Eur J Epidemiol. 2018;33(7):621–34. https://doi.org/10.1007/s10654-018-0392-x.
17. Wang H, O'Reilly ÉJ, Weisskopf MG, et al. Smoking and risk of amyotrophic lateral sclerosis: a pooled analysis of 5 prospective cohorts. Arch Neurol. 2011;68(2):207–13. https://doi.org/10.1001/archneurol.2010.367.
18. O'Reilly ÉJ, Wang H, Weisskopf MG, et al. Premorbid body mass index and risk of amyotrophic lateral sclerosis. Amyotroph Lateral Scler Front Degener. 2013;14(3):205–11. https://doi.org/10.3109/21678421.2012.735240.

19. Gallo V, Wark PA, Jenab M, et al. Prediagnostic body fat and risk of death from amyotrophic lateral sclerosis: the EPIC cohort. Neurology. 2013;80(9):829–38. https://doi.org/10.1212/WNL.0b013e3182840689.

20. Mariosa D, Beard JD, Umbach DM, et al. Body mass index and amyotrophic lateral sclerosis: a study of US military veterans. Am J Epidemiol. 2017;185(5):362–71. https://doi.org/10.1093/aje/kww140.

21. Julian TH, Glascow N, Barry ADF, et al. Physical exercise is a risk factor for amyotrophic lateral sclerosis: convergent evidence from Mendelian randomisation, transcriptomics and risk genotypes. EBioMedicine. 2021;68:103397. https://doi.org/10.1016/j.ebiom.2021.103397.

22. McCormick AL, Brown RH, Cudkowicz ME, Al-Chalabi A, Garson JA. Quantification of reverse transcriptase in ALS and elimination of a novel retroviral candidate. Neurology. 2008;70(4):278–83. https://doi.org/10.1212/01.wnl.0000297552.13219.b4.

23. Li W, Lee MH, Henderson L, et al. Human endogenous retrovirus-K contributes to motor neuron disease. Sci Transl Med. 2015;7(307):307ra153. https://doi.org/10.1126/scitranslmed.aac8201.

24. Bellmann J, Monette A, Tripathy V, et al. Viral infections exacerbate FUS-ALS phenotypes in iPSC-derived spinal neurons in a virus species-specific manner. Front Cell Neurosci. 2019;13:480. https://doi.org/10.3389/fncel.2019.00480.

25. Neumann M, Sampathu DM, Kwong LK, et al. Ubiquitinated TDP-43 in frontotemporal lobar degeneration and amyotrophic lateral sclerosis. Science. 2006;314(5796):130–3. https://doi.org/10.1126/science.1134108.

26. Olney NT, Spina S, Miller BL. Frontotemporal dementia. Neurol Clin. 2017;35(2):339–74. https://doi.org/10.1016/j.ncl.2017.01.008.

27. de Carvalho M, Matias T, Coelho F, Evangelista T, Pinto A, Luís ML. Motor neuron disease presenting with respiratory failure. J Neurol Sci. 1996;139(Suppl):117–22. https://doi.org/10.1016/0022-510x(96)00089-5.

28. Brooks BR. El Escorial World Federation of Neurology criteria for the diagnosis of amyotrophic lateral sclerosis. Subcommittee on Motor Neuron Diseases/Amyotrophic Lateral Sclerosis of the World Federation of Neurology Research Group on Neuromuscular Diseases and the El Escorial "Clinical limits of amyotrophic lateral sclerosis" workshop contributors. J Neurol Sci. 1994;124(Suppl):96–107. https://doi.org/10.1016/0022-510x(94)90191-0.

29. Brooks BR, Miller RG, Swash M, Munsat TL. El Escorial revisited: revised criteria for the diagnosis of amyotrophic lateral sclerosis. Amyotroph Lateral Scler Other Motor Neuron Disord. 2000;1(5):293–9. https://doi.org/10.1080/146608200300079536.

30. Vucic S, Ferguson TA, Cummings C, et al. Gold Coast diagnostic criteria: implications for ALS diagnosis and clinical trial enrollment. Muscle Nerve. 2021;64(5):532–7. https://doi.org/10.1002/mus.27392.

31. Shefner JM, Al-Chalabi A, Baker MR, et al. A proposal for new diagnostic criteria for ALS. Clin Neurophysiol. 2020;131(8):1975–8. https://doi.org/10.1016/j.clinph.2020.04.005.

32. Pugdahl K, Camdessanché JP, Cengiz B, et al. Gold Coast diagnostic criteria increase sensitivity in amyotrophic lateral sclerosis. Clin Neurophysiol. 2021;132(12):3183–9. https://doi.org/10.1016/j.clinph.2021.08.014.

33. Shen D, Yang X, Wang Y, et al. The Gold Coast criteria increases the diagnostic sensitivity for amyotrophic lateral sclerosis in a Chinese population. Transl Neurodegener. 2021;10(1):28. https://doi.org/10.1186/s40035-021-00253-2.

34. Roche JC, Rojas-Garcia R, Scott KM, et al. A proposed staging system for amyotrophic lateral sclerosis. Brain J Neurol. 2012;135(Pt 3):847–52. https://doi.org/10.1093/brain/awr351.

35. Chiò A, Hammond ER, Mora G, Bonito V, Filippini G. Development and evaluation of a clinical staging system for amyotrophic lateral sclerosis. J Neurol Neurosurg Psychiatry. 2015;86(1):38–44. https://doi.org/10.1136/jnnp-2013-306589.

36. Fang T, Al Khleifat A, Stahl DR, et al. Comparison of the King's and MiToS staging systems for ALS. Amyotroph Lateral Scler Front Degener. 2017;18(3–4):227–32. https://doi.org/10.1080/21678421.2016.1265565.

37. Al-Chalabi A, Chiò A, Merrill C, et al. Clinical staging in amyotrophic lateral sclerosis: analysis of Edaravone Study 19. J Neurol Neurosurg Psychiatry. 2021;92(2):165–71. https://doi.org/10.1136/jnnp-2020-323271.

38. Cedarbaum JM, Stambler N, Malta E, et al. The ALSFRS-R: a revised ALS functional rating scale that incorporates assessments of respiratory function. BDNF ALS Study Group (Phase III). J Neurol Sci. 1999;169(1–2):13–21. https://doi.org/10.1016/s0022-510x(99)00210-5.

39. Rooney J, Burke T, Vajda A, Heverin M, Hardiman O. What does the ALSFRS-R really measure? A longitudinal and survival analysis of functional dimension subscores in amyotrophic lateral sclerosis. J Neurol Neurosurg Psychiatry. 2017;88(5):381–5. https://doi.org/10.1136/jnnp-2016-314661.

40. Westeneng HJ, Debray TPA, Visser AE, et al. Prognosis for patients with amyotrophic lateral sclerosis: development and validation of a personalised prediction model. Lancet Neurol. 2018;17(5):423–33. https://doi.org/10.1016/S1474-4422(18)30089-9.

41. Fournier CN, Bedlack R, Quinn C, et al. Development and validation of the Rasch-Built Overall Amyotrophic Lateral Sclerosis Disability Scale (ROADS). JAMA Neurol. 2020;77(4):480–8. https://doi.org/10.1001/jamaneurol.2019.4490.

42. Bensimon G, Lacomblez L, Meininger V. A controlled trial of riluzole in amyotrophic lateral sclerosis. ALS/Riluzole Study Group. N Engl J Med. 1994;330(9):585–91. https://doi.org/10.1056/NEJM199403033300901.

43. Edaravone (MCI-186) ALS 16 Study Group. A post-hoc subgroup analysis of outcomes in the first phase III clinical study of edaravone (MCI-186) in amyotrophic lateral sclerosis. Amyotroph Lateral Scler Front Degener. 2017;18(sup1):11–9. https://doi.org/10.1080/21678421.2017.1363780.

44. Shefner J, Heiman-Patterson T, Pioro EP, et al. Long-term edaravone efficacy in amyotrophic lateral sclerosis: post-hoc analyses of Study 19 (MCI186-19). Muscle Nerve. 2020;61(2):218–21. https://doi.org/10.1002/mus.26740.

45. Writing Group, Edaravone (MCI-186) ALS 19 Study Group. Safety and efficacy of edaravone in well defined patients with amyotrophic lateral sclerosis: a randomised, double-blind, placebo-controlled trial. Lancet Neurol. 2017;16(7):505–12. https://doi.org/10.1016/S1474-4422(17)30115-1.

46. Tosolini AP, Sleigh JN. Motor neuron gene therapy: lessons from spinal muscular atrophy for amyotrophic lateral sclerosis. Front Mol Neurosci. 2017;10:405. https://doi.org/10.3389/fnmol.2017.00405.

47. Boros BD, Schoch KM, Kreple CJ, Miller TM. Antisense oligonucleotides for the study and treatment of ALS. Neurother J Am Soc Exp Neurother. 2022;19(4):1145–58. https://doi.org/10.1007/s13311-022-01247-2.

48. Meininger V, Genge A, van den Berg LH, et al. Safety and efficacy of ozanezumab in patients with amyotrophic lateral sclerosis: a randomised, double-blind, placebo-controlled, phase 2 trial. Lancet Neurol. 2017;16(3):208–16. https://doi.org/10.1016/S1474-4422(16)30399-4.

49. Giovannelli I, Heath P, Shaw PJ, Kirby J. The involvement of regulatory T cells in amyotrophic lateral sclerosis and their therapeutic potential. Amyotroph Lateral Scler Front Degener. 2020;21(5–6):435–44. https://doi.org/10.1080/21678421.2020.1752246.

50. Trias E, Ibarburu S, Barreto-Núñez R, et al. Post-paralysis tyrosine kinase inhibition with masitinib abrogates neuroinflammation and slows disease progression in inherited amyotrophic lateral sclerosis. J Neuroinflammation. 2016;13(1):177. https://doi.org/10.1186/s12974-016-0620-9.

51. Mora JS, Genge A, Chio A, et al. Masitinib as an add-on therapy to riluzole in patients with amyotrophic lateral sclerosis: a randomized clinical trial. Amyotroph Lateral Scler Front Degener. 2020;21(1–2):5–14. https://doi.org/10.1080/21678421.2019.1632346.

52. Dimos JT, Rodolfa KT, Niakan KK, et al. Induced pluripotent stem cells generated from patients with ALS can be differentiated into motor neurons. Science. 2008;321(5893):1218–21. https://doi.org/10.1126/science.1158799.

53. Körner S, Sieniawski M, Kollewe K, et al. Speech therapy and communication device: impact on quality of life and mood in patients with amyotrophic lateral sclerosis. Amyotroph Lateral Scler Front Degener. 2013;14(1):20–5. https://doi.org/10.3109/17482968.2012.692382.
54. Desport JC, Preux PM, Truong TC, Vallat JM, Sautereau D, Couratier P. Nutritional status is a prognostic factor for survival in ALS patients. Neurology. 1999;53(5):1059–63. https://doi.org/10.1212/wnl.53.5.1059.
55. Marin B, Desport JC, Kajeu P, et al. Alteration of nutritional status at diagnosis is a prognostic factor for survival of amyotrophic lateral sclerosis patients. J Neurol Neurosurg Psychiatry. 2011;82(6):628–34. https://doi.org/10.1136/jnnp.2010.211474.
56. Crockford C, Newton J, Lonergan K, et al. ALS-specific cognitive and behavior changes associated with advancing disease stage in ALS. Neurology. 2018;91(15):e1370–80. https://doi.org/10.1212/WNL.0000000000006317.
57. Beeldman E, Govaarts R, de Visser M, et al. Progression of cognitive and behavioural impairment in early amyotrophic lateral sclerosis. J Neurol Neurosurg Psychiatry. 2020;91(7):779–80. https://doi.org/10.1136/jnnp-2020-322992.
58. Pender N, Pinto-Grau M, Hardiman O. Cognitive and behavioural impairment in amyotrophic lateral sclerosis. Curr Opin Neurol. 2020;33(5):649–54. https://doi.org/10.1097/WCO.0000000000000862.
59. Rascovsky K, Hodges JR, Knopman D, et al. Sensitivity of revised diagnostic criteria for the behavioural variant of frontotemporal dementia. Brain J Neurol. 2011;134(Pt 9):2456–77. https://doi.org/10.1093/brain/awr179.
60. Rosen HJ, Allison SC, Schauer GF, Gorno-Tempini ML, Weiner MW, Miller BL. Neuroanatomical correlates of behavioural disorders in dementia. Brain J Neurol. 2005;128(Pt 11):2612–25. https://doi.org/10.1093/brain/awh628.
61. Seeley WW, Crawford R, Rascovsky K, et al. Frontal paralimbic network atrophy in very mild behavioral variant frontotemporal dementia. Arch Neurol. 2008;65(2):249–55. https://doi.org/10.1001/archneurol.2007.38.
62. Ringholz GM, Appel SH, Bradshaw M, Cooke NA, Mosnik DM, Schulz PE. Prevalence and patterns of cognitive impairment in sporadic ALS. Neurology. 2005;65(4):586–90. https://doi.org/10.1212/01.wnl.0000172911.39167.b6.
63. Ahmed RM, Newcombe REA, Piper AJ, et al. Sleep disorders and respiratory function in amyotrophic lateral sclerosis. Sleep Med Rev. 2016;26:33–42. https://doi.org/10.1016/j.smrv.2015.05.007.
64. Bourke SC, Tomlinson M, Williams TL, Bullock RE, Shaw PJ, Gibson GJ. Effects of non-invasive ventilation on survival and quality of life in patients with amyotrophic lateral sclerosis: a randomised controlled trial. Lancet Neurol. 2006;5(2):140–7. https://doi.org/10.1016/S1474-4422(05)70326-4.
65. Atalaia A, De Carvalho M, Evangelista T, Pinto A. Sleep characteristics of amyotrophic lateral sclerosis in patients with preserved diaphragmatic function. Amyotroph Lateral Scler. 2007;8(2):101–5. https://doi.org/10.1080/17482960601029883.
66. Hood S, Amir S. Neurodegeneration and the circadian clock. Front Aging Neurosci. 2017;9:170. https://doi.org/10.3389/fnagi.2017.00170.
67. Lo Coco D, La Bella V. Fatigue, sleep, and nocturnal complaints in patients with amyotrophic lateral sclerosis. Eur J Neurol. 2012;19(5):760–3. https://doi.org/10.1111/j.1468-1331.2011.03637.x.
68. Li X, Liu Q, Niu T, et al. Sleep disorders and white matter integrity in patients with sporadic amyotrophic lateral sclerosis. Sleep Med. 2023;109:170–80. https://doi.org/10.1016/j.sleep.2023.07.003.
69. Limousin N, Blasco H, Corcia P, Arnulf I, Praline J. The high frequency of restless legs syndrome in patients with amyotrophic lateral sclerosis. Amyotroph Lateral Scler. 2011;12(4):303–6. https://doi.org/10.3109/17482968.2011.557736.
70. Liu S, Shen D, Tai H, et al. Restless legs syndrome in Chinese patients with sporadic amyotrophic lateral sclerosis. Front Neurol. 2018;9:735. https://doi.org/10.3389/fneur.2018.00735.

71. Lo Coco D, Piccoli F, La Bella V. Restless legs syndrome in patients with amyotrophic lateral sclerosis. Mov Disord. 2010;25(15):2658–61. https://doi.org/10.1002/mds.23261.

72. Raheja D, Stephens HE, Lehman E, Walsh S, Yang C, Simmons Z. Patient-reported problematic symptoms in an ALS treatment trial. Amyotroph Lateral Scler Front Degener. 2016;17(3–4):198–205. https://doi.org/10.3109/21678421.2015.1131831.

73. Panda S, Gourie-Devi M, Sharma A. Sleep disorders in amyotrophic lateral sclerosis: a questionnaire-based study from India. Neurol India. 2018;66(3):700–8. https://doi.org/10.4103/0028-3886.232327.

74. Lo Coco D, Mattaliano P, Spataro R, Mattaliano A, La Bella V. Sleep-wake disturbances in patients with amyotrophic lateral sclerosis. J Neurol Neurosurg Psychiatry. 2011;82(8):839–42. https://doi.org/10.1136/jnnp.2010.228007.

75. Diaz-Abad M, Buczyner JR, Venza BR, et al. Poor sleep quality in patients with amyotrophic lateral sclerosis at the time of diagnosis. J Clin Neuromuscul Dis. 2018;20(2):60–8. https://doi.org/10.1097/CND.0000000000000234.

76. Lechtzin N, Wiener CM, Clawson L, Chaudhry V, Diette GB. Hospitalization in amyotrophic lateral sclerosis: causes, costs, and outcomes. Neurology. 2001;56(6):753–7. https://doi.org/10.1212/wnl.56.6.753.

77. EFNS Task Force on Diagnosis and Management of Amyotrophic Lateral Sclerosis, Andersen PM, Abrahams S, et al. EFNS guidelines on the clinical management of amyotrophic lateral sclerosis (MALS)—revised report of an EFNS task force. Eur J Neurol. 2012;19(3):360–75. https://doi.org/10.1111/j.1468-1331.2011.03501.x.

78. Czaplinski A, Yen AA, Appel SH. Forced vital capacity (FVC) as an indicator of survival and disease progression in an ALS clinic population. J Neurol Neurosurg Psychiatry. 2006;77(3):390–2. https://doi.org/10.1136/jnnp.2005.072660.

79. Lechtzin N, Wiener CM, Shade DM, Clawson L, Diette GB. Spirometry in the supine position improves the detection of diaphragmatic weakness in patients with amyotrophic lateral sclerosis. Chest. 2002;121(2):436–42. https://doi.org/10.1378/chest.121.2.436.

80. De Troyer A, Borenstein S, Cordier R. Analysis of lung volume restriction in patients with respiratory muscle weakness. Thorax. 1980;35(8):603–10. https://doi.org/10.1136/thx.35.8.603.

81. Pinto S, Swash M, De Carvalho M. Mouth occlusion pressure at 100ms (P0.1) as a respiratory biomarker in amyotrophic lateral sclerosis. Amyotroph Lateral Scler Front Degener. 2021;22(1–2):53–60. https://doi.org/10.1080/21678421.2020.1821061.

82. Lechtzin N. Respiratory effects of amyotrophic lateral sclerosis: problems and solutions. Respir Care. 2006;51(8):871–81; discussion 881–4.

83. Lechtzin N, Scott Y, Busse AM, Clawson LL, Kimball R, Wiener CM. Early use of noninvasive ventilation prolongs survival in subjects with ALS. Amyotroph Lateral Scler. 2007;8(3):185–8. https://doi.org/10.1080/17482960701262392.

84. Fitting JW, Paillex R, Hirt L, Aebischer P, Schluep M. Sniff nasal pressure: a sensitive respiratory test to assess progression of amyotrophic lateral sclerosis. Ann Neurol. 1999;46(6):887–93.

85. Tilanus TBM, Groothuis JT, TenBroek-Pastoor JMC, et al. The predictive value of respiratory function tests for non-invasive ventilation in amyotrophic lateral sclerosis. Respir Res. 2017;18(1):144. https://doi.org/10.1186/s12931-017-0624-8.

86. Quaranta VN, Carratù P, Damiani MF, et al. The prognostic role of obstructive sleep apnea at the onset of amyotrophic lateral sclerosis. Neurodegener Dis. 2017;17(1):14–21. https://doi.org/10.1159/000447560.

87. Elman LB, Siderowf AD, McCluskey LF. Nocturnal oximetry: utility in the respiratory management of amyotrophic lateral sclerosis. Am J Phys Med Rehabil. 2003;82(11):866–70. https://doi.org/10.1097/01.PHM.0000091985.22659.30.

88. Gonzalez-Bermejo J, Morélot-Panzini C, Tanguy ML, et al. Early diaphragm pacing in patients with amyotrophic lateral sclerosis (RespiStimALS): a randomised controlled triple-blind trial. Lancet Neurol. 2016;15(12):1217–27. https://doi.org/10.1016/S1474-4422(16)30233-2.

89. Pinto A, De Carvalho M, Evangelista T, Lopes A, Sales-Luís L. Nocturnal pulse oximetry: a new approach to establish the appropriate time for non-invasive ventilation in ALS patients. Amyotroph Lateral Scler Other Motor Neuron Disord. 2003;4(1):31–5. https://doi.org/10.1080/14660820310006706.

90. Vitacca M, Clini E, Facchetti D, et al. Breathing pattern and respiratory mechanics in patients with amyotrophic lateral sclerosis. Eur Respir J. 1997;10(7):1614–21. https://doi.org/10.1183/09031936.97.10071614.

91. Quigg KH, Wilson MW, Choi PJ. Transcutaneous CO_2 monitoring as indication for inpatient non-invasive ventilation initiation in patients with amyotrophic lateral sclerosis. Muscle Nerve. 2022;65(4):444–7. https://doi.org/10.1002/mus.27457.

92. Shefner JM, Bedlack R, Andrews JA, et al. Amyotrophic lateral sclerosis clinical trials and interpretation of functional end points and fluid biomarkers: a review. JAMA Neurol. 2022;79(12):1312–8. https://doi.org/10.1001/jamaneurol.2022.3282.

93. Sales de Campos P, Olsen WL, Wymer JP, Smith BK. Respiratory therapies for amyotrophic lateral sclerosis: a state of the art review. Chron Respir Dis. 2023;20:14799731231175915. https://doi.org/10.1177/14799731231175915.

94. Miller RG, Jackson CE, Kasarskis EJ, et al. Practice parameter update: the care of the patient with amyotrophic lateral sclerosis: drug, nutritional, and respiratory therapies (an evidence-based review): report of the Quality Standards Subcommittee of the American Academy of Neurology. Neurology. 2009;73(15):1218–26. https://doi.org/10.1212/WNL.0b013e3181bc0141.

95. Braun AT, Caballero-Eraso C, Lechtzin N. Amyotrophic lateral sclerosis and the respiratory system. Clin Chest Med. 2018;39(2):391–400. https://doi.org/10.1016/j.ccm.2018.01.003.

96. Hill NS. Noninvasive ventilation. Does it work, for whom, and how? Am Rev Respir Dis. 1993;147(4):1050–5. https://doi.org/10.1164/ajrccm/147.4.1050.

97. Spittel S, Maier A, Kettemann D, et al. Non-invasive and tracheostomy invasive ventilation in amyotrophic lateral sclerosis: utilization and survival rates in a cohort study over 12 years in Germany. Eur J Neurol. 2021;28(4):1160–71. https://doi.org/10.1111/ene.14647.

98. Berlowitz DJ, Howard ME, Fiore JF, et al. Identifying who will benefit from non-invasive ventilation in amyotrophic lateral sclerosis/motor neurone disease in a clinical cohort. J Neurol Neurosurg Psychiatry. 2016;87(3):280–6. https://doi.org/10.1136/jnnp-2014-310055.

99. Hirose T, Kimura F, Tani H, et al. Clinical characteristics of long-term survival with noninvasive ventilation and factors affecting the transition to invasive ventilation in amyotrophic lateral sclerosis. Muscle Nerve. 2018;58(6):770–6. https://doi.org/10.1002/mus.26149.

100. Heiman-Patterson TD, Cudkowicz ME, De Carvalho M, et al. Understanding the use of NIV in ALS: results of an international ALS specialist survey. Amyotroph Lateral Scler Front Degener. 2018;19(5–6):331–41. https://doi.org/10.1080/21678421.2018.1457058.

101. Morgan RK, McNally S, Alexander M, Conroy R, Hardiman O, Costello RW. Use of sniff nasal-inspiratory force to predict survival in amyotrophic lateral sclerosis. Am J Respir Crit Care Med. 2005;171(3):269–74. https://doi.org/10.1164/rccm.200403-314OC.

102. Hiwatani Y, Sakata M, Miwa H. Ultrasonography of the diaphragm in amyotrophic lateral sclerosis: clinical significance in assessment of respiratory functions. Amyotroph Lateral Scler Front Degener. 2013;14(2):127–31. https://doi.org/10.3109/17482968.2012.729595.

103. Hansen-Flaschen J, Ackrivo J. Practical guide to management of long-term noninvasive ventilation for adults with chronic neuromuscular disease. Respir Care. 2023;68(8):1123–57. https://doi.org/10.4187/respcare.10349.

104. Crescimanno G, Greco F, Arrisicato S, Morana N, Marrone O. Effects of positive end expiratory pressure administration during non-invasive ventilation in patients affected by amyotrophic lateral sclerosis: a randomized crossover study. Respirology. 2016;21(7):1307–13. https://doi.org/10.1111/resp.12836.

105. Kleopa KA, Sherman M, Neal B, Romano GJ, Heiman-Patterson T. Bipap improves survival and rate of pulmonary function decline in patients with ALS. J Neurol Sci. 1999;164(1):82–8. https://doi.org/10.1016/s0022-510x(99)00045-3.

106. Pinto AC, Evangelista T, Carvalho M, Alves MA, Sales Luís ML. Respiratory assistance with a non-invasive ventilator (Bipap) in MND/ALS patients: survival rates in a controlled trial. J Neurol Sci. 1995;129(Suppl):19–26. https://doi.org/10.1016/0022-510x(95)00052-4.

107. Vrijsen B, Buyse B, Belge C, et al. Noninvasive ventilation improves sleep in amyotrophic lateral sclerosis: a prospective polysomnographic study. J Clin Sleep Med. 2015;11(5):559–66. https://doi.org/10.5664/jcsm.4704.

108. Mitsumoto H, Rabkin JG. Palliative care for patients with amyotrophic lateral sclerosis: "prepare for the worst and hope for the best". JAMA. 2007;298(2):207–16. https://doi.org/10.1001/jama.298.2.207.

109. Chiò A, Calvo A, Ghiglione P, et al. Tracheostomy in amyotrophic lateral sclerosis: a 10-year population-based study in Italy. J Neurol Neurosurg Psychiatry. 2010;81(10):1141–3. https://doi.org/10.1136/jnnp.2009.175984.

110. Vianello A, Arcaro G, Palmieri A, et al. Survival and quality of life after tracheostomy for acute respiratory failure in patients with amyotrophic lateral sclerosis. J Crit Care. 2011;26(3):329.e7–14. https://doi.org/10.1016/j.jcrc.2010.06.003.

111. Tagami M, Kimura F, Nakajima H, et al. Tracheostomy and invasive ventilation in Japanese ALS patients: decision-making and survival analysis: 1990-2010. J Neurol Sci. 2014;344(1–2):158–64. https://doi.org/10.1016/j.jns.2014.06.047.

112. Glenn WW, Holcomb WG, Hogan J, et al. Diaphragm pacing by radiofrequency transmission in the treatment of chronic ventilatory insufficiency. Present status. J Thorac Cardiovasc Surg. 1973;66(4):505–20.

113. DiMarco AF, Onders RP, Kowalski KE, Miller ME, Ferek S, Mortimer JT. Phrenic nerve pacing in a tetraplegic patient via intramuscular diaphragm electrodes. Am J Respir Crit Care Med. 2002;166(12 Pt 1):1604–6. https://doi.org/10.1164/rccm.200203-175CR.

114. Onders RP, Elmo M, Khansarinia S, et al. Complete worldwide operative experience in laparoscopic diaphragm pacing: results and differences in spinal cord injured patients and amyotrophic lateral sclerosis patients. Surg Endosc. 2009;23(7):1433–40. https://doi.org/10.1007/s00464-008-0223-3.

115. Onders RP, Carlin AM, Elmo M, Sivashankaran S, Katirji B, Schilz R. Amyotrophic lateral sclerosis: the Midwestern surgical experience with the diaphragm pacing stimulation system shows that general anesthesia can be safely performed. Am J Surg. 2009;197(3):386–90. https://doi.org/10.1016/j.amjsurg.2008.11.008.

116. Gonzalez-Bermejo J, Morélot-Panzini C, Salachas F, et al. Diaphragm pacing improves sleep in patients with amyotrophic lateral sclerosis. Amyotroph Lateral Scler. 2012;13(1):44–54. https://doi.org/10.3109/17482968.2011.597862.

117. McDermott CJ, Bradburn MJ, Maguire C, et al. DiPALS: diaphragm pacing in patients with amyotrophic lateral sclerosis—a randomised controlled trial. Health Technol Assess. 2016;20(45):1–186. https://doi.org/10.3310/hta20450.

118. Chatwin M, Toussaint M, Gonçalves MR, et al. Airway clearance techniques in neuromuscular disorders: a state of the art review. Respir Med. 2018;136:98–110. https://doi.org/10.1016/j.rmed.2018.01.012.

119. Homnick DN. Mechanical insufflation-exsufflation for airway mucus clearance. Respir Care. 2007;52(10):1296–305; discussion 1306–7.

120. Sancho J, Servera E, Bañuls P, Marín J. Effectiveness of assisted and unassisted cough capacity in amyotrophic lateral sclerosis patients. Amyotroph Lateral Scler Front Degener. 2017;18(7–8):498–504. https://doi.org/10.1080/21678421.2017.1335324.

121. Morrow B, Zampoli M, van Aswegen H, Argent A. Mechanical insufflation-exsufflation for people with neuromuscular disorders. Cochrane Database Syst Rev. 2013;(12):CD010044. https://doi.org/10.1002/14651858.CD010044.pub2.

122. Hanayama K, Ishikawa Y, Bach JR. Amyotrophic lateral sclerosis. Successful treatment of mucous plugging by mechanical insufflation-exsufflation. Am J Phys Med Rehabil. 1997;76(4):338–9. https://doi.org/10.1097/00002060-199707000-00017.

123. Yaguchi H, Sakuta K, Mukai T, Miyagawa S. Fiberoptic laryngoscopic neurological examination of amyotrophic lateral sclerosis patients with bulbar symptoms. J Neurol Sci. 2022;440:120325. https://doi.org/10.1016/j.jns.2022.120325.
124. Boentert M. Sleep and sleep disruption in amyotrophic lateral sclerosis. Curr Neurol Neurosci Rep. 2020;20(7):25. https://doi.org/10.1007/s11910-020-01047-1.
125. Andersen T, Sandnes A, Brekka AK, et al. Laryngeal response patterns influence the efficacy of mechanical assisted cough in amyotrophic lateral sclerosis. Thorax. 2017;72(3):221–9. https://doi.org/10.1136/thoraxjnl-2015-207555.
126. Rafiq MK, Bradburn M, Proctor AR, et al. A preliminary randomized trial of the mechanical insufflator-exsufflator versus breath-stacking technique in patients with amyotrophic lateral sclerosis. Amyotroph Lateral Scler Front Degener. 2015;16(7–8):448–55. https://doi.org/1 0.3109/21678421.2015.1051992.
127. Suri P, Burns SP, Bach JR. Pneumothorax associated with mechanical insufflation-exsufflation and related factors. Am J Phys Med Rehabil. 2008;87(11):951–5. https://doi.org/10.1097/ PHM.0b013e31817c181e.
128. Bach JR. Update and perspective on noninvasive respiratory muscle aids. Part 2: the expiratory aids. Chest. 1994;105(5):1538–44. https://doi.org/10.1378/chest.105.5.1538.
129. Lechtzin N, Wolfe LF, Frick KD. The impact of high-frequency chest wall oscillation on healthcare use in patients with neuromuscular diseases. Ann Am Thorac Soc. 2016;13(6):904–9. https://doi.org/10.1513/AnnalsATS.201509-597OC.
130. Dorst J, Ludolph AC, Huebers A. Disease-modifying and symptomatic treatment of amyotrophic lateral sclerosis. Ther Adv Neurol Disord. 2018;11:1756285617734734. https://doi. org/10.1177/1756285617734734.
131. Van den Berg JP, Kalmijn S, Lindeman E, et al. Multidisciplinary ALS care improves quality of life in patients with ALS. Neurology. 2005;65(8):1264–7. https://doi.org/10.1212/01. wnl.0000180717.29273.12.
132. Blackhall LJ. Amyotrophic lateral sclerosis and palliative care: where we are, and the road ahead. Muscle Nerve. 2012;45(3):311–8. https://doi.org/10.1002/mus.22305.
133. Gotesman RD, Lalonde E, McKim DA, et al. Laryngospasm in amyotrophic lateral sclerosis. Muscle Nerve. 2022;65(4):400–4. https://doi.org/10.1002/mus.27466.
134. Llieva H, Vullaganti M, Kwan J. Advances in molecular pathology, diagnosis, and treatment of ALS. BMJ. 2023;383:075037.
135. Benditt JO, Boitano LJ. Pulmonary issues in patients with chronic neuromusuclar disease. Am J Respir Crit Care Med. 2013;187(10):1046–55.

Chapter 11
Respiratory Care in Spinal Cord Injury

Philip Wexler and David Quintero

Introduction

Spinal cord injury (SCI) is a significant life-altering event which frequently results in severe and permanent disability [1]. SCI occurs most often as a direct consequence of traumatic injuries, mainly automobile crashes and falls [2]. Non-traumatic etiologies like tumors, myelopathy, infections, and vascular damage are responsible for a lower proportion of SCI cases [3].

The American Spinal Injury Association (ASIA) has advanced the standard approach for the classification of the level of injury and extent of impairment in SCI (Fig. 11.1). The motor level of injury is defined as the most caudal muscle group that can be moved against gravity. For nerve roots that do not have muscles to test, such as T2 and L1, sensation is tested to estimate motor levels. This determines the ASIA neurologic level of injury. The completeness of injury is assessed, as well. Complete motor SCI refers to AIS (ASIA Impairment Scale) A which is defined by no sensory or motor function below the level of injury. Sensory incomplete, AIS B, refers to sensory but no motor function is preserved below the neurologic level. Incomplete injuries are graded AIS C, where motor function is preserved for voluntary anal contraction and there is some sparing of motor function more than three levels below the neurologic level in less than half of the muscles. AIS D is similar to AIS C, but half or more of the muscles below the neurologic level have motor function against gravity. In general, the more cephalad and complete the motor level of injury to the spinal cord, the greater the respiratory dysfunction [4].

Pulmonary complications are common in SCI patients. The most common cause of death in SCI is related to respiratory illnesses. Patients are most vulnerable to respiratory illness in the first year after injury but continue to suffer from respiratory

P. Wexler (✉) · D. Quintero
Shepherd Center, Atlanta, GA, USA
e-mail: Philip.wexler@shepherd.org; David.quintero@shepherd.org

N. Lechtzin (ed.), *Pulmonary Complications of Neuromuscular Disease*, Respiratory Medicine, https://doi.org/10.1007/978-3-031-65335-3_11

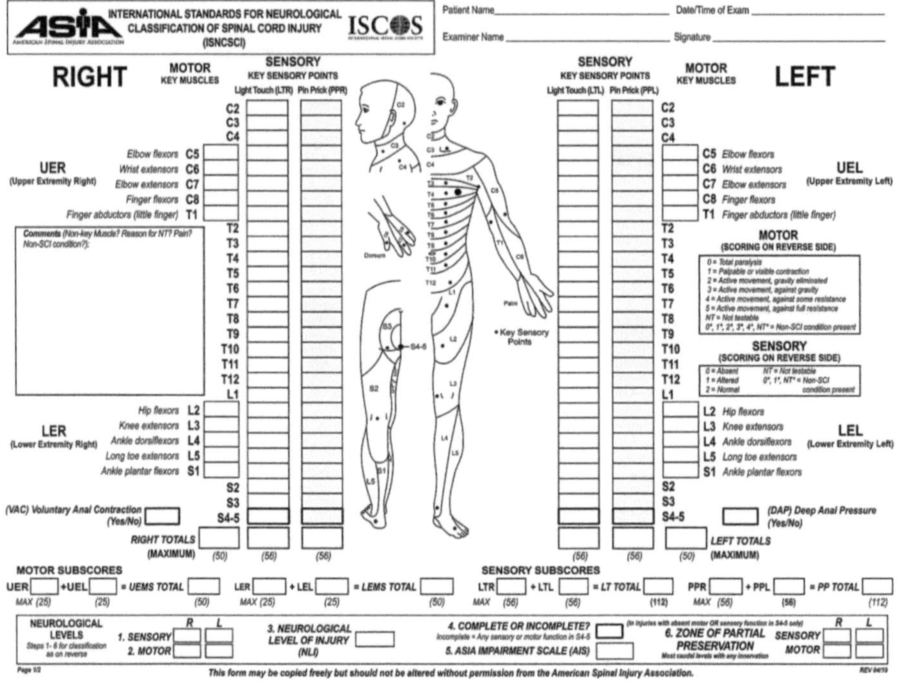

Fig. 11.1 ASIA scoring chart for SCI

complications throughout life [5]. Respiratory dysfunction in SCI is due to the inadequacy or failure of the muscles of respiration, ineffective cough, increased production of bronchial secretions, bronchospasm, and pulmonary edema [6]. Loss of the muscles of inspiration, with the inability to take a deep breath or sigh, can lead to atelectasis with right to left shunting of blood through alveoli that are not ventilated. This results in hypoxemia as well as the loss of lung compliance. Loss of the muscles of expiration leads to impaired cough with inadequate secretion clearance leading to atelectasis, increased airway resistance, and recurrent infection. These factors, individually or in combination, can lead to atelectasis, hypercapnia, hypoxemia, infection, respiratory failure, and death.

Epidemiology

The National Spinal Cord Injury Statistical Center (NSCISC) monitors ongoing changes in epidemiological data in the United States. As of 2021, the estimated number of people living in the United States with SCI is approximately 299,000 persons. There are approximately 18,000 new SCI cases each year, mostly secondary to traumatic injuries. Since 2015, most cases are male (78%), and the average

age at injury is 43. Incomplete tetraplegia is the most common type of SCI (46.8%), followed by complete paraplegia (20.1%), incomplete paraplegia (19.7%), and complete tetraplegia (12.8%) [7, 8]. Pulmonary complications are the leading cause of morbidity and mortality following SCI, particularly at the cervical and thoracic level [6]. The most common complications during the first 5 days post injury are atelectasis (36.4%), pneumonia (31.4%), and ventilatory failure (22.6%) [9].

Anatomy and Pathophysiology

In SCI, the degree of respiratory dysfunction correlates with the neurologic level of injury [10]. The muscles innervated by the nerve roots caudal to the level of injury are affected. Cervical and thoracic injuries carry higher risk of respiratory complications.

Inspiration is an active process that involves a forceful contraction of the diaphragm, the external intercostal muscles and the sternocleidomastoid, the upper trapezius, and the scalenes. These muscles act in a coordinated contraction that allows the chest cavity to expand. Expiration at rest is a passive process. During forced expiration, however, such as with exercise or in the generation of a cough, the muscles that depress the ribs and reduce the size of the thoracic cavity are recruited. The muscles of expiration include the internal intercostals, the rectus abdominis, and the external and internal obliques [11].

It is useful to review the muscles of respiration, their usual function, and innervation to comprehend the respiratory dysfunction in SCI. The anatomy and physiology of the respiratory muscles will also help illuminate the foundations of the therapies employed to address the underlying issues.

Muscles of Inspiration

Diaphragm

The diaphragm is the most important muscle of inspiration. It is innervated by the phrenic nerve which originates from the third to fifth cervical roots. The muscle is dome-shaped with a centrally located tendon and a zone of apposition abutting the inner aspect of the lower ribs. The vertebral portion inserts in the anterolateral aspect of the first three lumbar vertebrae and the costal portion inserts on the xiphoid process of the sternum and the upper margins of the lower six ribs. During inspiration, the muscle fibers shorten, the apposed area decreases, and the dome descends. This increases the thoracic cavity volume and displaces the abdominal contents caudally [11].

External Intercostal Muscles and the Accessory Muscles of Inspiration

The external intercostals attach from the inferior border of one rib to the superior border of the rib directly below it. These muscles are superficial to the internal intercostals, and the two are separated by an aponeurotic membrane. Both the external and internal intercostals are innervated by the corresponding thoracic spinal nerves. The external intercostals and the parasternal internal intercostals work in accord with the diaphragm during inspiration. The external intercostals work to elevate the second to 12th ribs at the sternocostal and costospinal joints [11, 12]. These muscles prevent the internal collapse of the ribs and contributes to lung expansion [13].

The accessory muscles of inspiration include the sternocleidomastoid and the upper trapezius, both innervated by cranial nerve XI, and the scalenes which are innervated by C2–C7. These muscles are recruited for forceful inspiration during times of increased respiratory demands. They work to elevate the upper ribs and the sternum.

Muscles of Expiration

Internal Intercostal Muscles

The internal intercostals are located in the rib spaces between ribs 1 and 12. These muscles orient in the opposing direction to the external intercostals. During expiration, the internal intercostals work to lower the 2nd to 12th ribs at the sternocostal and costospinal joints.

Rectus Abdominis and External and Internal Obliques

The rectus abdominis and the obliques participate in forced expiration. The rectus abdominis originates from the fifth, sixth, and seventh costal cartilages and the sternum and spans to the crest of the pubic bone. It is innervated by the lower thoracic nerves T5–T12 [11]. The rectus abdominis flexes the trunk and increases the intra-abdominal pressure which assists in forced expiration.

The external and internal obliques originate from the lower eight ribs and span to the iliac crest. The fibers of the external oblique run in an oblique line inferiorly and posteriorly. It is innervated by the lower six intercostal nerves. The internal oblique fibers run perpendicular to the external oblique. It is innervated by the lower intercostal nerves. The obliques function in opposition to the diaphragm. The obliques work to flex the trunk by pulling the chest downward and compress the abdominal cavity in concert to the rectus abdominis.

Pectoralis Major

The pectoralis major is innervated by C5–C7. The clavicular portion is inserted on the medial half of the clavicle. It works to contract the upper rib cage as an accessory muscle of expiration [14].

Bulbar-Innervated Muscles

The bulbar muscles refer to the muscles of the face, pharynx, and tongue that are innervated by the upper motor neurons of the cranial nerves, the corticobulbar system. The corticobulbar system includes the following: cranial nerve V, the trigeminal nerve, controls the muscles of mastication; cranial nerve VII, the facial nerve, controls the muscles of the face; cranial nerve X, the vagus nerve, innervates muscles of the pharynx and larynx; cranial nerve XI, the accessory nerve, controls the sternocleidomastoid and trapezius muscles; and cranial nerve XII, the glossopharyngeal nerve, controls the muscles of the tongue [15]. The corticobulbar system is spared in SCI unless there is extension into the brainstem. However, these muscles are frequently damaged by intubation, tracheotomy, and initial traumatic injury that led to SCI. This interferes with the ability to phonate and swallow. Glossopharyngeal breathing (GPB) is a maneuver that individuals with upper cervical-level SCI can use to "gulp" air to stack breaths to assist in tolerating time spent breathing off a ventilator and in coughing and swallowing. It is described further below. It is dependent on the bulbar-innervated muscles.

Injury Patterns and Timing

Tetraplegia

C1–C4 Injury

Persons with C1 and C2 complete injury have complete loss of the muscles of inspiration and expiration. They are noted to be apneic at the time of injury. If the initial injury is survived, these patients require long-term ventilation. Sixty percent of patients in this category can be eventually weaned off ventilatory support, but it may take up to 8 years [16]. Diaphragmatic pacing, cough assistance, and glossopharyngeal breathing may allow for periods of ventilator-free breathing (VFB).

C5–C8 Injury

Inspiratory muscle function is variable in the individuals with C5 to C8 injury. The diaphragm is intact in injuries below C5. The expiratory muscles are significantly impaired as is the effectiveness of a cough. The abdominal muscles and intercostal muscles remain absent. With gradual improvement in the respiratory muscle function over time, ventilator liberation is an achievable goal.

Paraplegia

T1–T12

Thoracic-level SCI is associated with intact diaphragm function. Cough effectiveness improves as the level of thoracic injury moves caudally [17].

Temporal Patterns in Spinal Cord Injury

SCI can be separated temporally into an initial phase, during the period immediately post injury through the next year, and a later, chronic phase through the rest of the life of the individual [18]. In the initial phase, there is an acute reduction in lung compliance. This early reduction in lung compliance is presumed to be due to muscle weakness and alterations in surfactant production as well. Chest wall compliance is reduced in tetraplegia, whereas the abdominal compliance is increased. The chest wall is stiff because of muscle spasticity and poor inspiratory muscle performance which leads to abnormalities of the rib articulations with the spine and sternum [18]. Partial recovery of respiratory muscle performance does occur over the first year. The improvement is noted in pulmonary function tests, as mentioned below. The performance of the diaphragm, the intercostals, and the accessory muscles of the neck appears to improve over the first year post injury [18, 19].

After the initial period of partial respiratory function improvement, there is a decline that may exceed the age-related decline in the non-injured population. The decline has been described in the SCI population after rehabilitation and is significantly worse when associated with cigarette smoking, higher BMI, lower inspiratory muscle strength, and declined physical fitness [20–22].

Assessment of Respiratory Function: Pulmonary Function Tests

Spirometry

Spirometry in SCI demonstrates a restrictive pattern with a reduction in forced vital capacity (FVC) and forced expiratory volume in 1 s (FEV_1). In comparison with other neuromuscular diseases, the inspiratory muscle function driven by the function of the diaphragm is generally preserved in SCI (outside of upper cervical SCI) versus the compromise and loss of function of the intercostal and abdominal muscles, the expiratory muscles. This is notable as there is a disproportionate reduction in the percent predicted values of FVC in comparison to the total lung capacity (TLC) [23]. There is noted correlation between the level and completeness of the spinal cord injury and the reduction in the FVC and FEV_1 [24–26].

Spirometry in people with cervical SCI is measurably increased in the supine versus the erect position [26, 27]. The use of an abdominal binder improves FVC by decreasing the compliance of the abdominal compartment. This restores the expanding effect of the diaphragm at the zone of apposition [28].

The FVC and FEV_1 are noted to be the lowest measured value in the period immediately post injury to the spinal cord. There is an initial improvement in FVC and FEV_1 that is noted over the 5 weeks post injury. This initial improvement is hypothesized to be due to resolution of spinal cord edema above the level of injury with subsequent return to functional capacity of muscles of respiration [29]. Throughout the next five months, the FVC and FEV_1 continue to improve gradually with improved diaphragm and accessory muscle function [23]. During the first year post injury, there is an overall improvement in spirometry [30, 31].

It has been observed that in chronic SCI there is a lung function decline with increased duration from SCI. The FVC and level of injury maintain an inverse relationship. A predictive model based on pooled spirometric data from SCI centers in New York and Los Angeles has been created and demonstrates that in high cervical SCI, the FVC is noted to be approximately 50% of preinjury predicted values with a 9% increase in FVC noted for each level below C5. For thoracic injury, the FVC prediction increases by 1% for each level drop from T1. Cigarette smoking is associated with reduced FVC [25]. Overall, this predictive model and others have proven inaccurate in predicting respiratory function over time [22, 32]. In SCI, there is an observed loss in lung function over time that may be in excess of that documented in the uninjured population. There was not an observed relationship between the level of injury and the rate of FVC decline [21].

Smoking, obesity, lower inspiratory muscle strength, declined physical fitness, and longer duration since injury are all associated with loss of lung function in SCI [22, 26, 33–35]. Spirometry is important to follow in persons with SCI to identify modalities to preserve lung function and to intervene in those at risk for respiratory compromise. Respiratory muscle strength training, treatment programs that aim at weight control, and maintaining physical fitness after inpatient rehabilitation may be beneficial to prevent the decline of pulmonary function and therewith decrease the risk of morbidity and mortality [21].

Airway Hyperreactivity and Bronchodilator Responsiveness in Spinal Cord Injury

Numerous studies have demonstrated that in people with cervical SCI there is a significantly increased prevalence in airway hyperreactivity and bronchodilator responsiveness [36]. The significant response in FEV_1 to bronchodilators in cervical SCI patients was noted despite baseline normal FEV_1/FVC ratios. This phenomenon is not noted in thoracic SCI or in other neuromuscular diseases with similar comparable muscle weakness. This suggests that there is an obstructive ventilatory impairment with an increased resting airway tone [37].

Methacholine challenge testing in subjects with cervical SCI demonstrated significant airway hyperresponsiveness [37]. A potential mechanism for this airway hyperresponsiveness in cervical SCI includes the interruption of sympathetic autonomic innervation. The vagus nerve, cranial nerve X, is intact in cervical cord injury. It innervates the autonomic ganglia in the airway walls and then throughout the lungs through postganglionic fibers. The parasympathetic nervous system is broncho-constrictive and increases the tone of the airway at baseline. Opposing the bronchoconstriction of the parasympathetic innervation is the sympathetic innervation of the lung that regulates the airway tone and reduces the airway caliber. The sympathetic nerves arrive to the lungs from the upper six thoracic nerve roots. In cervical SCI, the sympathetic innervation to the lungs is lost. The sympathetic innervation serves to counteract and modulate the parasympathetic nerves [23]. Without sympathetic innervation there is an unopposed parasympathetic tone. This can explain the increase in airway tone and decrease in caliber. In addition, low circulating epinephrine levels resulting from adrenal gland denervation, which also leads to unopposed vagal airway tone, has also been demonstrated [36–39].

Pretreatment with ipratropium bromide, a cholinergic antagonist, has been shown to block the airway response to methacholine in patients with cervical SCI [38]. Further, ipratropium bromide used in pulmonary function testing of bronchodilator response in cervical SCI subjects demonstrated improved airflow [37]. The results of testing of ipratropium bromide demonstrating improved resting airway tone and eliminating the airway response to methacholine in subjects with cervical SCI give further credence to the understanding that unopposed parasympathetic activity is the cause of this phenomenon.

Maximal Inspiratory Pressure/Maximal Expiratory Pressure

Measured at the mouth, the maximal inspiratory pressure (MIP or PImax) and the maximal expiratory pressure (MEP or PEmax) are non-invasive functional measures of global or aggregate respiratory muscle strength. Testing measures the generation of pressure against a blocked airway [11]. In many cases of SCI, the muscles of inspiration are generally preserved in comparison to the muscles of expiration, and therefore, the MIP is generally higher than the MEP. The MEP is impaired at all cervical and thoracic levels of spinal cord injury [40]. There is a direct correlation between the level of injury and the measure of the MIP and MEP in subjects with complete motor lesions. The MIP was generally preserved in subjects with low thoracic (below T7) and lumbar SCI [40].

Lung Volumes

Cervical SCI produces a restrictive ventilatory defect. Resulting from respiratory muscle weakness and inability to distend and expand the lungs and rib cage, the vital capacity (VC), the total lung capacity (TLC), the inspiratory capacity (IC), and the expiratory reserve volume (ERV) are reduced [24, 41]. The TLC is reduced as the level of injury ascends. The expiratory reserve volume (ERV) is the volume of gas maximally exhaled after end-inspiratory tidal breathing and is zero or near zero in subjects with all levels of cervical SCI. The residual volume (RV), the volume of gas in the airways after a maximal exhalation, is increased. The functional residual capacity (FRC), the sum of ERV and RV, is also reduced. The reduced FRC occurs due to the loss of ERV, although is partly compensated by the increase in RV. The denervation and weakness of the muscles of expiration explain the loss of ERV and increase in RV. The ability to forcefully exhale a volume of air beyond tidal breathing is significantly compromised or absent [31, 41, 42]. Over the first year of injury, the FRC remains constant and reduced; however, the ERV increases with improved expiration, and the RV is decreased [31, 43].

Peak Cough Flow

Peak cough flow (PCF) is the measure of the maximum expiratory flow generated during a normal cough. A cough consists of three phases: inspiratory, compressive, and expiratory. The first phase, inspiratory, consists of an initial deep inspiration. This is followed by a very brief closure of the glottis to maintain lung volumes as intrathoracic pressure builds due to isometric contraction of the expiratory muscles against a closed glottis. The expiratory phase is defined by an opening of the glottis with a rapid forceful expulsion created by the contraction of the abdominal muscles.

The initial component of the forced expulsion of the cough is marked by a supra-maximal flow of air known as the "cough spike." Subsequent lower flow rates over a slightly longer period complete the cough. Dynamic compression of the airways occurs during the expiratory phase, and the high-velocity expulsion of gas (air) sweeps airway debris along [44, 45]. During the measurement of PCF, the subject is instructed to inspire deeply to the TLC. The glottis is closed, and the subject is instructed to give maximal expiratory effort on opening the glottis [46]. Generally, a portable flowmeter is used to measure the peak expiratory flow during the cough. PCF below 160 L/min is considered ineffective to remove secretions, while less than 270 L/min increases the risk of respiratory complications [45].

Symptoms of Respiratory Dysfunction in Spinal Cord Injury

In a survey of 180 SCI subjects, 68% of SCI patients report at least one respiratory symptom. The level of injury is correlated with the symptoms of respiratory insufficiency in SCI. The most common reported respiratory symptom in subjects with SCI is breathlessness or dyspnea. Approximately half of the responders to a survey reported dyspnea. Cough, wheeze, and phlegm were also reported symptoms in subjects with SCI. Smoking was associated with increases in all respiratory symptoms [47].

Dyspnea

The subjective reporting of shortness of breath or breathlessness is common in people with SCI and occurs more frequently in those with higher levels of injury [48, 49]. It has been noted that those who require a motorized wheelchair had significantly more dyspnea with daily activities versus those with a hand-propelled wheelchair or walked with an aid or without assistance. There was no difference in the pulmonary function tests between the two groups. Dyspnea is more prevalent during talking, eating, dressing, and undressing. A proposed mechanism for the cause dyspnea during eating and speaking is related to impaired respiratory muscles with the suppression of breathing during the increased respiratory drive. There is a hypothesized difficulty in interrupting breathing to manipulate speaking volumes and phrasing [18, 49]. A hypothesis for dyspnea that occurs during dressing and undressing may be related to weakened respiratory muscles and the activity that uses the limb muscles that would otherwise be used as accessory muscles for breathing [49]. Active cigarette smoking is a significant risk factor for dyspnea, while exercise serves to attenuate the symptoms of dyspnea in SCI. In subjects undergoing an exercise program and in wheelchair athletes, improvements in reported dyspnea were noted. Significant change in FEV_1 or in other tests of respiratory muscle strength was not noted. Rather, it is more likely an effect of improved cardiovascular fitness that explains the improvement in dyspnea with exercise [50, 51].

Dyspnea has been described due to spasticity of chest wall and abdominal muscles interfering with regular inspiration. Muscle spasticity is a common symptom from injury to the upper motor neurons. "Spasticity is a motor disorder characterized by a velocity dependent increase in tonic stretch reflexes (muscle tone) with exaggerated tendon jerks, resulting from the hyperexcitability of the stretch reflex as one component of the upper motor neuron syndrome" [52]. About 65–78% of individuals with chronic SCI (>1 year post injury) have symptoms of spasticity. Spasticity occurs more frequently in cervical than thoracic SCI. Individuals diagnosed as ASIA A are more likely to have spasticity than ASIA B–D, as well. Spasticity negatively impacts the quality of life and activities of daily living [53]. As with limb muscles, the muscles of respiration are also affected by spasticity. Unintended contractions and increased tone with continuous activation have been shown to affect the abdominal muscles. When there is a spastic contraction of the abdominal muscles, there was an imbalance in the load placed on the muscles of inspiration and the capacity of those muscles to draw a breath. Using electromyography (EMG) recordings of the abdominal muscles, it was noted that spastic contractions of the abdominal muscles led to increased abdominal pressures which need to be overcome by the inspiratory muscles for the generation of a breath. Further, the subjects noted associated dyspnea with the spasm [11, 54]. There is no association between limb spasticity and pulmonary function [55].

Cough

Cough is a common and significant symptom in SCI. However due to muscle weakness, the cough is often inadequate. Cough involves stimulation of sensory receptors within the respiratory tract, whose afferent impulses to the brainstem activate the cough center. The afferent fibers of the cough reflex are carried by the vagus nerve. The vagus nerve, CN X, is not affected in SCI and remains intact [56]. Cough can trigger spasticity leading to dyspnea, pain, and discomfort.

Bronchial Mucus Hypersecretion

As mentioned above, in cervical SCI there is a loss of the sympathetic innervation to the lungs. Thus, there is unopposed vagal tone. The parasympathetic dominance is postulated to be a cause of increased airway mucus production. With copious secretions and ineffective cough, there is pooling of secretions, plugging of airways that often require assistance to clear.

Respiratory Complications of Spinal Cord Injury

Atelectasis

The most common respiratory complication after SCI, atelectasis, generally results from mucus plugging. The obstruction of a lobar bronchus results in more complete atelectasis than that of a subsegmental bronchus because of collateral ventilation. Low lung volumes and ineffective cough are significant components to mucus plugging and atelectasis. The inspiration of higher FiO_2 gas mixtures leads to more atelectasis because of the reduction in the fraction of inhaled nitrogen. The left lower lobe is most affected because of the geometric anatomy of the left mainstem bronchus. The angle of take-off of the left lower lobe from the left mainstem is more horizontal than the right lower lobe [57]. Secretions tend to pool in this left-sided airway and over time, with ineffective clearing, become thicker and harder to clear. This often results in atelectasis. Atelectasis increases the risk of pneumonia, dyspnea, cough, chest pain, and pleural effusions. It causes a pulmonary shunt from right to left leading to hypoxemia.

Pneumonia

Pneumonia occurs in half of all patients with acute SCI and is the most common cause of mortality in both acute and chronic SCI. Community-acquired, hospital-acquired, and ventilator-associated pneumonia are common. Aspiration pneumonia occurs in the setting of dysphagia, especially in patients with tracheostomy.

Sleep-Disordered Breathing

Sleep-disordered breathing (SDB) is common in the SCI population. It is characterized by collapse of the upper airway during sleep with poor, fragmented sleep and periodic hypoxemia. Symptoms include loud snoring, daytime hypersomnolence, nocturnal choking and gasping, and apneas [39]. Sleep apnea has been noted to occur in 62% of subjects with cervical SCI within 2 weeks of injury and persisted throughout the first year post injury. Of note, few of the patients were suspected of clinically having sleep apnea [58]. Sankari et al. [59] assessed the SDB and ventilation changes using in-laboratory polysomnography (PSG) comparing cervical and thoracic SCI. There was a higher prevalence of SDB in cervical SCI, 93% compared with 55% in thoracic SCI. SDB in patients with thoracic SCI was mainly obstructive, whereas SDB in patients with cervical SCI seemed to be both obstructive and centrally mediated. One in four patients with cervical SCI have Cheyne-Stokes respiration pattern or central sleep apnea (CSA) without evidence of heart failure [16, 59]. CSA is more common in SCI patients than in the general population [60].

Obstructive sleep apnea (OSA) has been associated with neurocognitive decline in persons with tetraplegia. In particular, nocturnal hypoxemia events in subjects with OSA are associated with decreased measures of verbal attention and concentration, immediate and short-term memory, cognitive flexibility, internal scanning, working memory, visual perception, attention, and concentration [61]. It has been well established in the general population that sleep apnea is directly related to an increase in the incidence of myocardial infarction, stroke, and metabolic dysfunction [60].

The pathophysiology of obstructive sleep apnea in persons with SCI is multifactorial. The proposed mechanisms include impaired respiratory muscle function that causes decreased respiratory efforts. This leads to the failure of effective airflow during sleep [16]. There is also poor coordination between the upper airway pharyngeal muscles and thoracic muscles, increased upper airway resistance due to sympathetic nervous system disruption, reduced lung volumes, and disrupted reflex responses from rib cage receptors. It has also been reported that increased nasal resistance may contribute to SDB in people with tetraplegia [62, 63]. In addition, SCI patients generally sleep in a supine position and cannot change body position by themselves and have a preferential supine sleeping position increasing upper airway stress due to gravity. In addition, the same risk factors for SDB in the general population also affect the SCI population, such as obesity, aging, and male gender [16]. The use of muscle relaxants are also possible risk factors for SDB in SCI [39].

Central sleep apnea is thought to be the result of hypoventilation (hypercapnia) or a consequence of post-hyperventilation (hypocapnia) [16]. Adequate ventilation during sleep depends on levels of arterial CO_2 ($PaCO_2$). The apneic threshold is the level of $PaCO_2$ that needs to be reached to generate a signal to breathe. If the $PaCO_2$ is above the apneic threshold, there is a signal for inspiration, whereas below the threshold apnea occurs. Fluctuations in the response of the ventilatory system to changing $PaCO_2$ (the chemoreflex sensitivity) and the effectiveness of the lung/respiratory system in decreasing $PaCO_2$ in response to hyperventilation lead to CSA. Changes in either parameter, the CO_2 receptor function or the effectiveness of the response to a low $PaCO_2$, change the level of hypocapnia to reach central apnea. In cervical SCI, the $PaCO2$ level resides at a level close to the apneic threshold. It seems that patients with cervical SCI are more susceptible than patients with thoracic SCI to develop CSA because of a baseline smaller FRC and alveolar hypoventilation. A small change in ventilation results in a larger change in CO_2 further from the apneic threshold. The large change in CO_2 is below the apnea threshold and leads to CSA [16].

Respiratory Failure

Hypoxemia in SCI is due to ventilation/perfusion mismatch and shunt from retained secretions, atelectasis, and pneumonia. Hypercarbia occurs due to respiratory muscle weakness. The risk of respiratory failure correlates with the level of injury. In the setting of respiratory failure after acute SCI, the standard of care is endotracheal intubation and mechanical ventilation. This is often followed by tracheostomy tube placement. The presence of the airway tubes increases the likelihood of pneumonia. Respiratory failure is the most important contributor to hospital length of stay and hospital costs [31].

Interventions

Respiratory management in people with SCI focuses on the prevention of secretion retention, atelectasis, and lower respiratory tract infection and ventilation-independent breathing. Airway clearance is a key component of the respiratory care of patients with SCI. Ineffective cough and lack of secretion clearance will cause atelectasis, pneumonia, and acute respiratory failure.

Chest Physiotherapy/Postural Drainage/Manually Assisted Cough

Positional chest physiotherapy with percussion or vibration is a commonly utilized procedure to assist in the migration of peripheral secretions centrally. Position changes utilize gravity to move secretions centrally. Once central, the secretions can be removed with an effective cough, which remains elusive in the cervical and thoracic SCI patient. Numerous positions targeting gravity drainage can be utilized including Trendelenburg, supine, prone, and left and right lateral. Each position should be held for at least 5 to 10 min as tolerated [64]. The Trendelenburg position presses the abdominal contents against their diaphragm; this can severely limit deep inspiration and may increase gastroesophageal reflux or emesis. SCI patients with a cervical collar or a halo immobilization device can have severely limited positioning [65].

Manually assisted cough also known as a "quad cough" is an effective maneuver for airway clearance. The maneuver is performed in the supine or slightly upright position with a therapist who straddles the patient. The patient inhales to TLC. A patient-initiated cough is begun, and at the same time, the therapist applies vigorous pressure to the abdomen under the left and right costal margins [18]. Breath stacking to a higher inspired volume using lung volume recruitment (LVR) with glossopharyngeal breathing or with a manual resuscitator bag can increase cough peak flows and assist in effective cough. The maneuver can be used as needed and more frequently during respiratory tract infections with increased secretion production [66].

Contraindications to chest physiotherapy and postural drainage include unstable spine and chest wall injuries, abdominal aortic aneurysm or stent, and the presence of an inferior vena cava filter.

Glossopharyngeal Breathing

Glossopharyngeal breathing (GPB) or "frog breathing" is a maneuver of autonomous positive pressure breath stacking. GPB is performed using the tongue and muscles of the pharynx as a piston to generate boluses, or gulps, of air past the glottis into the lungs. It can be used as lung volume recruitment and can generate increased volumes of air to improve voice and cough. It can allow for ventilator-free breathing for several hours in those that are ventilator dependent. Intact bulbar innervated muscles are needed for GPB, and this cannot be performed with a tracheostomy tube in place [66, 67]. In a 2011 study of 25 subjects with cervical spinal cord injury, the subjects were taught GPB. They performed four training sessions of ten GPB breaths per week for 8 weeks. Five subjects were unable to perform the maneuver. After the 8-week period, the participants were able to insufflate an additional 28% of their VC, increasing chest expansion both while doing GPB and at rest. The VC, ERV, FRC, and TLC increased significantly. The subjects were able to inhale and exhale more air. Lightheadedness was noted and three patients had syncope. This was believed to be due to a reduction in preload as a result of the increased intrathoracic pressure when the participants perform GPB [68].

Lung Volume Recruitment

In SCI, cough is ineffective. Loss of the muscles of inspiration in cervical SCI leads to the inability to take a large inspiratory volume. In both cervical and thoracic spinal cord injuries, the expiratory muscles are weak or ineffective and unable to generate forceful compressive and expiratory phases of cough [44, 46]. Over time, in SCI as in other neuromuscular diseases, the chest wall compliance decreases, and with muscle spasticity, the lung compliance and capacity decrease.

The lung volume recruitment (LVR) maneuver is an intervention that uses stacking of breaths delivered by a manual handheld resuscitation bag or via a mechanical ventilator. The maneuver begins with the subject taking a deep breath. The subject is instructed to hold that breath and then deliver additional stacked breaths until the maximum volume that can be retained with a closed glottis and with bulbar innervated muscle integrity is reached. This is the maximum insufflation capacity (MIC) [69]. With routine use of LVR, the volumes become easier to stack, and higher volumes, i.e., higher MIC, can be achieved. It has been noted that LVR is important to maintain pulmonary toilet, lung compliance, and lung volumes and increase forced vital capacity, cough peak flow, and an improvement in atelectasis and vocalization [66]. LVR can be administered via a mouthpiece and nasal/oral interfaces or with non-invasive ventilators. In subjects who cannot maintain a closed glottis or with impaired bulbar innervated muscles, LVR can be delivered via a manual resuscitator with blocked exhalation valve until MIC is achieved. Increased resistance to breath delivery in the manual resuscitator notes an adequate volume delivered. This is termed "passive LVR." Mechanical insufflation-exsufflation (MIE) devices can be used to provide passive LVR. For those on continuous mechanical ventilation, sighs can be utilized for passive LVR.

The LVR maneuver, when combined with abdominal compression (manually assisted coughing), has been shown to generate significantly improved PCF in cervical SCI [45, 70]. When LVR is done routinely with several repetitions performed daily over several weeks, the FVC has been shown to increase in addition to PCF [71]. In another study combining LVR, incentive spirometer use and glossopharyngeal muscle exercises over the course of 4–8 weeks led to significant improvements in FVC and PCF [72].

Respiratory Muscle Strength Training

Impaired respiratory muscle function in patients with high-level SCI impairs cough, inspiration, and expiration. Respiratory muscle strength training (RMST) uses resistive loading devices, or pressure-threshold devices, and is a useful treatment for respiratory muscle fatigue and improved exercise performance. The resistive trainer uses a small diameter hole that limits (resists) airflow and increases the training load on the muscle. Pressure-threshold trainers utilize a spring-loaded valve that requires sufficient force to overcome and allow airflow. Both types of trainers have a valve system that allows targeting of inspiratory and expiratory muscles selectively [73]. For a significant exercise effect, a vigorous and forceful effort is required. In SCI patients, the accessory respiratory muscles such as the pectoralis major can be strengthened and improved with exercise [14, 74]. Patients with cervical SCI have impaired inspiratory and expiratory muscles and can benefit from training of both muscle groups, while patients with thoracic SCI will have improvement by targeting expiratory muscles [75].

Trainer devices have shown benefit in the development of respiratory muscle strength and endurance in athletes, professional vocalists, instrumentalists; in individuals with COPD, Parkinson's disease, stroke, ALS, and MS, and in those who have been intubated for a prolonged period [76–78]. In patients with SCI, the training of the respiratory muscles results in improved endurance capacity and a concomitant increase in the aerobic exercise performance of these muscles [79]. Notable increases in peak inspiratory pressures, FVC and TLC, and MIP and MEP and increases in peak oxygen consumption during exercise and hypertrophy of the diaphragm have been documented [18, 79, 80].

There are several different RMST devices in the market. Incentive spirometers have insufficient resistance for training as they do not provide sufficient resistance and are influenced by airflow rates. They are not able to effectively target respiratory muscle strength [78]. Resistive trainers are devices with small-diameter open holes that are used to inspire or expire through. These devices are also impacted by airflow rate and are subject to changes in a user's breathing pattern and airflow rate. This may minimize the training effect [78]. Pressure-threshold devices are spring loaded and are flow independent. These devices provide a consistent pressure threshold that can be controlled and adjusted and must be overcome by a specific amount of inspiratory or expiratory pressure during respiration [81]. The user must maintain a constant pressure to overcome the pressure of the spring valve.

During inspiratory muscle training (IMT), the resistive trainer device is used to offer airflow resistance during inspiration. The diaphragm is the main target in IMT. Training can consist of using the device for 15–30 min two to three times per day. The exercise program generally begins with the lowest level of resistance until there is relative ease with performing the maneuver on at least three consecutive days. Subsequently, an increased level of resistance is chosen [80]. Expiratory muscle strength training (EMST) is used to strengthen the muscles of expiration including the intercostal muscles and the abdominals. The goal is to assist in improving force-generating capacity of expiration and in increasing MEP. There is evidence in the non-SCI population that EMST improves the effectiveness of cough and improves speech and swallow function [75, 82]. In a meta-analysis the pooled data demonstrated that RMST (with no delineation between studies of IMST, EMST, or device type) in SCI significantly improved FVC, PCF, MIP, and MEP [83].

Some contraindications for RMST include hiatal hernia and uncontrolled reflux, untreated hypertension, recent stroke, and recent pneumothorax.

Abdominal Binders

During inspiration, the diaphragm contracts, and the muscle fibers shorten displacing the muscle caudally. The descent of the diaphragm is opposed by the forces of the intra-abdominal contents and the tone of the abdominal wall. When the diaphragm contracts, the abdominal wall is displaced anterolaterally. The intra-abdominal pressure rises, opposing the movement of diaphragm, forcing an expansion of the rib cage which augments inspiration. The chest wall expands in a push laterally in the zone of apposition of the diaphragm and in a forced lift and expansion of the lower rib cage as the diaphragm is opposed to further downward descent. The compliance of the abdominal wall determines the extent of the rise in intra-abdominal pressure. With a stiff abdominal wall, the rib cage will expand more than if it were more compliant and flaccid. If the wall is compliant, it displaces easily, with slight pressure rise, and little elevation or expansion of the ribcage. In

SCI above the neurologic level T6, the innervation of the abdominal muscles is lost, and the abdominal wall becomes more compliant [84, 85].

Extrinsic abdominal support binders, used to cover the abdominal wall and not covering the lower rib cage and zone of diaphragm apposition, decrease the compliance of the abdominal wall. They increase intra-abdominal pressure forcing the diaphragm into a mechanically advantageous position to enhance rib cage expansion [85]. Abdominal binders have been demonstrated to improve VC, FVC, FEV_1, and inspiratory capacity (IC) in complete SCI patients versus measurements while the binder is off [86–88].

Concerns for prolonged use of the abdominal binder include increased inspiratory muscle fatigue. It is unclear if the use of the binder improves the effectiveness of cough. A contraindication to the abdominal binder is skin opening or pressure site at the region of the application of the binder [86].

Mechanical Insufflation-Exsufflation, Suction Catheters, and Bronchoscopy

In the setting of an ineffective cough, secretion pooling will occur. The pooled secretions are a nidus of infection and can lead to bronchitis and pneumonia. The secretions can obstruct the airways which can lead to atelectasis and respiratory failure. Cough augmentation and secretion removal remain the goal and are paramount to respiratory care. Manually assisted cough can help; however often mechanically assisted coughing is required to generate effective PCF.

Traditional suction catheters, inserted through an endotracheal or a tracheostomy tube, have limited effectiveness. They are limited in size and maneuverability. They do not pass the main bronchi and cannot readily be directed into the left mainstem, which as described above, due to the geometry of the airways, is the main locale of secretion pooling and atelectasis. Further, each insertion of an invasive plastic catheter introduces bacteria into the airways, increasing the risk of infection. Fiberoptic bronchoscopy is a significantly more effective tool in secretion clearance. It is significantly longer than traditional suction catheters and can be directed to the airways of concern. Using mechanical cough assist during bronchoscopy can help mobilize and clear secretions from distal airways. However, bronchoscopy is an invasive procedure with numerous associated risks. It is often reserved for hospital settings when other methods of secretion removal have failed [18].

Mechanical insufflation-exsufflation (MIE) overcomes the limitations of the suction catheter and bronchoscopy in secretion removal and is an effective device in cough augmentation. MIE clears both the right and left airways, uses the patient's weak cough to assist in the procedure, and expands the chest. MIE uses a device that forces passive inspiration to pressures of 40 to 70 cm H_2O and rapidly follows with a forced passive expiration in a cyclic fashion with negative pressures of -40 to -70 cm H_2O. The device can be used via an endotracheal tube, tracheostomy tube, mouthpiece, or facemask. Typically, a session of MIE includes three to five cycled insufflations and exsufflations timed with a patient-initiated cough, which can be further amplified with a manually assisted cough, followed by a brief rest to avoid hyperventilation. Symptoms and oxygen saturation improvements are monitored to assess the need for further cycles of MIE [66].

In a 1993 study of 46 ventilator-dependent subjects with neuromuscular disease who utilized MIE for airway clearance, five subjects had SCI. It was found that there was significant improvement in the FVC and PCF in the entire study group, but this was particularly noted in the SCI subgroup [89, 90]. In a separate study, compared to conventional chest physiotherapy, a group that received MIE in addition to routine treatment was also found to have significantly improved FVC, FEV_1, and peak expiratory flow [90].

In a survey of 18 subjects with SCI, when questioned regarding personal preference for secretion removal, a significant majority found MIE less irritating, less painful, less tiring, and less uncomfortable than endotracheal suctioning. Eighty-nine percent of patients preferred MIE to suctioning. The majority found MIE faster, more convenient, and more effective than suctioning. The study demonstrated that all measured aspects of patient experience are more positive for MIE than for suctioning [91].

Bronchodilators

Bronchodilator responsiveness has been observed in the chronic cervical SCI population, as noted previously. Approximately 45% of individuals had improvement in spirometry after inhalation of short-acting β_2-adrenergic agonist or a short-acting anticholinergic agent [17, 37, 92]. The effect was not seen in those with lower thoracic spine injury. Anticholinergic agents have a greater bronchodilator effect than β_2-adrenergic agonists [17]. The fact that this is prevalent in cervical, not thoracic, SCI and the greater effect from the anticholinergic agent indicates that the loss of sympathetic innervation and unopposed vagal tone is the etiology. Individuals with cervical SCI also demonstrate airway hyperreactivity in response to methacholine and histamine [38, 93].

The long-term implications of bronchodilator responsiveness and airway hyper-responsiveness are unknown. In a 2010 survey in Canada of greater than 60,000 subjects, 356 were noted to have SCI. It was found that after adjusting for age, sex, and smoking status, SCI was associated with a significant increased odds of asthma and chronic obstructive pulmonary disease [94]. This may indicate that SCI is an independent risk factor for chronic inflammatory airway disease.

β_2-Adrenergic Agonists

Forty percent of subjects with cervical SCI demonstrated significant improvement in FEV_1 following inhalation of metaproterenol sulfate, a short-acting β_2-adrenergic agonist [92]. The response was independent of smoking status. This was not present in the SCI patients with lower thoracic SCI. Pretreatment with a β_2-adrenergic receptor agonist has also been found to block nonspecific airway hyperreactivity [95].

Long-acting β_2-agonists have been shown to have beneficial effects on pulmonary function and possibly respiratory muscle strength. In a study of inhaled salmeterol, a long-acting β_2-adrenergic agonist, over a 4-week period noted improved FVC, FEV_1, PEF, MIP, and MEP. It is unclear if the improvements in pulmonary function tests and the measures of static mouth pressures may indicate improved bronchodilation or improved respiratory muscle strength [96].

β_2-Agonists are known to improve muscle strength because of anabolic properties. Given orally, β_2-agonists have been shown to improve muscle strength and size in subjects with cervical SCI [97]. Increase in exercise capacity and work output during functional electrical stimulation cycling increased with the use of salbutamol treatment in patients with SCI versus placebo. There was an increase in leg muscle size with the use of the β_2-agonist as well. However, side effects such as muscle spasms, headaches, anxiety, poor sleep, and palpitations were noted [98].

Anticholinergics

As discussed previously, in cervical SCI the loss of sympathetic innervation and unopposed vagal tone leads to increased airway tone, bronchodilator responsiveness, increased secretions, and hyperresponsive airways. The cholinergic innervation that causes constricted airways is responsive to anticholinergic inhaled medications. Ipratropium bromide led to a positive bronchodilator response in 50% of subjects with cervical SCI [37]. Ipratropium bromide has also been shown to attenuate the response to ultrasonically nebulized distilled water [93].

A study directly comparing ipratropium and albuterol was performed on subjects with chronic tetraplegia. Both groups demonstrated a significant bronchodilator response. While there was no statistically significant difference between the two groups in spirometry, the ipratropium group tended toward a more robust response. However, measures of airway conductance and resistance demonstrated a greater response to the ipratropium versus albuterol. It could be expected that the more vigorous bronchodilation induced by ipratropium in patients with cervical SCI would help improve cough and pulmonary clearance, resolve atelectasis, assist in the treatment of pneumonia and respiratory failure, and maximize lung function. It is also possible that the combined administration of ipratropium and albuterol to subjects with cervical SCI would cause further bronchodilation than either agent alone [17].

Non-invasive Ventilation

The goals of non-invasive ventilation (NIV) for neuromuscular disease, as described by Hansen-Flaschen et al., include enabling restful and restorative sleep, relieving breathlessness, and normalizing respiratory gas exchange [99]. NIV has demonstrated improved quality of life and survival in common chronic neuromuscular diseases. In SCI, further goals include an increase in cough flows, a maximizing of pulmonary compliance and lung volumes, and maintaining normal blood gases [66]. Monitoring symptoms, observing for the use of accessory muscles, and measuring the FVC routinely throughout the day and noting a decline can determine the need for NIV prior to frank respiratory failure [66]. Further monitoring of respiratory muscle strength, MIP and MEP, pulse oximetry, end-tidal or transcutaneous CO_2, and remote monitoring of the NIV device are used to track and assess progression of respiratory dysfunction over time [99].

Daytime Ventilation and Mouthpiece Ventilation

Intermittent non-invasive positive pressure ventilation interfaced via a mouthpiece, oronasal, or nasal mask can be used in cervical SCI. Daytime ventilation is utilized in the setting of hypercapnia, dyspnea, and fatigue and to assist with ventilation while napping. A nasal mask is generally preferred for continuous daytime ventilation. The nasal mask does allow for eating and drinking. Mouthpiece ventilation (MPV) utilizing an angled mouthpiece can be used to provide "sip ventilation" to deliver a large volume of air to be used as needed. It can be utilized in patients with intact bulbar innervated muscles, with the ability to manipulate the head neck and mouth to the mouthpiece and have adequate cognition. The as needed delivery of a large tidal volume is helpful in easing dyspnea and tachypnea which can interfere with eating and swallowing. It allows for generation of enough volumes for speech. It can be used for breath stacking to generate lung volume recruitment or cough. A breath cycle initiates via a flow trigger that detects any interruption of baseline airflow. Between breaths, flow is reduced to an undetectable rate. Typically, a volume-control mode of ventilation is utilized during MPV with a large tidal volume, 1000 to 1500 mL, with an inspiratory time of 1.5 s, respiratory rate, and positive end-expiratory pressure (PEEP) of 0. Pressure control mode is generally avoided since it does not allow for breath stacking as further inspired air is not delivered once the set pressure is reached [66, 99].

Nocturnal Non-invasive Ventilation

Symptomatic hypoventilation, with or without a diagnosis of sleep-disordered breathing, begins with sleep, and NIV is typically initiated during sleep. There are limited studies that examine the impact of therapy with continuous positive airway pressure (CPAP), in the SCI population with SDB. One case series documented improved sleep and oxygen saturation and decreased daytime sleepiness [100]. PSG titration of CPAP is performed to minimize or eliminate apneas and hypopneas. Bilevel positive airway pressure (BPAP) with a backup respiratory rate is required for the treatment of CSA. Nasal mask interface is most commonly utilized for CPAP and BPAP with sleep.

Invasive Mechanical Ventilation

Intubation and mechanical ventilation are common in the first few days following cervical SCI. Complete injuries above C3 frequently result in apnea and requires emergent intubation and ventilatory support [101, 102]. Traumatic SCI is often complicated by brain injury, coma, chest trauma, multiorgan failure, aspiration, and acute respiratory distress syndrome (ARDS) and often requires sedation for pain and anxiolysis and therefore intubation and mechanical ventilation [103]. More than 50% of patients with cervical spine injuries are intubated [103, 104]. For patients who do not require immediate invasive ventilatory support, elective intubation can be anticipated when there are signs of significant respiratory muscle fatigue. These include progressive decline of vital capacity, tachypnea, shallow breathing, hypercapnia, and increasing supplemental oxygen requirement [101].

Tidal Volumes

Acute SCI (less than 2 weeks) patients are at high risk for ARDS and death [105]. Additionally, in the acute setting, higher tidal volumes (TV) are associated with an increased risk of ventilator-associated pneumonia (VAP), when compared to standard TV [106]. There is no evidence of lung injury related to higher tidal volumes in the setting of subacute or chronic SCI. Therefore, the mechanical ventilation strategy during the acute phase should follow the principles of lung protective ventilation employing lower TV (6 to 8 mL per kg of predicted body weight (PBW)) are recommended [105, 106].

In contrast, during the post-acute (more than 2 weeks post injury) phase, the optimal mechanical ventilation strategy remains controversial. It has been reported that low TV ventilation in SCI patients not only increases the occurrence of atelectasis and mucous plugs, but there is also a notable decrease in alveolar surfactant production. Furthermore, low TV ventilation is associated with ventilator weaning failure [107, 108]. SCI patients during the subacute and chronic phase are generally at significantly less risk for developing ARDS. These patients might not need lung protective ventilation [109]. Large TV, up to 25 mL per kg of PBW, has been found to prevent closure of the small airways by stretching airway smooth muscle. The higher volumes reduce alveolar surface tension by increasing surfactant production. Overall, the higher volumes improve oxygenation [107, 108]. In addition, large TV ventilation appears to decrease weaning time. These volumes are often preferred by SCI patients because they help enhance speech, reduce work of breathing, and alleviate the sensation of breathlessness [110, 111] (see Fig. 11.2 as an example of improvement in atelectasis with the use of HTVV).

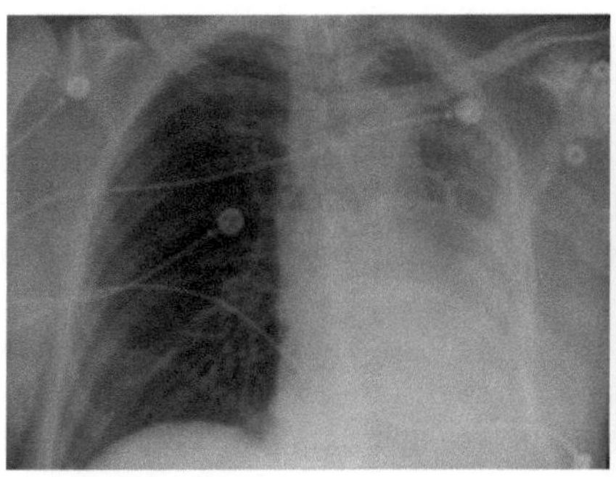
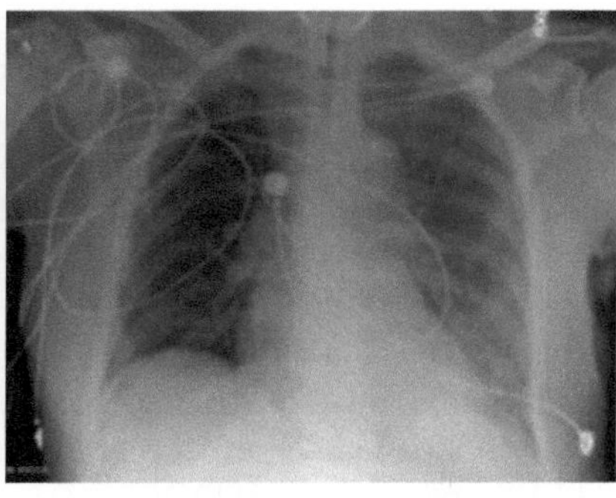

> CXR 01/17/2023
> Pt arrived to Shepherd Center on
> PSV 10/5. TV ~500
> Switched to AC VCV
> TV 750 ml (~10ml/Kg PBW)
> PIP 31-34

> CXR 01/19/2023
> AC: TV 950mL (13 mL/kg PBW)
> PIP 28-32

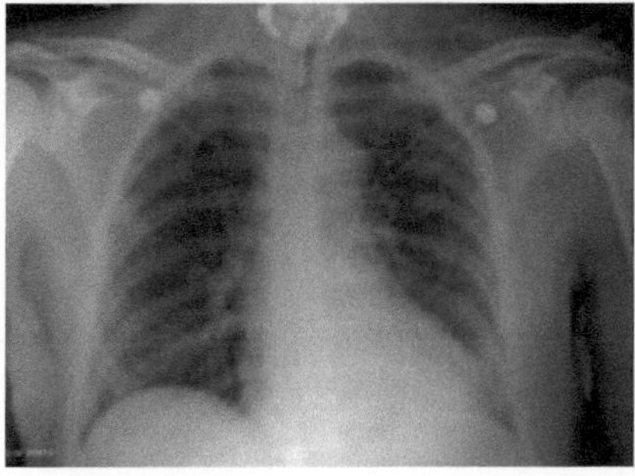

> CXR 01/22/2023
> AC: TV 950mL (~13 mL/kg PBW)
> PIP 20

> CXR 01/27/2023
> AC: TV 950mL (~13 mL/kg PBW)
> PIP 15

Fig. 11.2 A 62-year-old gentleman with C4 AIS A SCI that occurred on 12/23/2022. High tidal volume ventilation employed weaned off ventilator completely on 2/6/2023

In the absence of lung injury, in patients with "healthy lungs," high tidal volume ventilation (HTVV) between 10 and 25 mL per kg of PBW is widely used in clinical practice [64, 112, 113]. There is, however, no consensus in the level of TV that should be used [114]. Due to the flaccid chest muscle tone of individuals with early tetraplegia, the peak airway pressures while implementing HTVV usually remain within normal levels [108, 113]. There is mixed data regarding the safety of HTVV. No difference in pulmonary adverse events (barotrauma, VAP, ARDS) when using HTVV has been reported [108, 109]. In contrast, a recent publication suggested that HTVV is associated with an increased risk of pneumonia [115].

Positive End-Expiratory Pressure

There are few studies addressing the use of positive end-expiratory pressure (PEEP) in individuals with SCI. The standard practice has been to use 0 cm H_2O of PEEP to minimize the risk of air trapping. However, due to the benefit of PEEP in preventing cyclic closure and atelectrauma, using PEEP between 5 and 7 cm H_2O is a reasonable standard practice. Flow trigger is set at the lowest possible level to avoid auto triggering [64].

While there are conflicting data [108, 109, 111, 115], HTVV appears to be beneficial in stabilizing the pulmonary status and in expediting weaning from the ventilator in SCI patients. Further research is needed to determine the optimal level of TV, PEEP, and safety of HTVV.

Weaning Mechanical Ventilation

Ventilator weaning and extubation in the acute setting are outside the scope of this book chapter. Most patients with injuries below C3 can be partially to fully liberated from the ventilator. Though this process could be slow, requiring several months, it frequently occurs in the rehabilitation settings [116]. The process of weaning is a comprehensive one. It includes respiratory secretion management, inspiratory muscle training, lung volume recruitment, HTVV, and occasionally temporary diaphragmatic pacing for conditioning of the diaphragm. Additionally, nutritional optimization, evaluation of the upper airway by otolaryngologist, speech and swallowing evaluation, and evaluation by clinical psychologist and physiatrist are integral to the overall assessment of the SCI patients prior to discontinuation of mechanical ventilation [117–121].

When the patient is clinically stable, bronchial secretions are under control, and chest imaging shows significant resolution of atelectasis, the active weaning process should begin. The preferred and most commonly used method of weaning is progressive ventilator-free breathing (PVFB). Peterson and colleagues found that PVFB also known as T-piece was superior than intermittent mandatory ventilation

(IMV) in weaning patients from the ventilator (67.6% success compared to 34.6%) [122]. The process of spontaneous breathing for short periods with alternating rest periods on the ventilator aims to condition and strengthen the diaphragm while avoiding muscle fatigue. IMV, conversely, does not provide either prolonged periods of conditioning or adequate rest and has been shown to prolong the weaning process [122–126].

Ventilator-free breathing (VFB) trials can begin with periods as short as 1 min and are gradually increased in duration and frequency as tolerated. VFB trials of two or three times per day alternating with rest periods of 3 to 4 h in between trials have been used. VFB is progressively advanced until weaning is fully accomplished [109, 127]. Rest periods are supported by a variety of methods including controlled ventilation modes targeting HTVV, pressure support ventilation, IMV, continuous positive airway pressure, and non-invasive ventilation with the tracheostomy capped [102, 111, 113, 118, 128–130].

Every effort must be taken to discontinue mechanical ventilation. SCI patients who remain on the ventilator long term have a higher risk of dying [131]. The use of non-invasive ventilators or diaphragmatic pacing systems, as detailed in this chapter, may eventually allow SCI patients with injuries above C3 to be liberated from invasive mechanical ventilation.

Tracheostomy and Decannulation

The incidence of tracheostomy placement in cervical SCI tetraplegia is reported to be between 10% and 60%. A low FVC, a large volume of pulmonary secretions, and hypoxemia were found to be important predictors of the need for tracheostomy [132–134]. Tracheostomy is associated with fewer days on the ventilator and a shorter hospital stay in selected patients [5].

Complications related to the use of a tracheostomy tube include interruption of the natural barriers to infection and the mucociliary escalator. There are many other complications including atelectasis, infections, mucus plugs, chronic gram-negative colonization and chronic purulent bronchitis, tracheal granulations with stenosis and tracheal obstruction, tracheomalacia, stoma site infection, bleeding, and many others. The presence of the tube itself stimulates bronchial mucus production [128]. Decannulation should be the goal.

Cough effectiveness, patient cooperation, improved gas exchange, upcoming surgeries, active infections, and overall medical stability are important factors to consider when discussing removal of the tracheostomy tube. Interdisciplinary team evaluation and assessment have been noted to lead to successful decannulation [135]. Speech pathologist input is important to assess aspiration risk. The tube is generally changed from a cuffed to cuffless trach. A series of trach tube changes to smaller sized tubes is usually undertaken. Speaking valve use and tolerance are advanced to trach tube plugging. Ultimately, if tolerated and meeting criteria mentioned above, the tube is removed.

Respiratory Muscle Electrostimulation: Diaphragmatic Pacing

As discussed above, the diaphragm is the primary muscle of inspiration. It is innervated by the phrenic nerve which arises from the cervical nerve roots C3 to C5. Individuals with complete high cervical SCI (C1–C5) can suffer from complete diaphragmatic paralysis to partial dysfunction of the diaphragm [31, 93]. Patients with complete tetraplegia typically require mechanical ventilation following cervical SCI, and many of these patients may need ventilatory support for several months post injury [18, 101, 102]. While mechanical ventilation can be lifesaving, it can also carry deleterious effects on the diaphragm by inducing diaphragmatic atrophy. This harmful effect on the diaphragm caused by mechanical ventilation is known as ventilator-induced diaphragmatic dysfunction (VIDD) [136–138].

Respiratory electrostimulation was first described in 1970 by Glenn and colleagues [139]. Diaphragmatic pacing (DP) is a procedure for inducing diaphragmatic contractions. This technology may help ventilator-dependent quadriplegic individuals regain function of their inspiratory muscles, provide reliable minute ventilation, and eventually enable partial to full liberation from mechanical ventilation [140]. DP can be done by two different methods. The first technique, known as phrenic nerve pacing (PNP) directly stimulates the phrenic nerve at the level of the thorax. This procedure is done via open thoracotomy or video-assisted thoracoscopic surgery (VATS). PNP is more invasive than the sub-diaphragmatic approach and can be complicated by injury to the phrenic nerve during direct implantation. A second technique described in the early 2000s is a less invasive procedure known as diaphragmatic pacing system (DPS). This is performed by inserting two intramuscular electrodes into each hemidiaphragm near the phrenic nerve motor points via laparoscopic surgery. DPS is also a form of phrenic nerve pacing rather than direct diaphragmatic muscle pacing [18, 93, 141–144].

Intact phrenic nerve function is essential for successful DP. Evaluation of phrenic nerve function is a key step prior to implantation of the device. Ideal candidates for DP include patients with complete high cervical SCI usually above C4, with functional phrenic nerves and diaphragm, chest wall stability, and without significant airway or parenchymal lung disease [18, 64, 145]. Stable psychosocial settings, highly engaged patients, and a strong support structure within the family are other critical variables that can affect positive outcomes in DP [144, 146].

Diaphragmatic atrophy associated with prolonged mechanical ventilation is common. Hence, after DP implantation a period of reconditioning is necessary to restore diaphragmatic function. Pacing trials can begin with a few minutes of pacing every hour, and the pacing time is gradually increased as the patient tolerates. The length of the conditioning period varies and can range from a few weeks to several months. When compared to PNP, DPS is less expensive, patients can start pacing sooner (shortly after implantation) and wean faster [144, 147, 148]. DP is superior to traditional mechanical ventilation in that it improves the patient's mobility, comfort level, sense of smell, cost of medical treatment, and quality of life and reduces the frequency of lung infections [149–152]. Lastly, most patients with DP will require long-term tracheostomy due to upper airway obstruction associated with the asynchronous contraction of the upper airway muscles and the diaphragm [18, 144, 145].

Conclusion

Respiratory management in SCI has a significant overlap with other neuromuscular diseases. However, there are significant differences as the dysfunction in SCI occurs to muscles that are innervated via spinal cord levels caudal to the level of injury, not globally. Understanding the pathophysiology of SCI to predict complications and to provide appropriate care is necessary. The goals of care include liberation from mechanical ventilation, decannulation of tracheostomies, prevention of atelectasis, pneumonia and respiratory failure, and maximizing the individual's quality of life.

References

1. Marino RJ, Ditunno JF, Donovan WH, Maynard F. Neurologic recovery after traumatic spinal cord injury: data from the model spinal cord injury systems. Arch Phys Med Rehabil. 1999;80:1391–6. https://doi.org/10.1016/s0003-9993(99)90249-6.
2. Chen Y, Tang Y, Vogel LC, Devivo MJ. Causes of spinal cord injury. Top Spinal Cord Inj Rehabil. 2013;19:1–8. https://doi.org/10.1310/sci1901-1.
3. New PW, Rawicki HB, Bailey MJ. Nontraumatic spinal cord injury: demographic characteristics and complications. Arch Phys Med Rehabil. 2002;83:996–1001. https://doi.org/10.1053/apmr.2002.33100.
4. ASIA and ISCoS International Standards Committee, American Spinal Injury Association. International standards for neurological classification of spinal cord injury. Richmond, VA: American Spinal Injury Association; 2019.
5. Berlowitz DJ, Wadsworth B, Ross J. Respiratory problems and management in people with spinal cord injury. Breathe. 2016;12:328–40. https://doi.org/10.1183/20734735.012616.
6. Berlly M, Shem K. Respiratory management during the first five days after spinal cord injury. J Spinal Cord Med. 2007;30:309–18. https://doi.org/10.1080/10790268.2007.11753946.
7. National Spinal Cord Injury Statistical Center. 2021 annual statistical report for the spinal cord injury model systems—complete public version. Birmingham, AL: University of Alabama at Birmingham; 2021. https://www.nscisc.uab.edu/PublicDocuments/AR2021_public_version.pdf.
8. National Spinal Cord Injury Statistical Center, Traumatic spinal cord injury facts and figures at a glance, 2022. https://www.nscisc.uab.edu/public/Facts-and-Figures_2022-English-Final.pdf.
9. Jackson AB, Groomes TE. Incidence of respiratory complications following spinal cord injury. Arch Phys Med Rehabil. 1994;75:270–5. https://doi.org/10.1016/0003-9993(94)90027-2.
10. Como JJ, Sutton ERH, McCunn M, Dutton RP, Johnson SB, Aarabi B, Scalea TM. Characterizing the need for mechanical ventilation following cervical spinal cord injury with neurologic deficit. J Trauma Inj Infect Crit Care. 2005;59:912–6. https://doi.org/10.1097/01.ta.0000187660.03742.a6.

11. Terson De Paleville DGL, Mckay WB, Folz RJ, Ovechkin AV. Respiratory motor control disrupted by spinal cord injury: mechanisms, evaluation, and restoration. Transl Stroke Res. 2011;2:463–73. https://doi.org/10.1007/s12975-011-0114-0.

12. Han JN, Gayan-Ramirez G, Dekhuijzen R, Decramer M. Respiratory function of the rib cage muscles. Eur Respir J. 1993;6:722–8. https://doi.org/10.1183/09031936.93.06050722.

13. De Troyer A, Kirkwood PA, Wilson TA. Respiratory action of the intercostal muscles. Physiol Rev. 2005;85:717–56. https://doi.org/10.1152/physrev.00007.2004.

14. Estenne M, Knoop C, Vanvaerenbergh J, Heilporn A, De Troyer A. The effect of pectoralis muscle training in tetraplegic subjects. Am Rev Respir Dis. 1989;139:1218–22. https://doi.org/10.1164/ajrccm/139.5.1218.

15. Bhardwaj N, Yadala S. Neuroanatomy, corticobulbar tract. In: StatPearls. Treasure Island, FL: StatPearls; 2023. http://www.ncbi.nlm.nih.gov/books/NBK555891/. Accessed 21 Jun 2023.

16. Daoud A, Haider S, Sankari A. Noninvasive ventilation and spinal cord injury, sleep. Med Clin. 2020;15:461–70. https://doi.org/10.1016/j.jsmc.2020.08.006.

17. Schilero GJ, Hobson JC, Singh K, Spungen AM, Bauman WA, Radulovic M. Bronchodilator effects of ipratropium bromide and albuterol sulfate among subjects with tetraplegia. J Spinal Cord Med. 2018;41:42–7. https://doi.org/10.1080/10790268.2016.1235753.

18. Brown R, DiMarco AF, Hoit JD, Moh EG. Respiratory dysfunction and management in spinal cord injury. Respir Care. 2006;51:853–70.

19. Oo T, Watt JWH, Soni BM, Sett PK. Delayed diaphragm recovery in 12 patients after high cervical spinal cord injury. A retrospective review of the diaphragm status of 107 patients ventilated after acute spinal cord injury. Spinal Cord. 1999;37:117. https://doi.org/10.1038/sj.sc.3100775.

20. Mueller G, de Groot S, van der Woude L, Hopman MTE. Time-courses of lung function and respiratory muscle pressure generating capacity after spinal cord injury: a prospective cohort study. J Rehabil Med. 2008;40:269–76. https://doi.org/10.2340/16501977-0162.

21. Postma K, Haisma JA, de Groot S, Hopman MT, Bergen MP, Stam HJ, Bussmann JB. Changes in pulmonary function during the early years after inpatient rehabilitation in persons with spinal cord injury: a prospective cohort study. Arch Phys Med Rehabil. 2013;94:1540–6. https://doi.org/10.1016/j.apmr.2013.02.006.

22. Raab AM, de Groot S, Berlowitz DJ, Post MWM, Adriaansen J, Hopman M, Mueller G. Development and validation of models to predict respiratory function in persons with long-term spinal cord injury. Spinal Cord. 2019;57:1064–75. https://doi.org/10.1038/s41393-019-0313-1.

23. Schilero GJ, Spungen AM, Bauman WA, Radulovic M, Lesser M. Pulmonary function and spinal cord injury. Respir Physiol Neurobiol. 2009;166:129–41. https://doi.org/10.1016/j.resp.2009.04.002.

24. Baydur A, Adkins RH, Milic-Emili J. Lung mechanics in individuals with spinal cord injury: effects of injury level and posture. J Appl Physiol. 2001;90:405.

25. Linn WS, Spungen AM, Gong J, Adkins RH, Bauman A, Waters RL. Forced vital capacity in two large outpatient populations with chronic spinal cord injury. Spinal Cord. 2001;39:263. https://doi.org/10.1038/sj.sc.3101155.

26. Linn WS, Adkins RH, Gong H, Waters RL. Pulmonary function in chronic spinal cord injury: a cross-sectional survey of 222 Southern California adult outpatients. Arch Phys Med Rehabil. 2000;81:757–63. https://doi.org/10.1016/S0003-9993(00)90107-2.

27. Estenne M, De Troyer A. Mechanism of the postural dependence of vital capacity in Tetraplegie subjects. Am Rev Respir Dis. 1987;135:367–71. https://doi.org/10.1164/arrd.1987.135.2.367.

28. Hart N, Laffont I, de La Sota AP, Lejaille M, Macadou G, Polkey MI, Denys P, Lofaso F. Respiratory effects of combined truncal and abdominal support in patients with spinal cord injury. Arch Phys Med Rehabil. 2005;86:1447–51. https://doi.org/10.1016/j.apmr.2004.12.025.

29. Haas F, Axen K, Pineda H, Gandino D, Haas A. Temporal pulmonary function changes in cervical cord injury. Arch Phys Med Rehabil. 1985;66:139–44.
30. Ledsome JR, Sharp JM. Pulmonary function in acute cervical cord injury. Am Rev Respir Dis. 1981;124:41–4. https://doi.org/10.1164/arrd.1981.124.1.41.
31. Winslow C, Rozovsky J. Effect of spinal cord injury on the respiratory system. Am J Phys Med Rehabil. 2003;82:803–14. https://doi.org/10.1097/01.PHM.0000078184.08835.01.
32. Mueller G, de Groot S, van der Woude LH, Perret C, Michel F, Hopman MTE. Prediction models and development of an easy to use open-access tool for measuring lung function of individuals with motor complete spinal cord injury. J Rehabil Med. 2012;44:642–7. https://doi.org/10.2340/16501977-1011.
33. Jain NB, Brown R, Tun CG, Gagnon D, Garshick E. Determinants of forced expiratory volume in 1 second (FEV1), forced vital capacity (FVC), and FEV1/FVC in chronic spinal cord injury. Arch Phys Med Rehabil. 2006;87:1327–33. https://doi.org/10.1016/j.apmr.2006.06.015.
34. Stepp EL, Brown R, Tun CG, Gagnon DR, Jain NB, Garshick E. Determinants of lung volumes in chronic spinal cord injury. Arch Phys Med Rehabil. 2008;89:1499–506. https://doi.org/10.1016/j.apmr.2008.02.018.
35. Stolzmann KL, Gagnon DR, Brown R, Tun CG, Garshick E. Longitudinal change in FEV_1 and FVC in chronic spinal cord injury. Am J Respir Crit Care Med. 2008;177:781–6. https://doi.org/10.1164/rccm.200709-1332OC.
36. Schilero GJ, Grimm DR, Bauman WA, Lenner R, Lesser M. Assessment of airway caliber and bronchodilator responsiveness in subjects with spinal cord injury. Chest. 2005;127:149–55. https://doi.org/10.1378/chest.127.1.149.
37. Almenoff PL, Alexander LR, Spungen AM, Lesser MD, Bauman WA. Bronchodilatory effects of ipratropium bromide in patients with tetraplegia. Paraplegia. 1995;33:274–7. https://doi.org/10.1038/sc.1995.62.
38. Dicpinigaitis PV, Spungen AM, Bauman WA, Absgarten A, Almenoff PL. Bronchial hyperresponsiveness after cervical spinal cord injury. Chest. 1994;105:1073–6. https://doi.org/10.1378/chest.105.4.1073.
39. W. Sheel, D. Reid, A. Townson, N. Ayas, Respiratory management following spinal cord injury, 2014. https://www.semanticscholar.org/paper/Respiratory-Management-Following-Spinal-Cord-Injury-Sheel-Reid/ec3fed0352bd33f62c8851dac249456190dc3489. Accessed 6 Jun 2023.
40. Mateus SRM, Beraldo PSS, Horan TA. Maximal static mouth respiratory pressure in spinal cord injured patients: correlation with motor level. Spinal Cord. 2007;45:569–75. https://doi.org/10.1038/sj.sc.3101998.
41. Anke A, Aksnes AK, Stanghelle JK, Hjeltnes N. Lung volumes in tetraplegic patients according to cervical spinal cord injury level. Scand J Rehabil Med. 1993;25:73–7.
42. Ponce MC, Sankari A, Sharma S. Pulmonary function tests. In: StatPearls. Treasure Island, FL: StatPearls; 2023. Accessed 22 Jun 2023.
43. Loveridge B, Sanii R, Dubo HI. Breathing pattern adjustments during the first year following cervical spinal cord injury. Paraplegia. 1992;30:479–88. https://doi.org/10.1038/sc.1992.102.
44. Chang AB. The physiology of cough. Paediatr Respir Rev. 2006;7:2–8. https://doi.org/10.1016/j.prrv.2005.11.009.
45. Torres-Castro R, Vilaró J, Vera-Uribe R, Monge G, Avilés P, Suranyi C. Use of air stacking and abdominal compression for cough assistance in people with complete tetraplegia. Spinal Cord. 2014;52:354–7. https://doi.org/10.1038/sc.2014.19.
46. Braun SRMD, Giovannoni RBA, O'Connor MRRT. Improving the cough in patients with spinal cord injury. Am J Phys Med. 1984;63:1–10.
47. Spungen AM, Grimm DR, Lesser M, Bauman WA, Almenoff PL. Self-reported prevalence of pulmonary symptoms in subjects with spinal cord injury. Spinal Cord. 1997;35:652. https://doi.org/10.1038/sj.sc.3100489.

48. Ayas NT, Garshick E, Lieberman SL, Wien MF, Tun C, Brown R. Breathlessness in spinal cord injury depends on injury level. J Spinal Cord Med. 1999;22:97–101. https://doi.org/1 0.1080/10790268.1999.11719553.

49. Grandas NF, Jain NB, Denckla JB, Brown R, Tun CG, Gallagher ME, Garshick E. Dyspnea during daily activities in chronic spinal cord injury. Arch Phys Med Rehabil. 2005;86:1631–5. https://doi.org/10.1016/j.apmr.2005.02.006.

50. Garshick E, Mulroy S, Graves DE, Greenwald K, Horton JA, Morse LR. Active lifestyle is associated with reduced dyspnea and greater life satisfaction in spinal cord injury. Arch Phys Med Rehabil. 2016;97:1721–7. https://doi.org/10.1016/j.apmr.2016.02.010.

51. Wien MF, Garshick E, Tun CG, Lieberman SL, Kelley A, Brown R. Breathlessness and exercise in spinal cord injury. J Spinal Cord Med. 1999;22:297–302. https://doi.org/10.108 0/10790268.1999.11719583.

52. Lance JWMD. The control of muscle tone, reflexes, and movement: Robert Wartenbeg lecture. [Review]. Neurology. 1980;30:1303–13.

53. Adams MM, Hicks AL. Spasticity after spinal cord injury. Spinal Cord. 2005;43:577–86. https://doi.org/10.1038/sj.sc.3101757.

54. Laffont I, Durand M-C, Rech C, De La Sotta AP, Hart N, Dizien O, Lofaso F. Breathlessness associated with abdominal spastic contraction in a patient with C4 tetraplegia: a case report11No commercial party having a direct financial interest in the results of the research supporting this article has or will confer a benefit upon the author(s) or upon any organization with which the author(s) is/are associated. Arch Phys Med Rehabil. 2003;84:906–8. https:// doi.org/10.1016/S0003-9993(02)04898-0.

55. Roth EJ, Lu A, Primack S, Oken J, Nusshaum S, Berkowitz M, Powley S. Ventilatory function in cervical and high thoracic spinal cord injury. Relationship to level of injury and tone. Am J Phys Med Rehabil. 1997;76:262–7. https://doi.org/10.1097/00002060-199707000-00002.

56. Dicpinigaitis PV, Grimm DR, Lesser M. Cough reflex sensitivity in subjects with cervical spinal cord injury. Am J Respir Crit Care Med. 1999;159:1660.

57. Slonimski M, Aguilera EJ. Atelectasis and mucus plugging in spinal cord injury: case report and therapeutic approaches. J Spinal Cord Med. 2001;24:284–8. https://doi.org/10.108 0/10790268.2001.11753586.

58. Berlowitz DJ, Brown DJ, Campbell DA, Pierce RJ. A longitudinal evaluation of sleep and breathing in the first year after cervical spinal cord injury. Arch Phys Med Rehabil. 2005;86:1193–9. https://doi.org/10.1016/j.apmr.2004.11.033.

59. Sankari A, Bascom A, Oomman S, Badr MS. Sleep disordered breathing in chronic spinal cord injury. J Clin Sleep Med. 2014;10:65–72. https://doi.org/10.5664/jcsm.3362.

60. Chiodo AE, Sitrin RG, Bauman KA. Sleep disordered breathing in spinal cord injury: a systematic review. J Spinal Cord Med. 2016;39:374–82. https://doi.org/10.1080/10790268.201 5.1126449.

61. Sajkov D, Marshall R, Walker P, Mykytyn I, McEvoy RD, Wale J, Flavell H, Thornton AT, Antic R. Sleep apnoea related hypoxia is associated with cognitive disturbances in patients with tetraplegia. Spinal Cord. 1998;36:231. https://doi.org/10.1038/sj.sc.3100563.

62. Proserpio P, Lanza A, Sambusida K, Fratticci L, Frigerio P, Sommariva M, Stagni EG, Redaelli T, De Carli F, Nobili L. Sleep apnea and periodic leg movements in the first year after spinal cord injury. Sleep Med. 2015;16:59–66. https://doi.org/10.1016/j.sleep.2014.07.019.

63. Sankari A, Bascom AT, Badr MS. Upper airway mechanics in chronic spinal cord injury during sleep. J Appl Physiol. 2014;116:1390–5. https://doi.org/10.1152/japplphysiol.00139.2014.

64. Galeiras Vázquez R, Rascado Sedes P, Mourelo Fariña M, Montoto Marqués A, Ferreiro Velasco ME. Respiratory management in the patient with spinal cord injury. Biomed Res Int. 2013;2013:168757. https://doi.org/10.1155/2013/168757.

65. Kiser TS. Department of Physical Medicine and Rehabilitation/Trauma rehabilitation resources program. SPINAL CORD INJURY GUIDELINES 2021. SPINAL CORD INJURY CLINICAL GUIDELINE. Guidelines for respiratory management following spinal cord injury, 2021.

66. Bach JR, Burke L, Chiou M. Noninvasive respiratory management of spinal cord injury. Phys Med Rehabil Clin N Am. 2020;31:397–413. https://doi.org/10.1016/j.pmr.2020.03.006.
67. Maltais F. Glossopharyngeal breathing. Am J Respir Crit Care Med. 2011;184:381. https://doi.org/10.1164/rccm.201012-2031IM.
68. Nygren-Bonnier M, Wahman K, Lindholm P, Markström A, Westgren N, Klefbeck B. Glossopharyngeal pistoning for lung insufflation in patients with cervical spinal cord injury. Spinal Cord. 2009;47:418–22. https://doi.org/10.1038/sc.2008.138.
69. Kang S-W, Bach JR. Maximum insufflation capacity. Chest. 2000;118:61–5. https://doi.org/10.1378/chest.118.1.61.
70. Molgat-Seon Y, Hannan LM, Dominelli PB, Peters CM, Fougere RJ, McKim DA, Sheel AW, Road JD. Lung volume recruitment acutely increases respiratory system compliance in individuals with severe respiratory muscle weakness. ERJ Open Res. 2017;3:00135. https://doi.org/10.1183/23120541.00135-2016.
71. Jeong J, Yoo W. Effects of air stacking on pulmonary function and peak cough flow in patients with cervical spinal cord injury. J Phys Ther Sci. 2015;27:1951–2. https://doi.org/10.1589/jpts.27.1951.
72. Shin JC, Han EY, Cho KH, Im SH. Improvement in pulmonary function with short-term rehabilitation treatment in spinal cord injury patients. Sci Rep. 2019;9:17091. https://doi.org/10.1038/s41598-019-52526-6.
73. Berlowitz DJ, Tamplin J. Respiratory muscle training for cervical spinal cord injury. Cochrane Database Syst Rev. 2013;2013:CD008507. https://doi.org/10.1002/14651858.CD008507.pub2.
74. Fujiwara T, Hara YM, Chino NM. Expiratory function in complete tetraplegics: study of spirometry, maximal expiratory pressure, and muscle activity of pectoralis major and latissimus dorsi muscles. Am J Phys Med Rehabil. 1999;78:464–9.
75. Sapienza CM, Wheeler K. Respiratory muscle strength training: functional outcomes versus plasticity. Semin Speech Lang. 2006;27:236–44. https://doi.org/10.1055/s-2006-955114.
76. Lotters F, Van Tol B, Kwakkel G, Gosselink R. Effects of controlled inspiratory muscle training in patients with COPD: a meta-analysis. Eur Respir J. 2002;20:570–7. https://doi.org/10.1183/09031936.02.00237402.
77. Morgan DW, Kohrt WM, Bates BJ, Skinner JS. Effects of respiratory muscle endurance training on ventilatory and endurance performance of moderately trained cyclists*. Int J Sports Med. 1987;08:88–93. https://doi.org/10.1055/s-2008-1025647.
78. Sapienza CM. Respiratory muscle strength training applications. Curr Opin Otolaryngol Head Neck Surg. 2008;16:216–20. https://doi.org/10.1097/MOO.0b013e3282fe96bd.
79. Uijl SG, Houtman S, Folgering HT, Hopman MTE. Training of the respiratory muscles in individuals with tetraplegia. Spinal Cord. 1999;37:575. https://doi.org/10.1038/sj.sc.3100887.
80. Liaw M-Y, Lin M-C, Cheng P-T, Wong M-KA, Tang F-T. Resistive inspiratory muscle training: its effectiveness in patients with acute complete cervical cord injury. Arch Phys Med Rehabil. 2000;81:752–6. https://doi.org/10.1016/S0003-9993(00)90106-0.
81. Ray C, Trudeau MD, McCoy S. Effects of respiratory muscle strength training in classically trained singers. J Voice. 2018;32(644):e25–644.e34. https://doi.org/10.1016/j.jvoice.2017.08.005.
82. Kim J, Davenport P, Sapienza C. Effect of expiratory muscle strength training on elderly cough function. Arch Gerontol Geriatr. 2009;48:361–6. https://doi.org/10.1016/j.archger.2008.03.006.
83. Wang X, Zhang N, Xu Y. Effects of respiratory muscle training on pulmonary function in individuals with spinal cord injury: an updated meta-analysis. Biomed Res Int. 2020;2020:7530498. https://doi.org/10.1155/2020/7530498.
84. Goldman JM, Rose LS, Morgan MD, Denison DM. Measurement of abdominal wall compliance in normal subjects and tetraplegic patients. Thorax. 1986;41:513–8.
85. Goldman JM, Rose LS, Williams SJ, Silver JR, Denison DM. Effect of abdominal binders on breathing in tetraplegic patients. Thorax. 1986;41:940–5.

86. Cornwell PL, Ward EC, Lim Y, Wadsworth B. Impact of an abdominal binder on speech outcomes in people with tetraplegic spinal cord injury: perceptual and acoustic measures. Top Spinal Cord Inj Rehabil. 2014;20:48–57. https://doi.org/10.1310/sci2001-48.

87. McCool FD, Pichurko BM, Slutsky AS, Sarkarati M, Rossier A, Brown R. Changes in lung volume and rib cage configuration with abdominal binding in quadriplegia. J Appl Physiol. 1986;60:1198–202. https://doi.org/10.1152/jappl.1986.60.4.1198.

88. Wadsworth BM, Haines TP, Cornwell PL, Rodwell LT, Paratz JD. Abdominal binder improves lung volumes and voice in people with tetraplegic spinal cord injury. Arch Phys Med Rehabil. 2012;93:2189–97. https://doi.org/10.1016/j.apmr.2012.06.010.

89. Bach JR. Mechanical insufflation-exsufflation: comparison of peak expiratory flows with manually assisted and unassisted coughing techniques. Chest. 1993;104:1553–62. https://doi.org/10.1378/chest.104.5.1553.

90. Pillastrini P, Bordini S, Bazzocchi G, Belloni G, Menarini M. Study of the effectiveness of bronchial clearance in subjects with upper spinal cord injuries: examination of a rehabilitation programme involving mechanical insufflation and exsufflation. Spinal Cord. 2006;44:614–6. https://doi.org/10.1038/sj.sc.3101870.

91. Garstang SV, Kirshblum SC, Wood KE. Patient preference for in-exsufflation for secretion management with spinal cord injury. J Spinal Cord Med. 2000;23:80–5. https://doi.org/10.1080/10790268.2000.11753511.

92. Spungen AM, Dicpinigaitis PV, Almenoff PL, Bauman WA. Pulmonary obstruction in individuals with cervical spinal cord lesions unmasked by bronchodilator administration. Spinal Cord. 1993;31:404–7. https://doi.org/10.1038/sc.1993.67.

93. Schilero GJ, Bauman WA, Radulovic M. Traumatic spinal cord injury: pulmonary physiologic principles and management. Clin Chest Med. 2018;39:411–25. https://doi.org/10.1016/j.ccm.2018.02.002.

94. Cragg JJ, Warner FM, Kramer JK, Borisoff JF. A Canada-wide survey of chronic respiratory disease and spinal cord injury. Neurology. 2015;84:1341–5. https://doi.org/10.1212/WNL.0000000000001428.

95. Schilero GJ, Grimm D, Spungen AM, Lenner R, Lesser M. Bronchodilator responses to metaproterenol sulfate among subjects with spinal cord injury. J Rehabil Res Dev. 2004;41:59. https://doi.org/10.1682/JRRD.2004.01.0059.

96. Grimm DR, Schilero GJ, Spungen AM, Bauman WA, Lesser M. Salmeterol improves pulmonary function in persons with tetraplegia. Lung. 2006;184:335–9. https://doi.org/10.1007/s00408-006-0011-6.

97. Signorile JF, Banovac K, Gomez M, Flipse D, Caruso JF, Lowensteyn I. Increased muscle strength in paralyzed patients after spinal cord injury: effect of beta-2 adrenergic agonist. Arch Phys Med Rehabil. 1995;76:55–8. https://doi.org/10.1016/S0003-9993(95)80043-3.

98. Murphy RJ, Hartkopp A, Gardiner PF, Kjaer M, Béliveau L. Salbutamol effect in spinal cord injured individuals undergoing functional electrical stimulation training. Arch Phys Med Rehabil. 1999;80:1264–7. https://doi.org/10.1016/S0003-9993(99)90027-8.

99. Hansen-Flaschen J, Ackrivo J. Practical guide to management of long-term noninvasive ventilation for adults with chronic neuromuscular disease. Respir Care. 2023;68:1123. https://doi.org/10.4187/respcare.10349.

100. Biering-Sørensen M, Norup PW, Jacobsen E, Biering-Sørensen F. Treatment of sleep apnoea in spinal cord injured patients. Paraplegia. 1995;33:271–3. https://doi.org/10.1038/sc.1995.61.

101. Ball PA. Critical care of spinal cord injury. Spine. 2001;26:S27–30. https://doi.org/10.1097/00007632-200112151-00006.

102. Gardner BP, Watt JW, Krishnan KR. The artificial ventilation of acute spinal cord damaged patients: a retrospective study of forty-four patients. Paraplegia. 1986;24:208–20. https://doi.org/10.1038/sc.1986.30.

103. Bach JR, Burke L, Chiou M. Conventional respiratory management of spinal cord injury. Phys Med Rehabil Clin N Am. 2020;31:379–95. https://doi.org/10.1016/j.pmr.2020.04.004.

104. Seidl RO, Wolf D, Nusser-Müller-Busch R, Niedeggen A. Airway management in acute tetraplegics: a retrospective study. Eur Spine J. 2010;19:1073–8. https://doi.org/10.1007/s00586-010-1328-7.
105. Veeravagu A, Jiang B, Rincon F, Maltenfort M, Jallo J, Ratliff JK. Acute respiratory distress syndrome and acute lung injury in patients with vertebral column fracture(s) and spinal cord injury: a nationwide inpatient sample study. Spinal Cord. 2013;51:461–5. https://doi.org/10.1038/sc.2013.16.
106. Hatton GE, Mollett PJ, Du RE, Wei S, Korupolu R, Wade CE, Adams SD, Kao LS. High tidal volume ventilation is associated with ventilator-associated pneumonia in acute cervical spinal cord injury. J Spinal Cord Med. 2021;44:775–81. https://doi.org/10.1080/1079026 8.2020.1722936.
107. Massaro GD, Massaro D. Morphologic evidence that large inflations of the lung stimulate secretion of surfactant. Am Rev Respir Dis. 1983;127:235–6. https://doi.org/10.1164/arrd.1983.127.2.235.
108. Peterson P, Brooks C, Mellick D, Whiteneck G. Protocol for ventilator management in high tetraplegia. Top Spinal Cord Inj Rehabil. 1997;2:101–6.
109. Fenton JJ, Warner ML, Lammertse D, Charlifue S, Martinez L, Dannels-McClure A, Kreider S, Pretz C. A comparison of high vs standard tidal volumes in ventilator weaning for individuals with sub-acute spinal cord injuries: a site-specific randomized clinical trial. Spinal Cord. 2016;54:234–8. https://doi.org/10.1038/sc.2015.145.
110. Manning HL, Shea SA, Schwartzstein RM, Lansing RW, Brown R, Banzett RB. Reduced tidal volume increases "air hunger" at fixed PCO2 in ventilated quadriplegics. Respir Physiol. 1992;90:19–30. https://doi.org/10.1016/0034-5687(92)90131-f.
111. Peterson WP, Barbalata L, Brooks CA, Gerhart KA, Mellick DC, Whiteneck GG. The effect of tidal volumes on the time to wean persons with high tetraplegia from ventilators. Spinal Cord. 1999;37:284–8. https://doi.org/10.1038/sj.sc.3100818.
112. Consortium for Spinal Cord Medicine. Respiratory management following spinal cord injury: a clinical practice guideline for health-care professionals. J Spinal Cord Med. 2005;28:259–93. https://doi.org/10.1080/10790268.2005.11753821.
113. Wong SL, Shem K, Crew J. Specialized respiratory management for acute cervical spinal cord injury. Top Spinal Cord Inj Rehabil. 2012;18:283–90. https://doi.org/10.1310/sci1804-283.
114. Korupolu R, Stampas A, Jimenez IH, Cruz D, Giusto MLD, Verduzco-Gutierrez M, Davis ME. Mechanical ventilation and weaning practices for adults with spinal cord injury—an international survey. J Int Soc Phys Rehabil Med. 2021;4:131. https://doi.org/10.4103/JISPRM-000124.
115. Korupolu R, Stampas A, Uhlig-Reche H, Ciammaichella E, Mollett PJ, Achilike EC, Pedroza C. Comparing outcomes of mechanical ventilation with high vs. moderate tidal volumes in tracheostomized patients with spinal cord injury in acute inpatient rehabilitation setting: a retrospective cohort study. Spinal Cord. 2021;59:618–25. https://doi.org/10.1038/s41393-020-0517-4.
116. Schreiber AF, Garlasco J, Vieira F, Lau YH, Stavi D, Lightfoot D, Rigamonti A, Burns K, Friedrich JO, Singh JM, Brochard LJ. Separation from mechanical ventilation and survival after spinal cord injury: a systematic review and meta-analysis. Ann Intensive Care. 2021;11:149. https://doi.org/10.1186/s13613-021-00938-x.
117. Gutierrez CJ, Harrow J, Haines F. Using an evidence-based protocol to guide rehabilitation and weaning of ventilator-dependent cervical spinal cord injury patients. J Rehabil Res Dev. 2003;40:99–110. https://doi.org/10.1682/jrrd.2003.10.0099.
118. Atito- Narh E, Pieri-Davies S, Watt JWH. Slow ventilator weaning after cervical spinal cord injury. Br J Intensive Care. 2008;18:95–102.
119. Gundogdu I, Ozturk EA, Umay E, Karaahmet OZ, Unlu E, Cakci A. Implementation of a respiratory rehabilitation protocol: weaning from the ventilator and tracheostomy in difficult-to-wean patients with spinal cord injury. Disabil Rehabil. 2017;39:1162–70. https://doi.org/10.1080/09638288.2016.1189607.

120. Zhang B, Jiang H, Zhang C, Li Y, Zhao Z. Pulmonary rehabilitation throughout the weaning from mechanical ventilation for complete cervical spinal cord injury: a case report. Signa Vitae. 2020;16:210–4. https://doi.org/10.22514/sv.2020.16.0058.

121. Park J, Choi WA, Kang S-W. Pulmonary rehabilitation in high cervical spinal cord injury: a series of 133 consecutive cases. Spinal Cord. 2022;60:1014–9. https://doi.org/10.1038/s41393-022-00816-8.

122. Peterson W, Charlifue W, Gerhart A, Whiteneck G. Two methods of weaning persons with quadriplegia from mechanical ventilators. Paraplegia. 1994;32:98–103. https://doi.org/10.1038/sc.1994.17.

123. Sivak ED. Prolonged mechanical ventilation; an approach to weaning. Cleve Clin Q. 1980;47:89–96. https://doi.org/10.3949/ccjm.47.2.89.

124. Knebel AR. Weaning from mechanical ventilation: current controversies, heart lung. J Crit Care. 1991;20:321–31.

125. Brochard L, Rauss A, Benito S, Conti G, Mancebo J, Rekik N, Gasparetto A, Lemaire F. Comparison of three methods of gradual withdrawal from ventilatory support during weaning from mechanical ventilation. Am J Respir Crit Care Med. 1994;150:896–903. https://doi.org/10.1164/ajrccm.150.4.7921460.

126. Esteban A, Frutos F, Tobin MJ, Alía I, Solsona JF, Valverdú I, Fernández R, de la Cal MA, Benito S, Tomás R. A comparison of four methods of weaning patients from mechanical ventilation. Spanish Lung Failure Collaborative Group. N Engl J Med. 1995;332:345–50. https://doi.org/10.1056/NEJM199502093320601.

127. Wallbom A, Naran B, Thomas E. Acute ventilator management and weaning in individuals with high tetraplegia. Top Spinal Cord Inj Rehabil. 2005;10:1–7. https://doi.org/10.1310/K4Y4-YDXQ-9VNY-F562.

128. Bach JR. New approaches in the rehabilitation of the traumatic high level quadriplegic. Am J Phys Med Rehabil. 1991;70:13–9. https://doi.org/10.1097/00002060-199102000-00004.

129. Richard-Denis A, Feldman D, Thompson C, Albert M, Mac-Thiong J-M. The impact of a specialized spinal cord injury center as compared with non-specialized centers on the acute respiratory management of patients with complete tetraplegia: an observational study. Spinal Cord. 2018;56:142–50. https://doi.org/10.1038/s41393-017-0003-9.

130. Toki A, Nakamura T, Nishimura Y, Sumida M, Tajima F. Clinical introduction and benefits of non-invasive ventilation for above C3 cervical spinal cord injury. J Spinal Cord Med. 2021;44:70–6. https://doi.org/10.1080/10790268.2019.1644474.

131. Wicks AB, Menter RR. Long-term outlook in quadriplegic patients with initial ventilator dependency. Chest. 1986;90:406–10. https://doi.org/10.1378/chest.90.3.406.

132. Berney S, Bragge P, Granger C, Opdam H, Denehy L. The acute respiratory management of cervical spinal cord injury in the first 6 weeks after injury: a systematic review. Spinal Cord. 2011;49:17–29. https://doi.org/10.1038/sc.2010.39.

133. Berney SC, Gordon IR, Opdam HI, Denehy L. A classification and regression tree to assist clinical decision making in airway management for patients with cervical spinal cord injury. Spinal Cord. 2011;49:244–50. https://doi.org/10.1038/sc.2010.97.

134. Yugué I, Okada S, Ueta T, Maeda T, Mori E, Kawano O, Takao T, Sakai H, Masuda M, Hayashi T, Morishita Y, Shiba K. Analysis of the risk factors for tracheostomy in traumatic cervical spinal cord injury. Spine. 2012;37:E1633–8. https://doi.org/10.1097/BRS.0b013e31827417f1.

135. Ross J, White M. Removal of the tracheostomy tube in the aspirating spinal cord-injured patient. Spinal Cord. 2003;41:636–42. https://doi.org/10.1038/sj.sc.3101510.

136. Vassilakopoulos T, Petrof BJ. Ventilator-induced diaphragmatic dysfunction. Am J Respir Crit Care Med. 2004;169:336–41. https://doi.org/10.1164/rccm.200304-489CP.

137. Levine S, Nguyen T, Taylor N, Friscia ME, Budak MT, Rothenberg P, Zhu J, Sachdeva R, Sonnad S, Kaiser LR, Rubinstein NA, Powers SK, Shrager JB. Rapid disuse atrophy of diaphragm fibers in mechanically ventilated humans. N Engl J Med. 2008;358:1327–35. https://doi.org/10.1056/NEJMoa070447.

138. Petrof BJ, Jaber S, Matecki S. Ventilator-induced diaphragmatic dysfunction. Curr Opin Crit Care. 2010;16:19. https://doi.org/10.1097/MCC.0b013e328334b166.
139. Glenn WW, Holcomb WG, Gee JB, Rath R. Central hypoventilation; long-term ventilatory assistance by radiofrequency electrophrenic respiration. Ann Surg. 1970;172:755–73.
140. Onders RP, Khansarinia S, Ingvarsson PE, Road J, Yee J, Dunkin B, Ignagni AR. Diaphragm pacing in spinal cord injury can significantly decrease mechanical ventilation in multicenter prospective evaluation. Artif Organs. 2022;46:1980–7. https://doi.org/10.1111/aor.14221.
141. DiMarco AF, Onders RP, Kowalski KE, Miller ME, Ferek S, Mortimer JT. Phrenic nerve pacing in a tetraplegic patient via intramuscular diaphragm electrodes. Am J Respir Crit Care Med. 2002;166:1604–6. https://doi.org/10.1164/rccm.200203-175CR.
142. DiMarco AF, Onders RP, Ignagni A, Kowalski KE, Mortimer JT. Phrenic nerve pacing via intramuscular diaphragm electrodes in tetraplegic subjects. Chest. 2005;127:671–8. https://doi.org/10.1378/chest.127.2.671.
143. Onders RP, Dimarco AF, Ignagni AR, Aiyar H, Mortimer JT. Mapping the phrenic nerve motor point: the key to a successful laparoscopic diaphragm pacing system in the first human series. Surgery. 2004;136:819–26. https://doi.org/10.1016/j.surg.2004.06.030.
144. DiMarco AF. Diaphragm pacing. Clin Chest Med. 2018;39:459–71. https://doi.org/10.1016/j.ccm.2018.01.008.
145. Mansel JK, Norman JR. Respiratory complications and management of spinal cord injuries. Chest. 1990;97:1446–52. https://doi.org/10.1378/chest.97.6.1446.
146. Elefteriades JA, Quin JA, Hogan JF, Holcomb WG, Letsou GV, Chlosta WF, Glenn WWWL. Long-term follow-up of pacing of the conditioned diaphragm in quadriplegia. Pacing Clin Electrophysiol. 2002;25:897–906. https://doi.org/10.1046/j.1460-9592.2002.00897.x.
147. Ducko CT. Clinical advances in diaphragm pacing. Innovations (Phila). 2011;6:289–97. https://doi.org/10.1097/IMI.0b013e318237cc97.
148. Le Pimpec-Barthes F, Legras A, Arame A, Pricopi C, Boucherie J-C, Badia A, Panzini CM. Diaphragm pacing: the state of the art. J Thorac Dis. 2016;8:S376–86. https://doi.org/10.21037/jtd.2016.03.97.
149. Esclarín A, Bravo P, Arroyo O, Mazaira J, Garrido H, Alcaraz MA. Tracheostomy ventilation versus diaphragmatic pacemaker ventilation in high spinal cord injury. Paraplegia. 1994;32:687–93. https://doi.org/10.1038/sc.1994.111.
150. Hirschfeld S, Exner G, Luukkaala T, Baer GA. Mechanical ventilation or phrenic nerve stimulation for treatment of spinal cord injury-induced respiratory insufficiency. Spinal Cord. 2008;46:738–42. https://doi.org/10.1038/sc.2008.43.
151. Romero-Ganuza FJ, Gambarrutta-Malfatti C, Diez de la Lastra-Buigues E, Marín-Ruiz MÁ, Merlo-González VE, Sánchez-Aranzueque Pantoja AM, García-Moreno FJ, Mazaira-Álvarez J. Diaphragmatic pacemaker as an alternative to mechanical ventilation in patients with cervical spinal injury. Med Intensiva. 2011;35:13–21. https://doi.org/10.1016/j.medin.2010.10.003.
152. Romero FJ, Gambarrutta C, Garcia-Forcada A, Marín MA, Diaz de la Lastra E, Paz F, Fernandez-Dorado MT, Mazaira J. Long-term evaluation of phrenic nerve pacing for respiratory failure due to high cervical spinal cord injury. Spinal Cord. 2012;50:895–8. https://doi.org/10.1038/sc.2012.74.

Chapter 12
Approach to the Patient with Neuromuscular Diseases Causing Acute Respiratory Failure

Brandon Merical, Atul A. Kalanuria, and Matthew J. Michaels

Introduction

Neuromuscular respiratory failure is a commonly seen pathology in the intensive care unit (ICU). Patients with acute, subacute, acute on chronic, and chronic neuromuscular pathologies require prompt recognition and treatment to prevent morbidity and mortality. Patients with neuromuscular respiratory failure from neuromuscular diseases are at risk for additional intensive care unit-associated complications, including but not limited to infection, arrhythmia, electrolyte derangements, dysautonomia, and ileus, all of which should be anticipated by the clinician. The two most common causes of neuromuscular respiratory failure in the ICU setting are myasthenia gravis and Guillain-Barré syndrome [1, 2].

In addition to these two more common diagnoses, there are a variety of other infectious, inflammatory, endocrine, paraneoplastic, neoplastic, vasculitic, genetic, and mitochondrial diseases that can cause neuromuscular respiratory failure. Understanding of the underlying pathophysiology ensures that the clinical team promptly makes the correct diagnosis and initiates treatment while anticipating the potential complications and prognosis. The anticipation of these complications is crucial to reduce morbidity and mortality [3].

B. Merical
Neurocritical Care, Department of Neurology, The Hospital of The University of Pennsylvania, Philadelphia, PA, USA
e-mail: Brandon.Merical@pennmedicine.upenn.edu

A. A. Kalanuria · M. J. Michaels (✉)
Division of Neurocritical Care, Department of Neurology, Neurosurgery, Anesthesia and Critical Care, Penn Presbyterian Medical Center, The Hospital of The University of Pennsylvania, Philadelphia, PA, USA
e-mail: atul.kalanuria@pennmedicine.upenn.edu;
matthew.michaels@pennmedicine.upenn.edu

© The Author(s), under exclusive license to Springer Nature Switzerland AG 2024

N. Lechtzin (ed.), *Pulmonary Complications of Neuromuscular Disease*, Respiratory Medicine, https://doi.org/10.1007/978-3-031-65335-3_12

With specific focus on the clinical approach of obtaining a detailed history, the clinician can elucidate the most likely underlying pathology. In addition, the clinician can obtain a better understanding of the patient's location and velocity in their clinical trajectory. This is crucial for anticipating the patient's immediate and near-term clinical needs. Identification of the timeline is perhaps the most crucial piece of the history.

The neurologic examination is another powerful tool at the neurologist's disposal to confirm or deny the hypothesis generated from the history. Specific focus on the bulbar, motor, sensory, and reflex examination can not only elucidate the diagnosis but also shed light on the likelihood or severity of the impending neuromuscular respiratory failure [4]. There are a variety of special exam maneuvers that have high specificity for particular neuromuscular pathologies and are key components of the neurologist's diagnostic armamentarium. Additionally, there are a variety of tests that can be performed at the bedside that can reassure or worry the clinician about the strength of the patient's bulbar and respiratory systems. Understanding how to perform and interpret these exam maneuvers can be crucial for early recognition of impending neuromuscular respiratory failure.

Herein, we will discuss our diagnostic evaluation and clinical approach, including history, physical examination, special examination maneuvers to elucidate underlying pathology and respiratory strength including illustrations, laboratory evaluation, imaging, electromyography (EMG), nerve conduction study (NCS), and genetic testing. We will then discuss the acute and chronic neuromuscular pathologies along with their presentations and pathophysiology prior to shifting to disease-specific pathological states commonly encountered in the ICU. Following discussion of the pathologies, we will discuss the various treatment options and the data for each. We will conclude with discussion on ICU-specific management and support focused on the respiratory system and modes of ventilation.

Diagnostic Evaluation and Clinical Approach

History

> Listen to your patient; he is telling you the diagnosis.—William Osler, MD
> Patients present with symptoms that need careful evaluation before physical examinations which in turn should be firmly based on the diagnostic possibilities suggested by the history [5].

In the field of neurology, clinical history is the most valuable diagnostic tool. The ability to obtain the clinical history is equally as important and is a skill that must be learned and practiced frequently. For patients presenting with respiratory failure, the ability to identify that the patient's complaints are secondary to a neurologic problem, as opposed to a cardiac or pulmonary issue, can easily be obtained by a careful history. Clues regarding bulbar symptoms such as double vision or sensory phenomenon such as paresthesia should alert the clinician to the presence of a neurologic diagnosis, rather than that of cardiac or respiratory.

Often, in the intensive care unit, a patient is unable to provide you with the actual history due to respiratory failure. Despite this, history remains the most necessary tool within the diagnostic toolbox. Every effort must be made to obtain the history from the patient when able or from the relatives and friends.

Timeline

The timeline of symptom onset and progression is perhaps the most critical piece of clinical history to obtain. The initial onset of symptoms and their progression can differentiate between a variety of neuromuscular disorders and allow the clinician to rapidly move through the diagnostic algorithm to obtain the correct diagnosis. In addition to the clinical timeline assisting in identifying the diagnosis, the progression of symptoms is critical for the clinician in anticipating the illness's ultimate severity and need for an elevated level of care and monitoring. Specifically, for pathologies such as AIDP and MG, the rapidity of symptom onset and progression can alert the clinician to impending neuromuscular respiratory failure.

Provoking Illness and Provoking Factors

A thorough history will include investigating the events prior to the onset of symptoms. For patients with neurological conditions that could lead to neuromuscular respiratory failure, there is often a proceeding illness or immunologic stimulus prior to the onset of symptoms. Classically, for AIDP, patients will report a recent respiratory or GI illness within month of symptom onset in over 60% of cases [6]. Exposure to a viral or bacterial pathogen may trigger an immune response and typically occurs within 1–2 months of presentation. Less commonly, GBS can be triggered by noninfectious events such as trauma, vaccinations, immunosuppression, and pregnancy.

Myasthenia gravis can be associated with thymoma, an epithelial tumor originating in the anterior mediastinum. Additionally, myasthenia is seen in patients receiving immune checkpoint inhibitor therapy for cancer. Lambert-Eaton syndrome is classically associated with small-cell lung cancer.

Specific Symptoms to Focus on in the History

Many of the classic examination findings of a particular condition are not present early in the disease process or are difficult to objectively evaluate by examination maneuvers. Here, again obtaining a comprehensive history is extremely valuable.

Asking the patient about bulbar symptoms such as dysarthria and dysphagia may reveal pathology that is early or not obvious to the examiner. For example, the presence of chewing fatigue and ptosis that worsens throughout the day can clue the examiner into the diagnosis of myasthenia gravis. Diplopia is a subjective symptom, and its presence can clue the examiner into the presence of bulbar pathology even in the absence of obvious extraocular movement abnormalities on the physical examination.

Physical Examination: Neurologic

The neurologic examination is a valuable tool for assessing neurologic pathology. Once a thorough history is obtained, the examination can be focused on the appropriate realms to aid in the diagnosis. In this section, we will discuss the neurologic examination as it relates to the patient with a suspected neuromuscular disorder culminating in respiratory failure.

Mental Status

Classically, the most common neuromuscular pathologies do not involve the central nervous system (CNS). Mental status should be preserved assuming there is not a concomitant pathology. If the patient's level of arousal is affected in the setting of a suspected neuromuscular condition, this should alert the condition to the presence of hypercarbic respiratory failure or another secondary pathology. The presence of encephalopathy in the setting of neurologic symptoms should strongly suggest an alternative diagnosis.

Exceptions to the above include Bickerstaff's brainstem encephalitis where there is a concomitant encephalopathy [7]. Mitochondrial disorders can also present with both CNS and PNS manifestations. Toxic ingestions may also cause metabolic or toxic encephalopathy.

Cranial Nerve Examination

The cranial nerve examination is a critical component of the neurologic examination, especially in patients with neuromuscular conditions. A significant amount of the cranial nerve examination can be assessed while the patient is providing their history. The presence of dysarthria or nasal quality of speech suggests oropharyngeal weakness. Assessment of the patient's posture and neck position during the course of the history can suggest axial weakness and neck weakness. Observation of ptosis, drooling, and the ability to complete a sentence without taking a breath are all crucial components of the examination that are obtained while taking the patient's history.

Special Cranial Nerve Exam Maneuvers

Cogen's Lid Twitch

Cogen's lid twitch refers to a characteristic eyelid movement seen in some individuals with this neuromuscular disorder. It is named after Dr. David Cogen, who first described the phenomenon in 1965. Cogen's lid twitch is characterized by a momentary, repetitive upward movement of the upper eyelid, often occurring when the patient attempts to maintain sustained upward gaze. This is a common finding in myasthenia gravis, with specificity close to 99% and sensitivity of 75% [8].

Fatigable Upgaze

Fatigable upgaze is observed when the patient is asked to maintain upward gaze. Often ptosis will begin to develop, or the patient is unable to maintain the upward gaze after a brief period of time. This is a common finding in myasthenia gravis.

Tongue and Facial Weakness

This can be assessed by asking the patient to puff out their cheeks. Mild weakness can be assessed by pushing in on the cheek and the patient being unable to maintain the labial seal, allowing air to escape. Tongue strength can be assessed by asking the patient to push their tongue into their cheek against the examiner's pressure on the cheek. This is a common finding in many neuromuscular conditions and indicates bulbar weakness.

Extraocular Movement Abnormalities

Extraocular movement abnormalities are common in myasthenia gravis and a variety of neuromuscular conditions. The fatigable component and changes throughout the day support myasthenic pathology.

Motor Examination

The initial component of the motor examination involves observation by the examiner. Attention to atrophy, increased or decreased bulk, limb resting position, and additional movements of the muscles at rest are key features of the examination. In general, most acute neuromuscular disorders should have decreased tone without any obvious atrophy or additional movements. Exceptions include the observation of pseudoathetosis in patients with severe proprioceptive loss in sensory predominant neuropathies. Observations of fasciculation with atrophy in a patient with a more chronic presentation with upper motor neuron signs should suggest motor neuron disease. In addition to observation, a full motor examination should be performed in the standard fashion. Attention should be paid to the pattern of weakness, flexors versus extensors, and proximal versus distal. In addition to the full examination, some special tests can help the examiner support the suspected diagnosis and raise concern for impending respiratory muscle compromise.

Fatigable Weakness

Fatigable weakness in myasthenia refers to diminishing strength with repeated or sustained use, improving after periods of rest. Deltoid pumps are a specific method used to assess fatigability in myasthenia patients. In deltoid pumps, the patient's deltoid strength is initially tested and scored. The patient is then asked to repeatedly abduct their arm, typically 30 times. Initially, the muscle strength may appear normal, but as the activity continues, the muscles gradually weaken. After the repetitive activity, the patient's strength is tested again and scored, with a significant reduction of strength after 30 passive raises supportive of fatigable weakness. This same strategy can be applied to other muscle groups as well, such as wrist flexion, upgaze, and bicep flexion as alternative ways of testing fatigable weakness.

Neck Flexion and Extension

Neck flexion and extension are critical components of the neuromuscular examination and are considered surrogates for respiratory muscle strength. Findings of reduced neck flexion and extension on physical examination in a patient with a suspected neuromuscular condition should alert the clinician to the possibility of impending neuromuscular respiratory failure. The strength of the neck extensors can be tested by asking the patient to extend their neck against the examiner's hand holding the back of their head. For neck flexion, the patient should be asked to flex their neck to have their chin touch their chest. The examiner then applies pressure to their forehead evaluating for the ability to extend the patient's neck against the patient's flexion strength.

Single Breath Count

The single breath count test is a surrogate for a patient's vital capacity. This test can be done quickly and easily at the bedside by asking the patient to inhale maximally and count as high as they can in one single breath. If the patient can count above 20, this is reassuring. This test also allows the clinician to trend the patient's respiratory strength, or vital capacity, over time. This test is quite helpful for patients whose buccal and labial strength limits their ability to form a seal over the respiratory testing equipment with which vital capacity and negative inspiratory force are tested.

Objective Testing of Respiratory Strength and Reserve

In addition to the above bedside tests that can be performed without equipment, testing of a patient's negative inspiratory force (NIF) or maximal inspiratory pressure (MIP) and vital capacity (VC) are objective measures of a patient's respiratory strength and reserve which can be measured at the bedside, recorded, and followed overtime. These measures can aid the clinician in making clinical decisions about whether a patient is likely to need additional respiratory support and can even be useful in the decision about extubating a patient.

Negative Inspiratory Force (NIF) Testing

NIF or MIP (maximal inspiratory pressure) testing helps evaluate respiratory muscle weakness and the severity of neuromuscular respiratory failure. NIF testing is typically performed using a handheld device called a manometer or a portable spirometer. Below is typically how this is conducted:

1. The patient is seated in an upright position and instructed to breathe normally for a short period to establish a baseline.
2. The mouthpiece of the manometer or spirometer is placed in the patient's mouth, ensuring a tight seal to prevent air leakage. The patient's nose is often sealed using a clip, especially in patients with nasopharyngeal weakness.

3. The patient is then asked to take a deep breath in as forcefully as possible, trying to generate maximal inspiratory effort while keeping the mouthpiece in place.
4. During this process, the device measures the pressure generated by the inspiratory muscles. The patient may be coached and encouraged to achieve their maximum effort.
5. The test is usually repeated a few times to ensure consistent results, and the highest value obtained is recorded as the NIF or MIP.

The NIF is expressed as a negative value since it represents the strength of inspiratory muscles. A lower NIF indicates weaker respiratory muscles and can suggest respiratory muscle weakness. Increasingly negative values (more than $-20\,\text{cm}\,H_2O$) are considered concerning and may indicate a need for elective intubation or non-invasive positive pressure ventilation (NIPPV).

Vital capacity testing is a common pulmonary function test that measures the maximum amount of air a person can exhale forcefully after taking a full breath in. This test is reassuring when a patient has a vital capacity greater than 30 cc/kg. Values below this are concerning and may indicate the need for elective intubation or NIPPV.

Additional Considerations of the Neurologic Examination

The specifics of the complete neurologic examination relating to the diagnosis of a neuromuscular process are beyond this chapter's scope. Suffice it to say that the sensory, reflex, coordination, and gait examination are crucial components to the complete evaluation of a patient with a neuromuscular disorder. The examination components described above are tailored to the evaluation of a patient with suspected neuromuscular respiratory failure.

Many neuromuscular conditions involve the sensory fibers of the peripheral nervous system, while many others never involve the sensory fibers. The presence or absence of sensory symptoms is a crucial component of both the history and examination. The examination techniques for differentiating small or large fiber involvement are beyond the scope of this chapter but are important components of the neurologic examination that should be utilized in evaluating the patient with suspected neuromuscular disease. Spinal cord pathology is always on the differential for a patient presenting with bilateral weakness, and the ability to perform a competent sensory examination evaluating for a spinal cord level of sensory dysfunction is crucial. Additionally, in conditions like myasthenia gravis and motor neuron disease, for example, there should not be abnormal sensory findings.

General Examination

It is important to perform a complete physical examination to evaluate the patient's cardiopulmonary system, starting with the A, B, Cs as the initial part of the exam. A guide to the complete general physical examination is beyond the scope of this chapter, but it is important to be adept at evaluating a patient for subtle signs of respiratory distress, such as tachypnea, accessory muscle use, and paradoxical breathing. Additionally, in the patient with a presumed acute neuromuscular disease, a skin examination should be performed to evaluate for ticks (tick paralysis), rashes, and other stigmata of a rheumatologic-neurologic overlay condition.

History and Examination Summary

In the clinical approach to the patient with neuromuscular disease, the clinician is tasked with both obtaining the diagnosis and triaging the patient's likelihood of progression to or severity of neuromuscular respiratory failure. This progression's timeline is critical to both challenges and is critical for allowing the clinician to predict the patient's likelihood of neuromuscular respiratory failure. Obtaining an accurate and thorough history can guide the clinician to the likely diagnosis and assist in focusing the examination to the most critical parts to assess the patient's respiratory function. Specific examination maneuvers, as described above, in addition to simple observation of the patient, are crucial components to determining the diagnosis and assessing disease severity.

General Overview and Early Clinical Assessment

Patients with neuromuscular disease processes are most often admitted to medical ICUs or, in some cases, neurologic ICUs where available. Those with less severe or early manifestations of disease onset may be triaged to non-ICU medical or neurologic wards. In many patients, respiratory muscle weakness often goes undetected until a precipitating event triggers ventilatory failure, such as airway aspiration, pneumonia, or other new respiratory processes [9, 10]. Guillain-Barré syndrome is one of the most common neuromuscular disorders, with up to one-third of patients being admitted to the ICU setting for ventilatory support and monitoring. Other diseases with significant neuromuscular manifestations include CIDP, Charcot-Marie-Tooth, multifocal neuropathy, amyloidosis, sarcoidosis, Sjogren's, and phrenic neuropathy, all of which have been implicated in causing respiratory failure [11].

Weakness of the diaphragm and accessory muscles of respiration invariably impairs the ability of the lungs to ventilate, and bulbar weakness affects muscles that help control swallowing and clearance of secretions. Thus, neuromuscular disorders cause respiratory failure due to the inability to ventilate the lungs or to protect the airway, or in some cases, both. The diaphragm, being the primary muscle of respiration, contracts during inspiration and descends into the abdomen. This causes negative pressure within the thoracic cavity and thus ventilation of the lungs. The accessory muscles of the diaphragm include the abdominal rectus, intercostal, sternocleidomastoid, and scalene muscles. Hypoventilation typically occurs in the mid- to late stages of neuromuscular diseases, and with ensuing ventilation impairment, there is a resultant rise in CO_2 [12]. Hypoxia is a secondary result of ventilatory impairment in neuromuscular diseases, and normal compensation mechanisms such as increased respiratory rate may be blunted as the neuromuscular disease progresses. As such, clinicians may miss key clues of early ventilator failure and treat alveolar hypoventilation only with supplemental oxygen. Because of this, the clinical exam of the neuromuscular patient must take into consideration the status of the entire respiratory system, and clinicians must be vigilant for impending respiratory failure. The four main factors that contribute to complete respiratory failure are:

1. Upper-airway compromise

   Mouth, facial, oropharyngeal, and laryngeal muscle strength—risk of airway closure and aspiration syndrome

2. Weakness of the muscles of inspiration

   Diaphragm, intercostals, and accessory muscles resulting in inadequate lung expansion, atelectasis, and V/Q mismatch with eventual hypoxemia

3. Expiratory muscle weakness

   Inability to maintain cough reflex and inadequate secretion clearance

4. Complications of acute illness

   Pneumonia, ALI/ARDS, and pulmonary emboli

Often, the consequences of the initial three factors will contribute to acute illness such as persistent atelectasis, pneumonia, or pulmonary emboli, perpetuating the cycle of respiratory failure. Because of this, a high index of suspicion and close monitoring of respiratory parameters should always be undertaken. A more subjective assessment will consider the respiratory rate at rest, a clinical finding of sternal, dyspnea, or shallow respirations. Dysphonia and dysphagia are usually found later and are key clues that the neuromuscular disease is progressing [3]. Clinicians caring for neuromuscular patients should also monitor for the presence of rapid shallow breathing, abdominal paradoxical respirations, and cough after eating or drinking, as these are clues of diminishing respiratory and glottic function. Objective values that account for respiratory function should be followed closely and include vital capacity, maximal inspiratory pressure, and maximal expiratory pressure.

Significant limitations in inspiratory and expiratory flow translate into severe impairments with alveolar ventilation and inadequate respiratory flow needed to clear respiratory secretions, ultimately causing life-threatening mucous plugging or infection. When accounting for all ICU hospitalizations excluding neuromuscular disease processes, it has been shown that significant muscle impairment secondary to critical illness alone is not uncommon, affecting up to 62% of patients [13]. This severely impairs oxygenation and ventilation and further delays ventilator weaning efforts. As the innervation of motor units becomes increasingly impaired in critical illness, the diaphragm's ability to effectively generate force becomes severely diminished [14]. Even without considering the effect of neuromuscular diseases, factors that further affect the body's normal ability of ventilation include analgesia/sedation, malnutrition, and prolonged duration of mechanical ventilation. These entities are associated with ongoing critical illness, often implicated in ICU-acquired weakness, and further worsen respiratory failure in neuromuscular diseases [15].

ICU Assessment and Monitoring

As mentioned earlier, spirometry is a vital part of the clinical assessment in those with neuromuscular disease and must be considered frequently in the ICU environment. Maximal inspiratory force (MIP) indicates the strength of the inspiratory muscles, namely, the diaphragm, external intercostals muscles, and accessory muscles. Maximal expiratory pressure (MEP) represents the strength of the expiratory muscles, particularly the internal intercostals and the abdominal rectus muscles. The MEP is correlated to cough strength and ability to clear secretions from the airway. During clinical assessment, it is important to remember that each of these parameters are subject to error as they depend on the ability for the patient to maintain adequate mouth closure and lip seal with the spirometer. For intubated patients, the internal diameter and length of the endotracheal tube should be considered as this contributes to airway resistance. Using Ohm's law of resistance, one can surmise that a greater force will be required to generate a breath through an endotracheal tube with smaller inner diameter or longer length, thus impeding MIP and MEP values and contributing to overall increased work of breathing. Additionally, patient position should be taken into consideration, as physiologically normal patients in the supine position without neuromuscular weakness have approximately 10% decrease in vital capacity as compared to the upright position [16]. This reiterates that spirometry should always be evaluated in the upright seated position when fully awake to optimize respiratory mechanics and accuracy whenever possible.

Patients with long-standing neuromuscular disease, even with disease stability, should also be monitored closely with routine spirometry as above. In many of these patients, endotracheal intubation is not always necessary as non-invasive ventilation can be used for non-severe disease relapse [17]. When considering Guillain-Barré syndrome patients, it has been shown that those who progressed to requiring the ICU level of care and mechanical ventilation were more likely to have autonomic dysfunction, severe bulbar weakness, and especially rapid disease progression [3, 12]. These patients generally have spirometry values with a vital capacity lesser than 20 mL/kg with a reduction in greater than 30% of baseline in a relatively short period of time. Other clinical markers might include staccato speech and a single breath count of less than 15 (normal individuals are able to count to 50 with one single breath hold) [3]. These readily available tests and clinical findings are helpful to guide the decision for endotracheal intubation.

Review of Common Neuromuscular Pathology in the ICU

Myasthenia Gravis

Myasthenia gravis is the most common cause of neuromuscular respiratory failure encountered in the ICU [1]. Given its prevalence in the NICU patient population, it is important to understand the pathophysiology, diagnosis, and treatment of this condition. Myasthenia gravis is an antibody-mediated autoimmune disorder of the post-synaptic neuromuscular junction, specifically, acetylcholine receptors or their membrane-associated proteins. There are two clinically recognized forms: ocular and generalized. Its clinical manifestations are of fluctuating weakness in the ocular, bulbar, appendicular, and/or respiratory muscles. Myasthenia is classified based on the severity of symptoms as listed below [18]:

- Class I—Isolated extraocular muscle involvement.
- Class II—Mild generalized weakness.
- Class III—Moderate generalized weakness.
- Class IV—Severe generalized weakness.
- Class V—Neuromuscular respiratory failure requiring intubation.

The disease is caused by antibodies targeted to the post-synaptic acetylcholine receptors or their membrane-associated proteins (see Figs. 12.1 and 12.2). There are two subclasses of antibody targets in the disease. There are acetylcholine receptor-binding antibodies and muscle-specific receptor tyrosine kinase (MuSK). In addition to the action of blocking the acetylcholine receptor from being activated by acetylcholine, the antibodies have also demonstrated complement activation that can lead to destruction of the motor unit endplate over time (see Fig. 12.3) [19].

The diagnosis of myasthenia gravis is a clinical diagnosis supported by serologic and EMG/NCS testing. Testing for the presence of autoantibodies against the acetylcholine receptor (AChR) or against other muscle receptor-associated proteins (e.g., muscle-specific tyrosine kinase [MuSK] or low-density lipoprotein receptor-related protein 4 [LRP4]) can aid in confirmation of the diagnosis. In patients with generalized myasthenia, the overwhelming majority (85%) will have AChR antibodies. Less than 10% will have MuSK antibodies, while 1% will have LRP4 antibodies [20, 21]. The remainder, less than 10%, are seronegative patients [22].

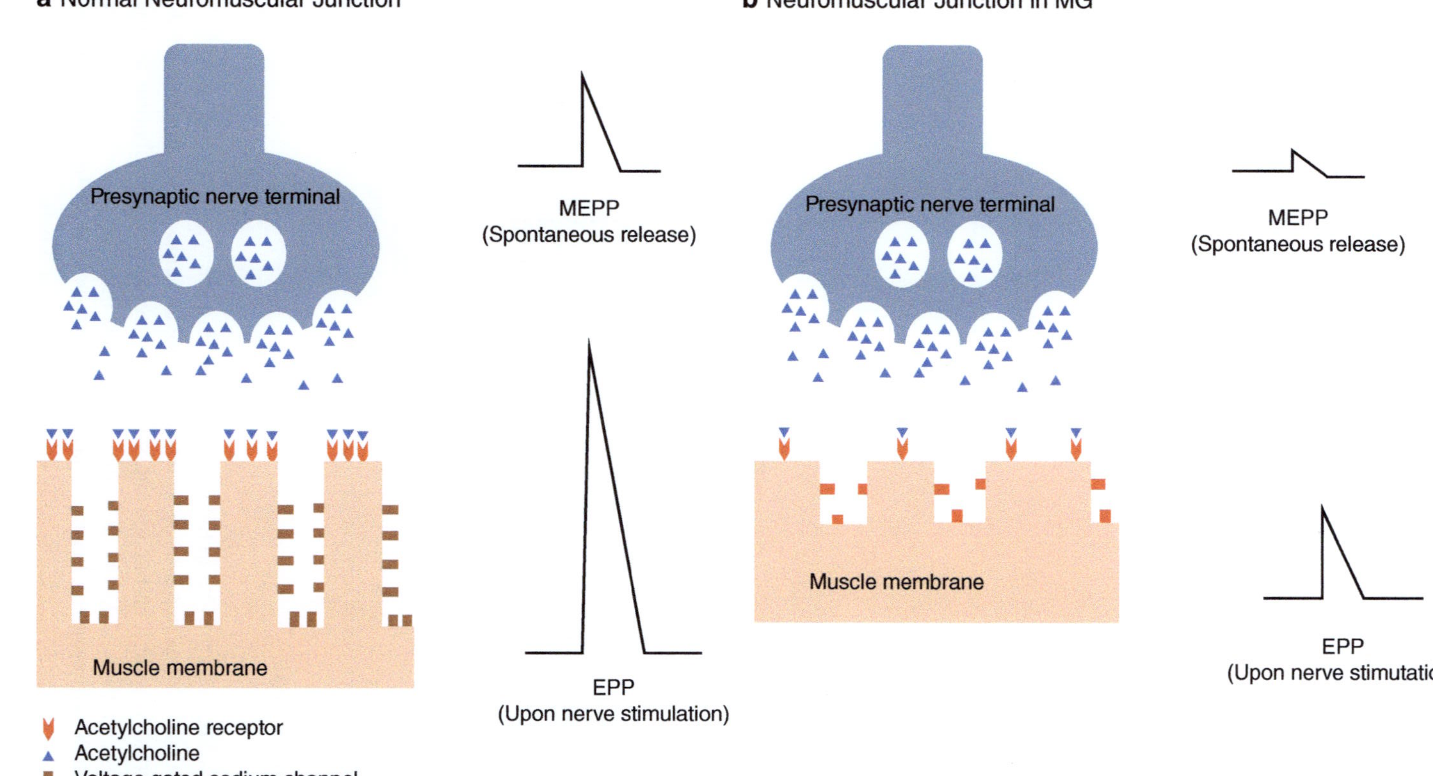

Fig. 12.1 Neuromuscular transmission in normal individuals (**a**) and in patients with MG (**b**). Decreased density of the AChR and complement-mediated damage to the post-synaptic membrane in MG patients result in decrease in miniature end-plate potential (MEPP), which occurs with spontaneous release of AChR vesicles, as well as end-plate potential (EPP) in response to nerve action potential of the presynaptic membrane. Diminished amplitude of EPP in MG results in impaired neuromuscular transmission [2]

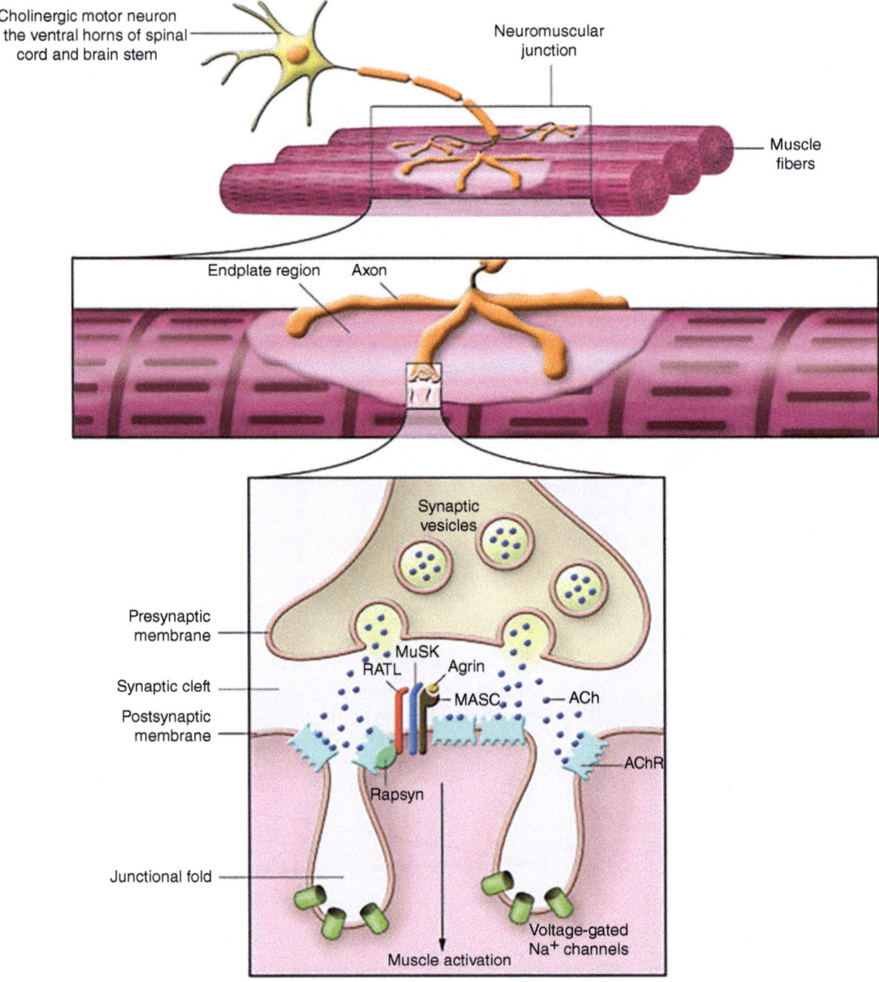

Fig. 12.2 Depiction of an α-motor neuron-innervating multiple muscle fibers, ultimately terminating in a neuromuscular junction. Depicted with the synaptic cleft, showing the presynaptic membrane-releasing acetylcholine onto the post-synaptic membrane resulting in activation of the muscle fiber through stimulation of the acetylcholine receptors [19]

Myasthenic Crisis

Patients with MG who present to the intensive care unit are typically suffering from myasthenic crisis. Myasthenic crisis is defined as myasthenic symptoms culminating in respiratory and/or bulbar muscle weakness necessitating intubation and/or mechanical ventilation [23, 24]. It is estimated that, of patients with myasthenia gravis, 10–20% will suffer at least one myasthenic crisis in their lifetime, with an annualized risk under 5% [25, 26]. It is not uncommon for a patient to present with

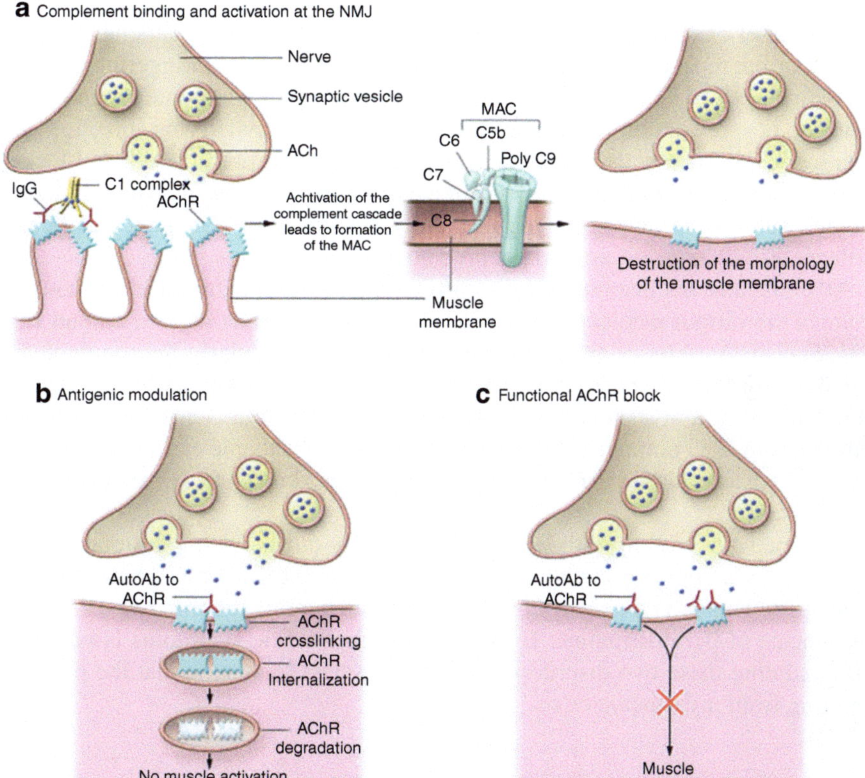

Fig. 12.3 (**a**) Demonstration of complement involvement in destruction of the motor endplate's morphology due to complement activation. (**b**) Acetylcholine receptor destruction through triggering internalization of receptors. (**c**) Functional block of acetylcholine receptors due to binding the acetylcholine receptor and blocking acetylcholine binding [19]

myasthenic crisis as their initial presentation of disease [27]. Epidemiologically, patients with MuSK-positive MG have a higher risk for the development of myasthenic crisis [28].

Clinical Presentation

Myasthenic crisis typically occurs concurrently with worsening generalized weakness, though respiratory muscle and bulbar weakness can be out of proportion to appendicular weakness in a minority of cases. The descent into respiratory failure can be precipitous, particularly when a patient's generalized weakness masks the clinician's ability to recognize accessory muscle use and overt tachypnea [29]. Hypercapnia can be a particularly late finding in these patients and suggests that intubation may be more urgent than the clinical exam might suggest [25, 30, 31]. The causes of exacerbation of myasthenia gravis resulting in myasthenic crisis are numerous, but most often there is an underlying infection that is triggering the acute worsening [32]. In a retrospective cohort analysis of 141 myasthenic exacerbations requiring hospitalization, 39.7% were found to have an underlying infection contributing to their presentation. Of additional note, patients prescribed beta-blockers were also associated with a higher risk of exacerbation [32]. Surgical intervention is another well-known culprit for triggering myasthenic crisis. Pregnancy and childbirth are also recognized as possible precipitants.

All clinicians, not just intensivists, caring for patients with myasthenia should be aware of the various medications that can worsen myasthenia (Tables 12.1 and 12.2) [33]. Specific antibiotics are particularly important, particularly fluoroquinolones, aminoglycosides, and macrolides. These antibiotics can unfortunately be picked for the treatment of a myasthenic patient's underlying infection causing exacerbation. This decision can compound the issue and lead to a myasthenic crisis. Cardiac medications such as beta-blockers and magnesium are also known to worsen myasthenic weakness.

Most patients with myasthenia are concurrently on acetylcholinesterase inhibitors. Overdose from this medication can mimic a myasthenic crisis, named cholinergic crisis. This is a rare entity not often seen with commonly prescribed doses and frequencies of pyridostigmine. Evaluation for cholinergic symptoms is helpful in differentiating these two disorders, though it is safest to assume that the patient is suffering from myasthenic crisis.

Table 12.1 Drugs reported to cause MG exacerbation via alteration of immune response

Drug	Mechanism	ADR probability	Comments
Immune checkpoint inhibitors	T cell activation, increased ratio of T effector to T regulatory cells, B cell activation, autoantibody production, cytokines (IL-17)	Definite	Avoid after emergence of life-threatening MG If to be used in MG patients, pretreat with steroids, IVIG, or plasmapheresis
D-Penicillamine	Modification of MHC on the surface of antigen-presenting cells	Definite	Discontinue and avoid if MG occurs
Interferons	Immune dysregulation through changes in cytokines, NK cells, alteration of lymphocyte profiles	Possible	Not contraindicated, association rarely reported
Statin	Shift in T cell polarization Superimposed myopathy Mitochondrial toxicity	Probable	Discontinue and avoid in rare cases of emergence or exacerbation of MG

[a] Adapted from Sheikh et al. [33]

Table 12.2 Drugs associated with MG-like symptoms, unmasking/exacerbation of MG via effect on neuromuscular transmission

Drug	Mechanism	ADR probability	Comments
Macrolides	Impair neuromuscular transmission, possibly at the presynaptic level	Definite	Avoid in MG patients if there is another alternative, otherwise closely monitor
Fluoroquinolones	Impair neuromuscular transmission, pre- and post-synaptic levels	Probable	Avoid in MG patients if there is another alternative, otherwise closely monitor
Aminoglycosides	Impair neuromuscular transmission, pre/post-synaptic levels	Definite	Avoid in MG patients if there is another alternative, otherwise closely monitor
Penicillins	Unclear, impaired neuromuscular transmission in an animal model	Probable	Can be used in MG patients as MG exacerbation is rare
β-Adrenergic blockers	Unclear effect on neuromuscular transmission	Probable	Can be used in stable MG patients, monitor closely, especially early after starting
L-type calcium channel blockers	Unclear effect on neuromuscular transmission	Probable	Can be used in stable MG patients, monitor closely, especially early after starting
Class Ia antiarrhythmics	Impair neuromuscular transmission, pre- and post-synaptic levels	Definite	Avoid in MG patients if there is another alternative, otherwise closely monitor
Magnesium	Presynaptic (blocks release of ACh) and post-synaptic	Definite	Caution and close monitoring are advised in magnesium replacement (especially IV)
Neuromuscular blockers and inhalation anesthetics	Post-synaptic neuromuscular block	Definite	Avoid nondepolarizing NMBs and inhalation anesthetics; if used, close monitoring, consider acetylcholinesterase inhibitor or sugammadex
Corticosteroids	Unknown; possible direct effect on neuromuscular transmission at high doses	Definite	Avoid starting high doses, consider pretreatment with IVIG or plasmapheresis
Botulinum toxin	Presynaptic reduction in ACh release	Definite	Avoid if possible, may offer with caution and slow dose titration in those with mild/stable MG with blepharospasm or cervical dystonia

[a] Adapted from Sheikh et al. [33]

Diagnosis

In most cases of neuromuscular respiratory failure secondary to myasthenia gravis, the diagnosis is already known. In a patient presenting with neuromuscular respiratory failure that is unable to provide history, the importance of history from family or loved ones becomes critical. Focusing on the neurologic examination to include reflexes is important as well. In cases where the diagnosis is unknown at the time of admission, a thorough diagnostic evaluation to exclude mimics (considering imaging and lumbar puncture) and confirm the diagnosis with urgent electrophysiologic testing and serum analysis for antibodies. Checkpoint inhibitor-associated myasthenia gravis should be suspected in patients presenting with neuromuscular failure on these medications.

Management

Patients with impending myasthenic crisis or myasthenic crisis should be admitted to the intensive care unit and frequently assessed for respiratory muscle strength as discussed previously in the physical examination section of this chapter. Patients determined to have myasthenic crisis should be electively intubated at the clinician's discretion. Considering that hypercapnia and hypoxemia are late findings in neuromuscular respiratory failure secondary to myasthenic crisis [34], the clinician's ability to evaluate several factors including clinical exam, MIP, and VC together along with their trend is critical in determining whether the patient warrants invasive or non-invasive ventilatory support. MIP and VC are typically trended every 2 or 4 h in the ICU setting, especially early in the course to establish an objective trend. These measures are important even while the patient is intubated to track response to therapy and safety for liberation from invasive ventilatory support.

Immediate Management of Myasthenic Crisis

Elective intubation is the ideal response to impending neuromuscular respiratory failure secondary to myasthenic crisis, as opposed to emergent intubation. The decision to intubate should be based on both the subjective measures of dyspnea and dysphagia but also the objective measurements of VC and MIP. The typical recommendation is to consider elective intubation for patients with a VC less than 20 cc/kg and/or a NIF less negative than -25 cm H_2O. Despite the above, many patients with values more reassuring than those above can have an inability to clear secretions or severe dyspnea that warrants intubation. Non-invasive ventilation (NIV) can be considered for a select group of patients with myasthenic crisis. It can be utilized early and may have benefit in avoiding mechanical ventilation. In a multicenter retrospective study of 250 patients with myasthenic crisis, invasive mechanical support was avoided in 38% of patients [27]. Consideration of NIV for patients with minimal secretion burden, with adequate cough, who can tolerate the interface may be of benefit in these patients. This method of ventilation should be avoided in patients with significant secretion burden due to the risk of upper-airway obstruction or impaction of secretions.

When choosing sedation and paralysis in these patients, attention should be paid to the choice of anesthetic and paralytic. A non-depolarizing neuromuscular blocking agent is preferred to a depolarizing agent. Depolarizing agents, such as succinylcholine, are not as effective in MG due to the reduced number of receptors present at the cell surface and would require a higher dosage. For the non-depolarizing agents, such as rocuronium, lower doses should be used.

Acetylcholinesterase Inhibitor Management

For patients with myasthenic crisis that are intubated or who have significant secretion burden, pyridostigmine is typically discontinued to avoid the complications of cholinergic stimulation, specifically increased airway secretions resulting in pneumonia and obstructive atelectasis. Once a patient has demonstrated a satisfactory recovery with the initiation of rapid immunotherapy, these medications can be gradually and cautiously restarted, mindful of significant cholinergic side effects. Typically, these medications are restarted prior to extubation in patients that have initiated immunotherapy and are demonstrating improvement.

Immediate Management of Myasthenic Crisis: Initiation of Immunotherapy

Both intravenous immunoglobulin (IVIG) infusion and plasma exchange (PLEX) are efficacious and commonly used treatments for myasthenic crisis [35–37]. The data comparing the two therapies are not substantial enough to demonstrate a significant advantage of one therapy versus the other. The major studies are mostly systematic reviews and retrospective cohort analysis demonstrating that there is no clear difference. In the Myasthenia Gravis Clinical Study Group trial, which randomly assigned patients with myasthenic crisis to either IVIG or PLEX, both groups had no difference in strength at day 15, though the PLEX group reached the study primary endpoint of target strength increase more quickly (9 days) than the IVIG cohort (12 days). Expert opinion suggests that PLEX onset is more rapid and therefore is preferred as first-line therapy. Consideration of availability of PLEX and additional complication of a central large-bore catheter to facilitate the procedure are important factors to consider. Some experts argue that IVIG is preferable due to the ease of administration, lower incidence of serious side effects (mainly related to line complications and infection but also including bleeding risk associated with PLEX-induced coagulopathy), and at least similar efficacy as demonstrated in the above reviews and trial. The consensus statement by the Myasthenia Gravis Foundation of America suggests that PLEX is more effective and works more quickly in the treatment of impending or manifest myasthenic crisis [23].

It is important to understand both the time of onset of the above therapies (typically within several days) and their duration of effect (a few weeks). If appropriate chronic immunotherapy is not administered concurrently with the immediate therapy, the patient is at risk for relapse. Typically, initiation of moderate- to high-dose oral (or by nasogastric tube) steroids is recommended. The benefit of these medications is typically recognized at the 2- to 4-week mark. This timeline is important as the benefit of the immediate immunotherapies begins to wane around this time. Many patients will experience an exacerbation of their MG despite being on glucocorticoids as their chronic regimen. Additionally, some patients may have a contraindication to high-dose glucocorticoids, and perhaps their initial admission was as a consequence of one of these side effects (infection, hyperglycemia, gastrointestinal bleed, etc.). Other immunosuppressive medications including azathioprine, mycophenolate mofetil (MMF), and rituximab can be considered in these patients. Alternatively, chronic therapy with maintenance IVIG infusion or some of the newer agents targeting complement activation are options that can be considered with neuromuscular specialist guidance.

Weaning from Mechanical Ventilation

Extubation failure is common in patients suffering from myasthenic crisis. In a small retrospective cohort analysis from J. Seneviratne and colleagues detailing 46 patients with myasthenic crisis, re-intubation occurred in nearly one-fourth of the patients [38]. In the retrospective cohort analysis by Thomas CE et al., 25% of patients were extubated by day 7, 50% by day 13, and 75% by 31 days (about 1 month) [39]. As such, the decision to extubate a patient undergoing treatment of myasthenic crisis is often challenging and still carries a significant likelihood of failure.

Given these challenges, there remains no set guideline or best practice for invasive ventilation weaning in this population. Regarding the general ICU population, daily spontaneous breathing trials (SBTs) are considered the preferred method for evaluating extubation readiness. Deciding when to initiate SBTs for patients with myasthenic crisis should include an understanding of the duration to the onset of the rapid immunotherapy choice (IVIG vs PLEX) in addition to the evaluation of objective evidence of improved respiratory muscle function (NIF and VC) and secretion burden. If a patient has been restarted on acetylcholinesterase inhibitor therapy, has initiated chronic immunotherapy, has tolerable secretion burden (not requiring excessive oral and or ETT suctioning), has VC greater than 20 cc/kg and NIF more negative than -30 cm H_2O, then extubation can be considered.

Guillain-Barré Syndrome (GBS)

Guillain-Barré syndrome (GBS) is the second most common cause of neuromuscular respiratory failure in the intensive care unit. GBS describes a variety of acute immune-mediated polyneuropathies including acute inflammatory demyelinating polyneuropathy (AIDP), Miller Fisher syndrome (MFS), Bickerstaff's brainstem encephalitis, and the axonal variants: acute motor axonal neuropathy (AMAN), acute motor and sensory axonal neuropathy (AMSAN), and pharyngeal-cervical-brachial weakness (see Fig. 12.4). These entities are discussed separately from their cousin illnesses—subacute inflammatory demyelinating polyneuropathy (SIDP) and chronic inflammatory demyelinating polyneuropathy (CIDP)—which are similar entities in pathophysiology but differ in timeline, severity, and pattern of weakness. Additional rare variants of GBS are described in the literature including acute pan-dysautonomia, pure sensory GBS, facial diplegia and distal limb paresthesia, and acute bulbar palsy which are beyond the scope of this chapter. Figure 12.5 provides an overview of the evaluation, management, and outcomes in GBS.

Approximately 10–30% of all patients with GBS require invasive ventilation during their disease course [42]. Studies support that half or even three-fourths of patients with GBS present with a recent respiratory or GI infection within 4 weeks [43]. *Campylobacter jejuni* infection is the most common precipitant of GBS and is identified in nearly one-fourth of cases [44]. It is also responsible for the majority of cases of AMAN. There is additional data to support that antecedent influenza-like illnesses, such as CMV [45], influenza A and B, COVID-19, and HIV, can precipitate GBS [46]. In addition to antecedent infections, vaccinations have been linked to increased incidence of GBS. The risks, according to numerous studies, suggest

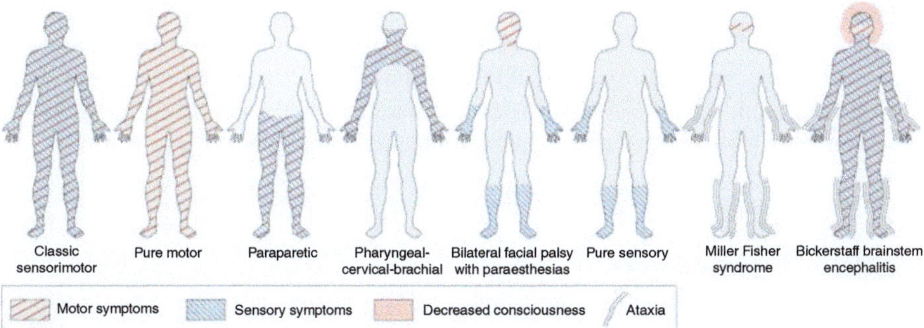

Fig. 12.4 Graphical depiction of the atypical presentations of acute inflammatory demyelinating polyneuropathy (AIDP) (adapted from diagnosis and management of Guillain-Barré syndrome in ten steps [40, 41])

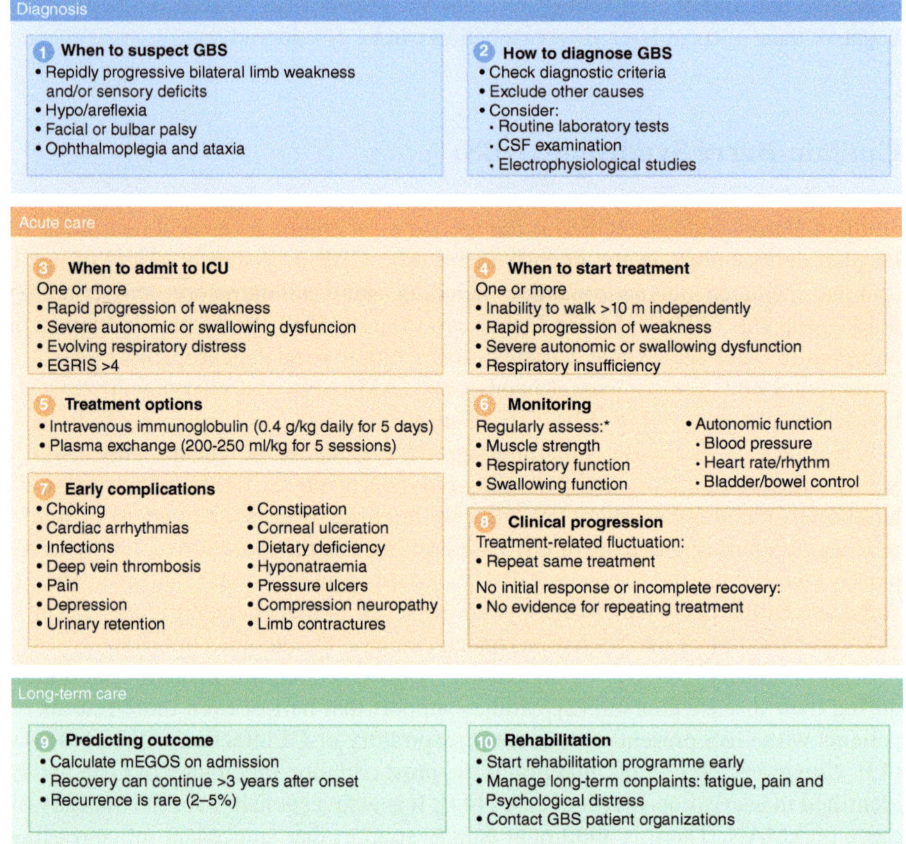

Fig. 12.5 A proposed ten-step approach to the holistic management of patients with suspected AIDP put forth by Leonhard et al. detailing the considerations in diagnosis, acute, and long-term care [41]

however that the risk of GBS following vaccination is lower than the risk of GBS following infection [47]. Discussion on the significance of the risk of GBS in the setting of recent vaccination is beyond the scope of this chapter, but data does demonstrate that both the risk of GBS from vaccination and the risk of GBS following infection from a vaccinated entity are significantly lower [48, 49].

Clinical Presentation

GBS typically presents with the acute onset of progressive and symmetric muscle weakness with or without sensory symptoms. As discussed earlier in this chapter, the time course of symptoms is a critical piece of information to obtain from the history and is integral in obtaining the diagnosis. As a rule, symptoms progress over a period of 2 weeks reaching a nadir. After 4 weeks, the nadir of symptoms should be reached [50]. If symptoms continue to progress beyond this point, the diagnosis should be questioned and re-evaluated.

Patients classically present with progressive symmetric flaccid proximal and distal arm and leg weakness. The weakness typically begins in the proximal (not distal) legs and then involves the remainder of the limbs and face. Most patients will experience diffuse weakness by the 2-week point in disease progression. Deep tendon reflexes are decreased or absent in over 90% of patients at the time of presentation. Findings of hyperreflexia should alert the clinician to an alternative diagnosis and warrant further evaluation of CNS pathology. Sensory symptoms are reported in most patients with GBS but are typically mild and involve the distal extremities at presentation. Pain is a common presenting symptom and typically is reported in the dorsal thighs and lower back.

Bowel and bladder dysfunction are known symptoms of GBS but are typically observed later in the course. Patients presenting with early and significant bowel and bladder dysfunction with other atypical features should be evaluated for an alternative diagnosis. The sensory examination is a critical piece of the neurologic examination in these patients, and findings of a sensory level should alarm the clinician of spinal cord pathology.

Diagnosis

Diagnosis is initially based on the historical and clinical findings of the acute onset of progressive and symmetric weakness with hypo- or areflexia. The clinical diagnosis can be bolstered with further laboratory analysis of CSF and even electrodiagnostic testing. Classically, CSF studies demonstrate an albumino-cytologic dissociation. CSF protein elevation is typically >50 mg/dL up to 200 mg/dL, though early in the disease process the protein may be normal. CSF protein elevation is present within the first week of symptom onset in up to two-thirds of patients and is present in greater than three-fourths of patients in the third week [51, 52]. CSF cell count is classically normal, though can be elevated up to 50 cells/μL. In the retrospective cohort analysis by Fokke C et al. of 494 patients diagnosed with GBS, a pleocytosis of 5–50 cells/μL was present in 15% of patients, and none had more than 50 cells/μL.

Nerve conduction studies (NCS) and electromyography (EMG) are performed in many patients with GBS both to support the diagnosis and to prognosticate disease severity. Classically, findings of prolonged or absent F waves and absent H reflexes are the earliest findings. Prolonged distal latencies with conduction block of motor responses are also seen.

Differential Diagnosis

The differential diagnosis for GBS is broad and includes SIDP, CIDP, spinal cord pathology, diseases of the neuromuscular junction (MG and Lambert-Eaton myasthenic syndrome), myopathy, and other acute polyneuropathies. Findings that should cast doubt on the diagnosis of GBS include rapid onset of <24 h to symptom nadir, a sensory level, prominent early neuromuscular respiratory failure, early bowel and bladder dysfunction that is severe, early fever, and CSF findings of significant pleocytosis and/or neutrophilic or monocyte predominance. Additional polyneuropathies to consider include arsenic poisoning, Lyme disease, tick paralysis, acute intermittent porphyria, leptomeningeal carcinomatosis, paraneoplastic polyneuropathy, sarcoidosis, HIV/AIDS, hexane exposure, and thiamine deficiency.

Myopathies such as dermatomyositis, polymyositis, and critical illness myopathy or myoneuropathy can present similarly to GBS.

Important Complications of GBS in the ICU

Dysautonomia

Patients with GBS commonly experience dysautonomia which can be severe and should be anticipated by the intensivist. Dysautonomia prevalence is common and causes severe complications [53, 54]. Autonomic dysfunction is a significant source of mortality in patients with GBS [54, 55]. In a retrospective cohort analysis of 187 patients with the diagnosis of GBS by Chakraborty et al., ileus occurred in 42% of patients, fever in 27%, and tachycardia or bradycardia in 27% [54]. In a review of patients with GBS by Zaeem et al., mortality was increased in patients experiencing autonomic symptoms [56]. Ileus can be severe and may warrant consideration of post-pyloric feeding and motility agents in some patients with unremitting disease.

Syndrome of Inappropriate Antidiuretic Hormone Secretion

Syndrome of inappropriate antidiuretic hormone secretion (SIADH) is a well-described entity in GBS and is associated with increased severity of disease and autonomic symptoms [57, 58]. The SIADH can be severe in some patients and, according to the prospective study by Saifudheen et al., occurred in nearly half of their cohort of 50 patients experiencing severe SIADH. The severity of SIADH was also correlated with worse prognosis.

Management

Considerations for ICU-Level Care

This chapter focuses on the clinical approach to neuromuscular respiratory failure management, so we will focus on the manifestations of impending neuromuscular respiratory failure secondary to GBS. The initial evaluation and considerations of these patients are extremely similar to the evaluation described above for myasthenia gravis. Approximately 10–30% of patients with GBS will require mechanical ventilatory support during their hospital admission [42, 59]. The significant differences to consider, again, are the timeline and expected progression of disease. A knowledgeable clinician who evaluates a patient with severe weakness at day 3 or 4 of symptom onset can anticipate that at some point during their hospital course they will develop neuromuscular respiratory failure.

In addition to clinical acumen, the Erasmus GBS Respiratory Insufficiency Score (EGRIS) is used to predict the risk of respiratory failure within the first week of admission [59] (see Table 12.3). Patients with a score of 0–2 are at low risk (4% risk of respiratory failure), 3–4 are at intermediate risk (24% risk of respiratory failure), and 5–7 are at elevated risk (65% risk of respiratory failure). Other indications for ICU admission should include assessment of impending respiratory failure based on subjective dyspnea or difficulty with secretions in addition to clinical exam findings of neck extensor/flexor weakness and NIF less negative than -30 cm H_2O and VC of <20 cc/kg. Autonomic instability such as cardiac arrhythmias or severe tachycardia or bradycardia should also be considered for ICU admission.

Table 12.3 EGRIS scoring system

Predictor	Categories	Score
Time from the onset of weakness to hospital admission, days	>7	0
	4–7	1
	≤3	2
Facial and/or bulbar weakness at hospital admission	Absent	0
	Present	1
MRC sum score at hospital admission	51–60	0
	41–50	1
	31–40	2
	21–30	3
	≤20	4
EGRIS total score		0–7

EGRIS Erasmus Guillain-Barré Syndrome Respiratory Insufficiency Score, *MRC* Medical Research Council

Treatment: Immunosuppression

Like the above section on myasthenia gravis treatment, GBS can be treated with IVIG or PLEX. However, there is no role for corticosteroids in the treatment of GBS as numerous studies have demonstrated no benefit. For acute treatment of GBS, IVIG has shown similar efficacy to PLEX and therefore is considered the treatment of choice due to less adverse events associated with IVIG and ease of use. A Cochrane review described that PLEX improves recovery, as does IVIG [60]. Interestingly, they also found that PLEX followed by IVIG did not demonstrate extra benefit. Additionally, the guideline from the AAN, stemming from the "Evidence-based guideline: Intravenous immunoglobulin in the treatment of neuro-muscular disorders—report of the Therapeutics and Technology Assessment Subcommittee of the American Academy of Neurology" by Patwa HS et al. states that IVIG is as efficacious as plasmapheresis and should be offered for treating GBS as Level A evidence [61]. Evaluation of some of the more robust trials reveals that the time to initial improvement may be shortened by nearly 50% in non-ambulatory patients treated with either PLEX or IVIG [62].

Dysautonomia Monitoring and Management

Patients with more severe manifestations of GBS are more likely to have dysauto-nomia. Continuous telemetry and frequent blood pressure measurement should be utilized. Intra-arterial monitoring may be warranted in patients with fluctuating blood pressure requiring vasoactive medications. Severe tachycardia resulting in stress cardiomyopathy is a possibility. Additionally, severe hypertension resulting in PRES is an additional possibility in these patients. Many patients may have severely labile blood pressure that is hyper-responsive to adrenergic blockade or stimulation. As a result, the clinician should avoid utilizing long-acting medications and instead consider titratable options.

ICU Management: Additional Early Complications

Severe dysautonomia is detailed above and is perhaps the most important clinical consideration in the acute phase. Additional considerations include ileus, deep venous thrombosis, and pulmonary embolism. Patients should have aggressive bowel regimens to ensure regular defecation to prevent this, even including pro-motility agents when significant. Patients with significant bulbar manifestations will have reduced facial nerve tone, resulting in inability to close their eyes, especially during sedation or sleep. This can result in various degrees of corneal ulceration which can result in severe visual loss and even blindness. Care should be taken to ensure frequent moisturizing of the ocular membranes. Some patients may even require suturing of the eyelids. Nursing care and early physical therapy are also important aspects of care in these patients to prevent contractures, pressure-induced nerve palsies, and pressure ulcers.

ICU Management: Early Tracheostomy

The prolonged clinical timeline of GBS manifesting with neuromuscular respiratory failure requiring intubation makes tracheostomy a common occurrence. Specific variants of GBS, particularly AMAN and AMSAN, have a prolonged and more severe course and thus a higher likelihood of requiring tracheostomy to complete recovery. In their paper "Tracheostomy or not: Prediction of prolonged mechanical ventilation in GBS", Walgaard and colleagues demonstrated that predictors of prolonged mechanical ventilaton included evidence of axonal degeneration and inabiliy to lift the upper extremies of the bed at 7 days [63].

Intubation and Mechanical Ventilation

With worsening bulbar dysfunction comes poor glottic control and thus inability to maintain secretion clearance. In neuromuscular patients with oropharyngeal weakness, airway suction via the nose or mouth is frequently performed prior to intubation but is poorly tolerated and is generally ineffective at mobilizing deep lower respiratory tract secretions. Because of this, endotracheal intubation is usually needed, and a significant percentage of patients that do not experience at least partial recovery will require tracheostomy. Although tracheostomy has shown to be helpful in the elimination of upper-airway resistance involving the oropharyngeal membranes, lower airway tract secretions continue to be problematic. Ongoing suctioning via tracheostomy can be irritating and induce hypoxemia by severe bronchospasm [64]. Tracheal suctioning should be done with care and caution, and the use of small amounts of saline may be required for more tenacious secretions. It is worth noting that tracheal suctioning catheters introduced via tracheostomy rarely enter the left bronchus and as such will be ineffective in clearing much of the bronchial tree [64, 65]. Because of this, flexible bronchoscopy is often needed to clear life-threatening mucous plugs that occlude the airways. Some less routinely recognized secretion clearance methods include manually assisted cough and mechanical insufflation/exsufflation, which can also be used with non-invasive mechanical ventilation [11, 66].

Regarding Guillain-Barré and myasthenia syndromes, early intubation is recommended as positive pressure ventilation helps prevent progression of atelectasis and further gas exchange impairment [12]. Some studies have suggested that prevention of early atelectasis may allow for earlier liberation of mechanical ventilation [10,

67]. Appropriate preparation for intubation is important as many patients with neuromuscular disease have dysautonomia. The use of intravenous sedation and analgesia during rapid sequence intubation may further worsen hypotension, and peri-intubation complications may include vagally mediated cardiac arrhythmias. Manipulation of the airway has also been noted to diminish vagal tone and induce hypotension [12, 39]. Because of this, it is important to avoid excessive amounts of analgesia, sedation, and AV nodal blocking agents, and one should have vasoactive and antiarrhythmic medications ready for unexpected hypotension. Additionally, given the heightened risk of hypotension, it is worth assessing the patient's circulating vascular volume status and attempting to correct hypovolemia prior to intubation attempts.

Although often used early in disease course, non-invasive ventilation has been controversial in Guillain-Barré and myasthenia gravis patients and should only be considered if upper-airway muscular function is preserved. In these patients, the goal is to provide a state of rest and allow for lung expansion during mechanical ventilation [68]. NIV can be used in some cases to decrease the work of breathing; however extreme caution must be utilized as oropharyngeal secretions can be forced into the lower respiratory tract. Positive end-expiratory pressures are typically maintained around 5–15 cm H_2O, with goal plateau pressures less than 35 cm H_2O. For NIV measures, tidal volume should ideally be maintained at 8–10 mL/kg of ideal body weight with breaths of 8–10/min, keeping with normal minute ventilation [66, 68]. Patients with chronic CO_2 retention due to obstructive sleep apnea, obesity hypoventilation syndrome, hypothyroidism, or COPD may have elevated bicarbonate levels, and overventilation post intubation may induce renal bicarbonate wasting, contributing to acid-base disturbances that further complicate ventilator weaning [9, 12]. When initiating invasive mechanical ventilation, the aim is to allow physiologic rest, promote lung expansion, and limit further alveolar collapse [12, 39]. Tidal volumes can vary and again should range from 8 to 10 mL/kg of ideal body weight; however if ARDS or ALI is a concern, a low-stretch lung protective strategy should be employed with 4–6 mL/kg ideal body weight. Appropriate PEEP should be used to "stent" open distal airways, generally anywhere from 5 to 15 cm, and the amount used will also depend on the extent of thoracic restriction or extra-thoracic disease such as obesity.

Considerations for Ventilator Weaning, Mechanically Assisted Cough, and Sedation

Ventilator weaning is the gradual process of lowering ventilator settings to acceptable, near physiologic levels of support. Given the disease complexity and prolonged duration of many neuromuscular disorders, ventilator weaning of patients with neuromuscular disease is extremely challenging, and such patients are among those with the highest incidence of ventilator weaning failure [69]. Patients with

NMD requiring prolonged mechanical ventilation are at elevated risk of mortality and morbidity, and their long and often protracted hospital course can impose significant economic burden on the health system [70]. Conventional methods of ventilator weaning that would be applicable to the general critically ill population usually do not apply to neuromuscular disease patients. For those without NMD, the decision to discontinue mechanical ventilation is often based on the clinical assessment of wakefulness, hemodynamic stability, and adequate treatment of the underlying disease process. However, those with neuromuscular disease processes must reliably show that they can overcome the effective resistance of the respiratory system to meet the metabolic demands of the body and maintain carbon dioxide homeostasis. Factors that complicate ventilator weaning in NMD patients include advanced patient age, co-existing conditions such as chronic obstructive lung disease, idiopathic lung disease, or pneumonia. These conditions may prompt sooner consideration for tracheostomy to facilitate more rapid ventilator weaning [71]. The definition for difficult ventilator weaning has taken on many definitions, and some have proposed failure of at least three spontaneous breathing trials within a 7-day period [72].

The process of ventilator weaning frequently includes a combination of CPAP or pressure-support trials and T-piece breathing trials. Some have suggested that a successful weaning trial in NMD patients has been defined as complete ventilator liberation for 5 days and without the need of tracheostomy; however this remains controversial [73]. The process is typically initiated once there has been improvement or resolution of the neuromuscular disease process, and respiratory mechanics (including lung volume, lung compliance, and airway patency) are intact. Much like the decision to start mechanical ventilation, the tests that are necessary to consider ventilator weaning are forced expiratory volume, inspiratory force, and expiratory force. These simple bedside tests are useful in determining the ability to successfully come off invasive mechanical ventilation and rely on the muscles of respiration, especially the diaphragm, innervated by C3–C5 nerve roots. The intercostals, parasternal intercostals, and scalene muscles (T1–T11 innervation) contract in collaboration with the diaphragm and increase the anteroposterior and transverse diameters of chest wall, generating inspiratory force through the creation of negative pressure. If ventilator weaning is delayed, complications including ventilator-induced lung injury, ventilator-associated pneumonia, and ventilator-induced diaphragm injury are likely to occur [74, 75]. It is important to note that in many cases with NMD, the disease process will likely not have completely resolved, but has at least improved to a point to consider a trial of ventilator weaning [74]. Although many recommendations have been put forth, there remains no consensus as to what constitutes reversal of the underlying problem, and furthermore, a combination of objective and subjective criteria is generally used to determine appropriateness of ventilator weaning.

Some accepted objective criteria for ventilator weaning include [75–77]:

- Respiratory rate of <35 breaths/min
- Good tolerance to spontaneous breathing trials

- Heart rate of <140/min or heart rate variability of <20% of usual baseline
- Arterial oxygen saturation of >90% or PaO_2 of >60 mmHg on no more than 40% inspired oxygen
- FiO_2 equal to or less than 0.4 or 40% of inspired oxygen
- Systolic blood pressure of <180 mmHg or <20% change from baseline
- Absent signs of increased work of breathing

In addition to these, the clinician should rigorously evaluate accessory muscle use, paradoxical or asynchronous rib cage or abdominal movements, intercostal retractions, nasal flaring, profuse diaphoresis, or agitation. Removal of ventilator support prematurely often results in re-intubation, which is associated with lengthened ICU course, prolonged hospitalization, and increased incidence of tracheostomy [72]. Because of this, it is important to consider the patient's ability to protect their airway. In those with NMD, the ability to protect from excessive secretions via cough reflex is one of the most common barriers to safe extubation. For this reason, the cough and gag reflexes, amount of secretions, and frequency of suctioning should be considered prior to extubating [78]. For those with NMD who definitively require intubation, a pre-intubation NIV experience was a good predictor of successful extubation, and some literature suggests that prior exposure to NIV may benefit weaning in neuromuscular patients by improving tolerance [65].

The recent use and amount of sedation and analgesia must also be considered during ventilator weaning. Excess analgesia and sedation result in poor performance of spontaneous awakening and breathing trials, and the timing of sedation cessation must be considered when considering ventilator liberation. In many cases, the role of sedation might be less relevant as it is not uncommon to have such patients on mechanical ventilation without sedation. In many cases, low doses of analgesia can be used to suppress the gag reflex from endotracheal tubes or irritation of tracheostomy cannulas. The role of protocolized sedation weaning and daily spontaneous awakening and breathing trials is likely to be of greater use in the general (non-neuromuscular disease) critically ill population. Many studies on ICU patients in North America have indicated that daily sedation interruption reduced the total duration of mechanical ventilation; however the results were heterogeneous among studies [76].

After extubation and discontinuation of mechanical ventilation, patients must be closely monitored for labored respirations, rapid or shallow breaths, accessory muscle use, and paradoxical respiratory muscle movement. An arterial blood gas should also be done to determine if acidemia, hypercarbia, or hypoxemia is present. Other clinical factors that might be less obvious include depressed mental status, sweating, or restlessness. It is important to remember that in NMD, progression to hypercarbia is often gradual, and accessory muscle fatigue is less obvious making progression to impending acute respiratory failure more severe with higher morbidity when it does occur [79]. If any indicators of ensuing respiratory failure are present, evaluation for re-intubation may be necessary.

In select patients with prolonged or terminal NMD, some work has shown that those intubated for respiratory failure, specifically those that had respiratory muscle weakness and low vital capacity, could be successfully extubated using NIV, which could be continued after the resolution of their acute respiratory failure for which intubation was required [65]. In some cases, daily NIV use has been shown to help prevent intubation and tracheostomy and prolong survival in those with DMD, among other types of neuromuscular diseases [65]. Interval use of NIV may offer the benefit of also allowing the potential of some patients to eat when NIV is not in use. This of course requires careful scheduling of NIV around times of the day set aside for nutrition as the risk of aspiration will be increased after feeding. When trying to wean patients with neuromuscular disease, a tracheostomy eliminates a significant amount of upper-airway resistance presented by the nasopharynx, oropharynx, and tongue. For the patient on prolonged invasive mechanical ventilation, the transition from endotracheal tube often requires tracheostomy to facilitate ongoing ventilator weaning. The optimal timing for tracheostomy has been controversial, however postulated to be ideal within 14 days (about 2 weeks) after intubation. Despite performing tracheostomy, patients are often still faced with impaired secretion clearance, and tracheal suctioning frequently adds to airway irritation which can induce more secretions and resultant hypoxemia if not careful [80]. Airway clearance techniques have continued to focus primarily on tracheal suction and chest physiotherapy, both of which, even when combined, are often ineffective at clearing life-threatening mucous plugs [78]. Other techniques that have been used include chest percussion and postural drainage; however, these have also shown little benefit even when properly employed. The use of mechanical exsufflation and deep insufflation has been shown helpful for eliminating airway secretions and permitting safe extubation for neuromuscular disease patients with negligible peak cough flows and thus have been found beneficial when used with some of the techniques mentioned above [80, 81].

In patients with ongoing severe neuromuscular disease necessitating mechanical ventilation either by endotracheal tube or tracheostomy, some have shown that a peak cough flow greater than 160 L/min could be successfully extubated or, in the case of tracheostomy, decannulated [65, 78]. In some cases, if there is an ongoing need for mechanical ventilation, a mouthpiece can be used to facilitate ongoing NIV and coupled with a cough assist machine. This approach has been shown useful in Duchenne muscular dystrophy and other NMD patients to limit intubation and aid in secretion clearance [65, 66]. In a study by Bach and Saporito, the ability to generate at least 160 L/min of peak cough flow (PCF), whether unassisted or manually assisted, was found to be an important predictor of successful endotracheal extubation or tracheostomy decannulation [78]. It has also been shown that these techniques helped increase the vital capacity and oxygen saturation by clearing upper-airway mucus without tracheal suctioning maneuvers. However, it was noted that limitations to using mechanical insufflation-exsufflation exist, namely, when there is poor glottic stability during exsufflation, as in those with bulbar-onset amyotrophic lateral sclerosis (ALS) or small children with limited cooperation [78].

The Deconditioned Diaphragm

Diaphragm dysfunction is a consequence of diaphragm weakness and atrophy and is common in the ICU setting. The diaphragm, being the largest muscle of respiration, is subject to insults in the critical care setting including sepsis, hypoxia, and especially atrophy from deconditioning [82]. It has been proposed that mechanical ventilation in those with critical illness encounters diaphragm weakness by a mechanism of reduced force-generating capacity and is frequently underrecognized by clinicians in the ICU setting. Additionally, mechanical ventilation, a major part of the treatment for neuromuscular disease patients, is implicated in the pathogenesis of diaphragm dysfunction, making it more prone to atrophy [83]. Some clinicians have postulated quantifying diaphragm dysfunction by diagnostic tools such as video fluoroscopy, phrenic nerve conduction study, surface EMG (to assess electrical activity of the diaphragm), and more recently ultrasound techniques [83, 84]. Diaphragm ultrasound with M-mode has been useful to help clinicians better understand how diaphragm dysfunction complicates ventilator weaning; however, acceptable limits and cut-off values for diaphragm excursion and muscle thickness have yet to be determined [82]. It has also been suggested that even short durations (18–96 h) of mechanical ventilation can cause significant atrophy of the diaphragm, while longer courses of mechanical ventilation have revealed diminished muscle fiber cross-sectional area along with increased oxidative stress and structural injury of these muscle fibers [85]. The pressure-generating capacity of the diaphragm can be characterized by its ability to shorten and produce force, descending into the abdomen creating negative pressure within the thorax, thus allowing for alveolar ventilation. In mechanically ventilated patients, diaphragm excursion is poorly correlated with markers of pressure-generating capacity but has been associated with successful outcomes and ventilator weaning [14, 83].

Currently, there exists no consensus on diaphragm monitoring in the ICU setting; however point-of-care ultrasound has found use as a non-invasive tool which is commonplace in many ICUs. Ultrasound assessments have included measuring diaphragmatic excursion, diaphragm thickness, and speed of diaphragm contraction, all which can be done with good reproducibility among users [84, 86]. Some have advocated measuring diaphragm thickness fraction (DTF) as a percentage, calculated by thickness at end inspiration minus thickness measured at end expiration and then divided by thickness at end expiration. Calculating this fraction has been shown to correlate with pressure-generating capacity of the diaphragm, and when compared to healthy individuals, patients with neuromuscular disease tend to have significant reduction in diaphragm thickness as well as excursion during spontaneous respiration, as signified by lower DTF value [69]. Despite this, there have not been many studies that have considered the functional assessment of the diaphragm specifically in the ventilator weaning process of neuromuscular patients.

Extubation Failure

It is important for clinicians to identify the optimal timing of extubation and ventilator liberation. Untimely extubation, either too early or delayed, can be detrimental to patients, exposing to further respiratory muscle fatigue, excessive sedation, or increased risk of infection. Unfortunately, studies dedicated to extubation in those with neuromuscular disease continue to be limited. In the general critical care population, excluding neuromuscular disease, extubation failure has been associated with an 8-fold higher odds ratio for nosocomial pneumonia and an up to 12-fold increase overall mortality risk [74, 87]. Because of this, clinicians should balance aggressive ventilator liberation with extubation safety and appropriate timing to allow for appropriate recovery of the neuromuscular process when possible. There has been a debate over what is an acceptable failed extubation rate, with some arguing that a value too low suggests unnecessary delays in ventilator removal and values too high suggest untimely delay in extubation and ventilator removal. As reported from various studies, re-intubation rates are highly variable and have been noted to range from 4% to 23% across different ICU populations and possibly as high as 33% in patients with neurologic disease or impairment [13, 74, 87]. Although never subjected to rigorous cost/benefit analyses, re-intubation rates of 5–20% after extubation failure have typically been generally considered reasonably acceptable in the general ICU population [74]. It is worth noting that re-intubation in neuromuscular disease patients with neuromuscular blocking agents may introduce detrimental effects, as these medications can precipitate re-worsening of the neuromuscular disease process that might have been in recovery. The advent of systematic ventilator weaning protocols has helped integrate optimal timing of a spontaneous breathing trial with sedation weaning to form cost-effective spontaneous awakening and breathing trials. Other important weaning predictors include heart rate variability, sleep quality, hand grip strength, presence of diaphragmatic dysfunction, and markers of oxidative stress. Heart rate variability is common among patients with NMD, and studies have shown that such variability during spontaneous breathing trials has been associated with increased risk of extubation failure [88]. DiNino and colleagues found that measuring the differences between diaphragm thickness with ultrasound near the zone of apposition during inspiration and expiration was useful, suggesting that a difference of 30% or more could predict extubation failure with a sensitivity of 88% and a specificity of 71% [89].

Consideration for Tracheostomy

When considering tracheostomy, one of its long-term advantages is decreased risk of laryngotracheal injury which is often caused by prolonged use of endotracheal tubes [90]. Other benefits of tracheostomy include reduced dead space and enhanced patient comfort. Tracheostomy allows for gradual recovery of respiratory muscles that might not otherwise be possible when accounting for upper-airway resistance of the nasopharyngeal space. Although tracheostomy allows for improved pulmonary toileting, some have argued that tracheal suction may induce more bronchospasm complicating the overall weaning process [66]. Additionally, superficial tracheal lumen trauma can occur and may cause upper-airway bleeding, especially in patients on anticoagulation, platelet inhibitors, or those with coagulopathy. Because of this, overly frequent or aggressive deep tracheal suction should be minimized, and the potential benefits and risks of tracheostomy should be considered along with appropriate timing of the procedure.

Another significant advantage of a tracheostomy is reduction of airway resistance, which in turn decreases overall workload on the respiratory system, facilitating the weaning process. Other benefits include increased patient mobility and the opportunity for articulated speech [90]. Given their acute 90° angle, airflow turbulence is greater in tracheostomy tubes; however this is usually overcome due to the shorter length. The shorter length of a tracheostomy is less subject to occlusion, and ease of access to the lower respiratory tract allows for suction and clearance of secretions within the lumen. If the tracheostomy lumen does become occluded, the inner cannula can be replaced when secretions become hardened. The optimal timing of tracheostomy has not been established; however, some have recommended at least within a 14–21-day timeframe. Many clinicians feel that tracheostomy is reasonable before 2 weeks if the need for prolonged mechanical ventilation is anticipated. Regarding GBS patients, prolonged mechanical ventilation and tracheostomy were more likely to occur in the elderly and in those with the presence of preexisting pulmonary disease [70].

Tracheostomy should be considered after an initial period of stabilization on the ventilator, when it becomes apparent that the patient will require prolonged ventilator assistance. Previous studies showed that tracheostomy within 1 week after intubation was beneficial, also conveying lower rates of pneumonia and shortening the duration of mechanical ventilation [91, 92]. Risks associated with tracheostomy include local hemorrhage, tracheoinnominate fistula and tracheal stenosis, local bleeding, or hemorrhage secondary to ongoing cuff pressure and erosion. When patients require mechanical ventilation for 2–3 weeks, the benefits of tracheostomy begin to outweigh the risks, and if mechanical ventilation is anticipated beyond 2–3 weeks, then early tracheostomy should be considered, especially in those with limited response to IVIG and plasmapheresis. Also, tracheostomy may expose patients to perioperative complications related to surgery and long-term airway injury [90].

Conclusions

This chapter on the clinical approach to the patient with acute neuromuscular respiratory failure discusses the most common causes of acute neuromuscular respiratory failure and other less common clinical pathologies. We discussed the initial clinical approach, emphasizing the importance of obtaining an accurate and reliable history to guide the neurologic examination. We also discuss the two most commonly encountered neuromuscular pathologies in the intensive care unit, detailing the initial evaluation, diagnosis, pathophysiology, management, risk stratification, respiratory evaluation, common complications, and treatment considerations.

References

1. Serrano MC, Rabinstein AA. Causes and outcomes of acute neuromuscular respiratory failure. Arch Neurol. 2010;67:1089–94.
2. Dresser L, Wlodarski R, Rezania K, Soliven B. Myasthenia gravis: epidemiology, pathophysiology and clinical manifestations. J Clin Med. 2021;10:2235.
3. Mehta S. Neuromuscular disease causing acute respiratory failure. Respir Care. 2006;51:1016–23.
4. Kelly BJ, Luce JM. The diagnosis and management of neuromuscular diseases causing respiratory failure. Chest. 1991;99:1485–94.
5. Patten J. Neurological differential diagnosis. London: Springer; 1996.
6. Jacobs B, et al. The spectrum of antecedent infections in Guillain-Barré syndrome: a case-control study. Neurology. 1998;51:1110–5.
7. Yoshikawa K, et al. Bickerstaff brainstem encephalitis with or without anti-GQ1b antibody. Neurol Neuroimmunol Neuroinflamm. 2020;7:e889.
8. Singman EL, et al. Use of the Cogan lid twitch to identify myesthenia gravis. J Neuroophthalmol. 2011;31:239–40.
9. Racca F, et al. Practical approach to respiratory emergencies in neurological diseases. Neurol Sci. 2020;41:497–508.
10. Buyse B, et al. Respiratory dysfunction in multiple sclerosis: a prospective analysis of 60 patients. Eur Respir J. 1997;10:139–45.
11. Howard RS. Respiratory failure because of neuromuscular disease. Curr Opin Neurol. 2016;29:592–601.
12. Hill NS. Ventilator management for neuromuscular disease. Semin Respir Crit Care Med. 2002;23(3):293–306.
13. Epstein SK, Ciubotaru RL. Independent effects of etiology of failure and time to reintubation on outcome for patients failing extubation. Am J Respir Crit Care Med. 1998;158:489–93.
14. Dres M, Demoule A. Diaphragm dysfunction during weaning from mechanical ventilation: an underestimated phenomenon with clinical implications. Crit Care. 2018;22:1–8.
15. Kim SM, Kang S-W, Choi Y-C, Park YG, Won YH. Successful extubation after weaning failure by noninvasive ventilation in patients with neuromuscular disease: case series. Ann Rehabil Med. 2017;41:450–5.
16. Vilke GM, Chan TC, Neuman T, Clausen JL. Spirometry in normal subjects in sitting, prone, and supine positions. Respir Care. 2000;45:407–10.
17. Bach JR, Martinez D. Duchenne muscular dystrophy: continuous noninvasive ventilatory support prolongs survival. Respir Care. 2011;56:744–50.
18. Jaretzki A, et al. Myasthenia gravis: recommendations for clinical research standards. Neurology. 2000;55:16–23.
19. Conti-Fine BM, Milani M, Kaminski HJ. Myasthenia gravis: past, present, and future. J Clin Invest. 2006;116:2843–54.
20. McConville J, et al. Detection and characterization of MuSK antibodies in seronegative myasthenia gravis. Ann Neurol. 2004;55:580–4.
21. Higuchi O, Hamuro J, Motomura M, Yamanashi Y. Autoantibodies to low-density lipoprotein receptor–related protein 4 in myasthenia gravis. Ann Neurol. 2011;69:418–22.

22. Chan KH, Lachance DH, Harper CM, Lennon VA. Frequency of seronegativity in adult-acquired generalized myasthenia gravis. Muscle Nerve. 2007;36:651–8.
23. Sanders DB, et al. International consensus guidance for management of myasthenia gravis: executive summary. Neurology. 2016;87:419–25.
24. Bedlack RS, Sanders DB. On the concept of myasthenic crisis. J Clin Neuromuscul Dis. 2002;4:40–2.
25. Wendell LC, Levine JM. Myasthenic crisis. Neurohospitalist. 2011;1:16–22.
26. Berrouschot J, Baumann I, Kalischewski P, Sterker M, Schneider D. Therapy of myasthenic crisis. Crit Care Med. 1997;25:1228–35.
27. Neumann B, et al. Myasthenic crisis demanding mechanical ventilation: a multicenter analysis of 250 cases. Neurology. 2020;94:e299–313.
28. Nelke C, et al. Independent risk factors for myasthenic crisis and disease exacerbation in a retrospective cohort of myasthenia gravis patients. J Neuroinflammation. 2022;19:89.
29. Mier A, Laroche C, Green M. Unsuspected myasthenia gravis presenting as respiratory failure. Thorax. 1990;45:422–3.
30. Juel VC. Seminars in neurology. New York: Thieme Medical Publishers, Inc.; 2004. p. 75–81.
31. Rabinstein AA, Wijdicks EF. Seminars in neurology. New York: Thieme Medical Publishers, Inc.; 2002. p. 97–104.
32. Gummi RR, Kukulka NA, Deroche CB, Govindarajan R. Factors associated with acute exacerbations of myasthenia gravis. Muscle Nerve. 2019;60:693–9.
33. Sheikh S, et al. Drugs that induce or cause deterioration of myasthenia gravis: an update. J Clin Med. 2021;10:1537. https://doi.org/10.3390/jcm10071537.
34. Maramattom BV, Wijdicks EF. Acute neuromuscular weakness in the intensive care unit. Crit Care Med. 2006;34:2835–41.
35. Clark WF, et al. Therapeutic plasma exchange: an update from the Canadian Apheresis Group. Ann Intern Med. 1999;131:453–62.
36. Gajdos P, et al. Clinical trial of plasma exchange and high-dose intravenous immunoglobulin in myasthenia gravis. Ann Neurol. 1997;41:789–96.
37. Qureshi AI, et al. Plasma exchange versus intravenous immunoglobulin treatment in myasthenic crisis. Neurology. 1999;52:–629.
38. Seneviratne J, Mandrekar J, Wijdicks EF, Rabinstein AA. Predictors of extubation failure in myasthenic crisis. Arch Neurol. 2008;65:929–33.
39. Thomas C, et al. Myasthenic crisis: clinical features, mortality, complications, and risk factors for prolonged intubation. Neurology. 1997;48:1253–60.
40. Wakerley BR, Yuki N. Mimics and chameleons in Guillain–Barré and Miller Fisher syndromes. Pract Neurol. 2015;15:90–9.
41. Leonhard SE, et al. Diagnosis and management of Guillain–Barré syndrome in ten steps. Nat Rev Neurol. 2019;15:671–83.
42. Green C, Baker T, Subramaniam A. Predictors of respiratory failure in patients with Guillain–Barré syndrome: a systematic review and meta-analysis. Med J Aust. 2018;208:181–8.
43. Doets AY, et al. Regional variation of Guillain-Barré syndrome. Brain. 2018;141:2866–77.
44. Rees JH, Soudain SE, Gregson NA, Hughes RA. Campylobacter jejuni infection and Guillain–Barré syndrome. N Engl J Med. 1995;333:1374–9.
45. Orlikowski D, et al. Guillain–Barré syndrome following primary cytomegalovirus infection: a prospective cohort study. Clin Infect Dis. 2011;52:837–44.
46. Hao Y, et al. Antecedent infections in Guillain-Barré syndrome: a single-center, prospective study. Ann Clin Transl Neurol. 2019;6:2510–7.
47. Greene SK, et al. Guillain-Barré syndrome, influenza vaccination, and antecedent respiratory and gastrointestinal infections: a case-centered analysis in the Vaccine Safety Datalink, 2009–2011. PLoS One. 2013;8:e67185.
48. Kwong JC, et al. Risk of Guillain-Barré syndrome after seasonal influenza vaccination and influenza health-care encounters: a self-controlled study. Lancet Infect Dis. 2013;13:769–76.

49. Kuitwaard K, Bos-Eyssen ME, Blomkwist-Markens PH, Van Doorn PA. Recurrences, vaccinations and long-term symptoms in GBS and CIDP. J Peripher Nerv Syst. 2009;14:310–5.
50. Fokke C, et al. Diagnosis of Guillain-Barré syndrome and validation of Brighton criteria. Brain. 2014;137:33–43.
51. Willison HJ, Jacobs BC, van Doorn PA. Guillain-Barré syndrome. Lancet. 2016;388:717–27.
52. Wong AHY, et al. Cytoalbuminologic dissociation in Asian patients with Guillain-Barré and Miller Fisher syndromes. J Peripher Nerv Syst. 2015;20:47–51.
53. Flachenecker P. Autonomic dysfunction in Guillain-Barré syndrome and multiple sclerosis. J Neurol. 2007;254:II96–101.
54. Chakraborty T, Kramer CL, Wijdicks EF, Rabinstein AA. Dysautonomia in Guillain–Barré syndrome: prevalence, clinical spectrum, and outcomes. Neurocrit Care. 2020;32:113–20.
55. Hund EF, Borel CO, Cornblath DR, Hanley DF, McKhann G. Intensive management and treatment of severe Guillain-Barré syndrome. Crit Care Med. 1993;21:433–46.
56. Zaeem Z, Siddiqi ZA, Zochodne DW. Autonomic involvement in Guillain–Barré syndrome: an update. Clin Auton Res. 2019;29:289–99.
57. Hoffmann O, Reuter U, Schielke E, Weber JR. SIADH as the first symptom of Guillain–Barré syndrome. Neurology. 1999;53:1365–1365-a.
58. Saifudheen K, Jose J, Gafoor VA, Musthafa M. Guillain-Barré syndrome and SIADH. Neurology. 2011;76:701–4.
59. Doets AY, et al. International validation of the erasmus Guillain–Barré syndrome respiratory insufficiency score. Ann Neurol. 2022;91:521–31.
60. Hughes RA, Swan AV, Van Doorn P. Intravenous immunoglobulin for Guillain-Barré syndrome. Cochrane Database Syst Rev. 2014.
61. Patwa H, Chaudhry V, Katzberg H, Rae-Grant A, So Y. Evidence-based guideline: intravenous immunoglobulin in the treatment of neuromuscular disorders [RETIRED]: report of the Therapeutics and Technology Assessment Subcommittee of the American Academy of Neurology. Neurology. 2012;78:1009–15.
62. Plasmapheresis and acute Guillain-Barré syndrome. Neurology. 1985;35:1096–6.
63. Walgaard C, et al. Tracheostomy or not: prediction of prolonged mechanical ventilation in Guillain–Barré syndrome. Neurocrit Care. 2017;26:6–13.
64. Bach JR, Alba AS. Management of chronic alveolar hypoventilation by nasal ventilation. Chest. 1990;97:52–7.
65. Bach JR, Gonçalves MR, Hamdani I, Winck JC. Extubation of patients with neuromuscular weakness: a new management paradigm. Chest. 2010;137:1033–9.
66. Bach JR, Alba AS. Noninvasive options for ventilatory support of the traumatic high level quadriplegic patient. Chest. 1990;98:613–9.
67. Pilcher DV, et al. Outcomes, cost and long term survival of patients referred to a regional weaning centre. Thorax. 2005;60:187–92.
68. Mayer SA, Yavagal DR. Pulmonary complications of neuromuscular diseases. 2002.
69. Krishnakumar M, Muthuchellappan R, Chakrabarti D. Diaphragm function assessment during spontaneous breathing trial in patients with neuromuscular diseases. Neurocrit Care. 2021;34:382–9.
70. Windisch W, et al. Prolonged weaning from mechanical ventilation results from specialized weaning: Centers—a registry-based study from the WeanNet initiative. Dtsch Arztebl Int. 2020;117(12):197–204.
71. Rabinstein and Mueller-Kronast. Risk of extubation failure in patients with myesthenic crisis. Neurocrit Care. 2005;03:213–5.
72. Torres R, Lima Í, Resqueti VR, Fregonezi GA. Weaning from mechanical ventilation in people with neuromuscular disease: protocol for a systematic review. BMJ Open. 2019;9:e029890.
73. Zein H, Baratloo A, Negida A, Safari S. Ventilator weaning and spontaneous breathing trials; an educational review. Emerg (Tehran). 2016;4:65.
74. MacIntyre NR. Evidence-based assessments in the ventilator discontinuation process. Respir Care. 2012;57:1611–8.

75. Thille AW, Richard J-CM, Brochard L. The decision to extubate in the intensive care unit. Am J Respir Crit Care Med. 2013;187:1294–302.
76. Burry L, et al. Daily sedation interruption versus no daily sedation interruption for critically ill adult patients requiring invasive mechanical ventilation. Cochrane Database Syst Rev. 2014;2014(7):CD009176.
77. Boles J-M, et al. Weaning from mechanical ventilation. Eur Respir J. 2007;29:1033–56.
78. Bach JR, Saporito LR. Criteria for extubation and tracheostomy tube removal for patients with ventilatory failure: a different approach to weaning. Chest. 1996;110:1566–71.
79. Bernardes Neto SCG, Torres-Castro R, Lima I, et al. Weaning from mechanical ventilation in people with neuromuscular disease: a systematic review. BMJ Open. 2021;11:e047449.
80. Bach JR, Lee HJ. New therapeutic techniques and strategies in pulmonary rehabilitation. Yonsei Med J. 1993;34:201–11.
81. Bach JR, Wang DW. Mechanical insufflation-exsufflation to facilitate ventilator weaning and possible decannulation for patients with encephalopathic conditions. J Neurorestoratol. 2023;11:100031.
82. Kim WY, et al. Diaphragm dysfunction assessed by ultrasonography: influence on weaning from mechanical ventilation. Crit Care Med. 2011;39:2627–30.
83. Dres M, Demoule A. Monitoring diaphragm function in the ICU. Curr Opin Crit Care. 2020;26:18–25.
84. Matamis D, et al. Sonographic evaluation of the diaphragm in critically ill patients. Technique and clinical applications. Intensive Care Med. 2013;39:801–10.
85. Levine S, et al. Rapid disuse atrophy of diaphragm fibers in mechanically ventilated humans. N Engl J Med. 2008;358:1327–35.
86. Suttapanit K, et al. Ultrasonographic evaluation of the diaphragm in critically ill patients to predict invasive mechanical ventilation. J Intensive Care. 2023;11:40.
87. Frutos-Vivar F, et al. Outcome of reintubated patients after scheduled extubation. J Crit Care. 2011;26(5):502–9.
88. Huang CT, et al. Application of heart-rate variability in patients undergoing weaning from mechanical ventilation. Crit Care. 2014;18(1):R21.
89. DiNino E, et al. Diaphragm ultrasound as a predictor of successful extubation from mechanical ventilation. Thorax. 2014;69:423–7.
90. Hefner JE. The role of tracheostomy. Chest. 2001;120:477S–81.
91. Chorath K, Hoang A, Rajasekaran K, Moreira A. Association of early vs late tracheostomy placement with pneumonia and ventilator days in critically ill patients: a meta-analysis. JAMA Otolaryngol Head Neck Surg. 2021;147:450–9.
92. Hsu C, et al. Timing of tracheostomy as a determinant of weaning success in critically ill patients: a retrospective study. Crit Care. 2005;9:R46–52.

Chapter 13
The Global Perspective on Respiratory Care for Neuromuscular Disease

Anita K. Simonds

Trends in Prevalence and Global Impact of Neuromuscular Disorders

Prevalence estimates of neuromuscular disorders (NMD) have grown in accuracy over the last few decades as case ascertainment has been based on genetic evidence rather than clinical features. In addition, while the incidence is unlikely to have changed greatly, the prevalence number of those with many NMD conditions has increased as individuals are surviving longer. For example, in the UK [1] there has been a significant trend in the prevalence of NMD over time from 2000 to 2019, with a 66% increase in males and 61% increase in the prevalence of females, while overall incidence was unchanged. Lifetime prevalence increased across all age groups, and median age in prevalent cases rose by about 5 years from 52 in 2000 to 57 years in 2019. This equated to a NMD prevalence rate 223.6 per 100,000 persons. There was no regional variation. The survey group included those with amyotrophic lateral sclerosis (ALS), muscular dystrophies, inflammatory myopathies, sensory motor neuropathies, Guillain-Barre syndrome and myasthenia gravis.

Looking specifically at muscular dystrophies, Theadom et al. [2] carried out a systematic literature review identifying neuro-epidemiological studies from Northern America, Asia, Oceania and Europe. Crude prevalence rates per 100,000 for all muscular dystrophies varied widely, ranging from 3.8 in Japan to 26.8 in Egypt. However, when studies with low risk of bias were considered, the prevalence estimates narrowed to between 19.8 and 25.1 per 100,000. Myotonic dystrophy was

A. K. Simonds (✉)
Royal Brompton and Harefield Hospital, Guys and St Thomas' NHS Foundation Trust, London, UK

National Heart and Lung Institute, Imperial College, London, UK
e-mail: A.Simonds@rbht.nhs.uk

© The Author(s), under exclusive license to Springer Nature Switzerland AG 2024
N. Lechtzin (ed.), *Pulmonary Complications of Neuromuscular Disease*, Respiratory Medicine, https://doi.org/10.1007/978-3-031-65335-3_13

identified as the most prevalent muscular dystrophy at 0.5–18.1, followed by Duchenne muscular dystrophy (DMD) at 1.7–4.2 and facioscapulohumeral muscular dystrophy at 3.2–4.6 per 100,000. Unfortunately, no studies reported prevalence by age or gender. In view of discrepancies between case ascertainment and verification of diagnosis, the need for standardisation of conducting and reporting on epidemiological studies was emphasised.

Another systematic review and meta-analysis [3] of the prevalence of muscular dystrophies in 2016 found a worldwide prevalence of combined muscular dystrophies of 16.4 per 100,000 or 1 in 6200. Here too, myotonic dystrophy was most prevalent, followed by facioscapulohumeral muscular dystrophy (FSHMD) and then DMD—the latter being the dominant muscular dystrophy of childhood. Limitations in gathering data in these studies are clear in that there was lack of genetic testing in earlier studies, non-random geographical sampling and population-based registries which were limited to parts of Europe, Asia and North America.

A recent review [4] of the global epidemiology of Duchenne MD cumulated 44 studies. The pooled global prevalence of DMD was 7.1 cases per 100,000 males and 2.8 cases per 100,000 of the general population (95% CI 1.6–4.6). A caution is that few studies were of high quality.

Amyotrophic lateral sclerosis: variation in the worldwide incidence of ALS is under intensive investigation. Marin et al. carried out a meta-analysis [5] including 44 studies covering 45 geographical areas and 11 sub-continents, identifying a total of over 13,000 cases. The overall pooled crude ALS incidence was 1.75 (CI 1.55–1.96) per 100,000 and 1.68 (CI 1.50–1.85) per 100,000 following standardisation. Wide heterogeneity was found in ALS standardised incidence between North Europe and East Asia, China, Japan and South Asia. However more homogenous rates were reported in populations from Europe, North America and New Zealand. It should be noted that 24 studies (53.3%) originated from Europe and 14 (31.1%) from the American continent but far fewer from South and East Asia. The pooled standardised incidence of ALS in the USA was 1.68 (1.50–1.85) and for Europe 1.89 (1.46–2.32) per 100,000. The figures for New Zealand were 2.56 (2.22–2.90), North Africa 2.03 (1.16–2.91) and East Asia 0.83 (0.42–1.24) per 100,000, respectively. As the authors stress, from this information it is impossible to dissect out the impact of ancestral/genetic origin, from lifestyle and environmental features.

Relevance of Population Studies in ALS and Their Limitations

As population studies are limited by problems with accurate case ascertainment, registries have more recently assumed importance in gathering real-world data. The National ALS registry in the USA was launched in 2010 and collects data from national databases on trends, and risk factors, as well as incidence. The most recent report [6] in 2021 showed fairly stable figures for age-adjusted incidence rates of ALS at 1.8 in 2014, 1.6 in 2015 and 1.6 in 2016 per 100,000 US population. ALS was more common in white ethnic groups, males and persons aged 60–79 years.

These rates are somewhat lower than in European ALS registries (2.6 per 100,000), which has been attributed to wider population diversity in the USA. That may also explain a lower prevalence in the Southern USA but could also be explained by delays in diagnosis or lack of access to healthcare.

Origins of Geographical Gradient and Ethnic Diversity in ALS

Many studies have suggested that a latitude gradient (higher rates in north compared to south) may be a key factor in determining incidence as this has been reported not only globally but within countries, e.g. Finland, Sweden, Italy and Spain.

As far as known genetic influences, the C9orf72 gene is the most common gene associated with ALS and responsible for approximately 40% of familial cases and 8% of sporadic cases. The prevalence of this gene is much lower in the East, e.g. Japan, South Asia and Iran. The gene has a high incidence in Finland which has one of the highest ALS incidence rates in the world. Logroscino et al. [7] describe the variant arising as a mutation in Scandinavia around 1500 years ago and spreading across Northern Europe and the UK associated with Viking invasions. Pliner et al. [8] discuss the possibility of a MAPT mutation arising in Wales, UK, 500 years ago being exported to British colonies in British Columbia, Virginia, and Australasia. The second most commonly mutated gene in Europe associated with ALS is superoxide dismutase (SOD1).

Specific foci of ALS were identified in Guam in the 1950s, but the incidence here has subsequently dropped markedly, at a rate too great to be explained by genetic determinants. Here modifiable environmental factors are postulated to be responsible, such as the dietary intake of cyanobacterial toxin present in the traditional local Chamorro diet [7].

A further explanation for global difference in rates is age. Overall ALS tends to be a disease of older individuals with a peak at age 73 years, and while prevalence rates and maybe rising, age-adjusted rates have changed only a little. This means that with an increasingly ageing population prevalence rates will inevitably rise, and the highest growth in cases is likely to be in Africa, followed by Asia and South America.

Healthcare Impact of NMD

In terms of healthcare impact in the USA, NMD comprised 5% of hospital discharges and 2% of emergency department visits in 2013, and within ED visits 46% were admitted, although reasons for this were not given. Mean hospital charges with a neuromuscular diagnosis were $59,100, which was 38% higher than mean charge for any health condition, and discharges to other healthcare facilities were common [9].

Another study by the Muscular Dystrophy Association, USA, looked at medical, non-medical and lost income costs in ALS, DMD and myotonic dystrophy patients in the USA and came up with the figures below per patient, per annum [10]:

Disorder	Medical costs	Nonmedical costs	Lost income	Total
ALS	$31,121	$17,889	$14,628	$63,692
DMD	$22,533	$12,939	$15,481	$50,953
DM	$17,451	$5157	$9628	$32,236

For the care of NMD overall, some authors [11] have estimated that annual charges associated with medical care are more than $46 billion annually, with subgroups of neuromuscular junction disorders, peripheral nerve disease and myopathies costing around $10 billion in charges each.

Duchenne Muscular Dystrophy Health Burden

A more complex idea—the overall health burden of a disease—is a result of its prevalence, total healthcare costs and societal impact. This has not been quantitated in all NMD, but DMD is an example where these consequences have been analysed in detail. Landfeldt et al. [12] have examined the burden in an international cross-sectional study involving 770 DMD patients from Germany, Italy, the UK and the USA. They assessed the quality of life in patients and carers and estimated mean loss of quality of life compared to an age-matched unaffected population. In addition they measured per patient annual costs for medical care including hospital visits and consultations, medications, devices, informal care and indirect costs, e.g. loss of work and leisure time transport (see Fig. 13.1).

Mean per patient annual direct costs in dollars were $42,360 in Germany; $23,920 in Italy; $54,160 in the UK; and $54,270 in the USA which represents approximately 10, 8, 16 and 7 times the average per capita health expenditure in the countries, respectively.

Crucially over and above direct costs, DMD caused large losses in production for patients and caregivers. Between 27% and 49% of caregivers had decreased their working hours or stopped working because of their son's condition. It is clear from Fig. 13.1 that informal care from caregivers was a major cost factor. Without this, it is likely that patients would have to be accommodated in a long-stay care facility. Summating all the costs, the authors concluded that the total societal burden was between $80,120 and $120,910 annually per person, with this probably being a conservative estimate, as it does not include the wider family impact. It should be added the health-related quality-of-life scores were similar in DMD patients across countries, but there was a considerable impact on the quality of life of caregivers.

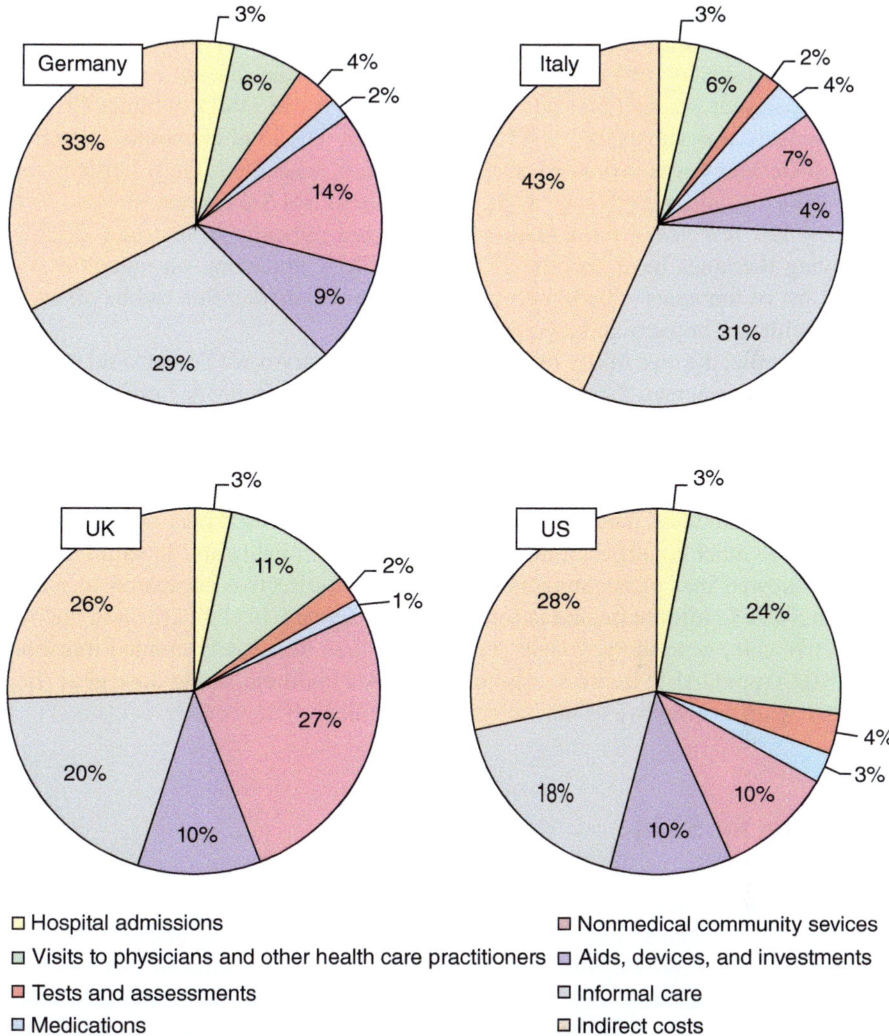

Fig. 13.1 International comparison of contributors to annual costs in Duchenne muscular dystrophy (Germany, Italy, the UK and the USA) (hospital admissions include emergency and respite care. Nonmedical community services include home help, personal assistants, nannies and transportation. Informal care is usually provided by families). (From Landfeldt et al. [12])

Spinal Muscular Atrophy (SMA) Disease Burden (Including the Impact of Nusinersen and Gene Therapy)

Prior to the introduction of disease-modifying approaches such as nusinersen, risdiplam and gene therapy, Klug et al. [13] evaluated the disease burden of SMA in Germany focusing on the cost of the illness (COI). They used the PedQL tool to analyse disease-specific quality of life and included 198 patients with a median age of 19 years. Importantly only 12 had SMA 1, 73 SMA 2 and 104 SMA 3. Ventilatory support was used by 13%. Overall direct COI across the disease categories was €54,721 per year but €99,664 per year in SMA 1. As in DMD, indirect COI for SMA patients was substantial at €15,845 per year. The total economic burden of SMA to Germany was estimated at €106.2 million, with the highest burden from SMA 2 (€41.4 million per year), as the prevalence of SMA 2 is greatest.

In the last few years, the situation has changed radically in that new disease-modifying therapies have become available in SMA impacting on outcomes and costs. Cost of therapies is high, but it is vital to know whether this can be offset by fewer healthcare impacts and a better quality of life.

For example, the cost utility of onasemnogene abeparvovec (Zolgensma) therapy compared to nusinersen therapy and best supportive care in SMA 1 children under 2 years has been compared using incremental quality-adjusted life year and incremental cost-effectiveness as the main outcome measures [14]. These analyses are complex and rely on the results of small trials and assumptions and extrapolations about future outcomes. The costings are also US based which may not be directly applicable to other countries, although relative costs probably are. In summary, the authors showed that onasemnogene therapy is cost-effective compared to nusinersen in SMA 1 children treated before the age of 2 years. In comparison to the best supportive care, gene therapy costs were higher than the usually applied threshold at $150,000 per QALY. In pre-symptomatic SMA 1 children, single-dose gene therapy was again as effective as nusinersen but significantly less costly.

Screening for SMA

The cost utility of newborn screening for SMA has been investigated [15], as such screening is essential to identify pre-symptomatic children. For example, with an incidence of 1:10,000 live births in England, it has been estimated that newborn screening would identify 96% of all '5q' cases of SMA per year, and this would save more than £62 million over the lifetime of an incident cohort, screened over 1 year. Newborn screening was also estimated to increase QALYs accrued by the yearly cohort over their lifetime by 529. So overall newborn screening was less costly and more effective than a scenario without newborn screening, taking into account all factors, including costs and patient outcomes.

Basic Research in NMD

Undoubtedly a better understanding of the molecular and genetic basis of a condition is likely to lead to better therapies and potentially a cure. Research on many neuromuscular conditions has previously been limited by the fact these are rare and less likely to attract investment by pharma companies. Recent rare disease initiatives have been successful in addressing these inequities. Cortial et al. [16] in 2020 reviewed national approaches to researching rare diseases in Germany, France, Spain, the UK, Europe as a whole, Canada and the USA. Using the definition that a rare disease affects fewer than 5 in 10,000 people, it is estimated that there are around 300 million people worldwide with rare disorders. Policies can be traced back to 1972 in Japan, with the USA passing the Orphan Drug Act in 1983. European regulation for orphan medicinal products dates from 2000. Of note Orphanet was initiated in France in 1997 to gather information on the diagnosis and management of rare diseases, and this has now evolved to a network of 41 countries globally. Within countries a range of policy processes occur related to research and clinical funding, centres of excellence and genomic programmes. It is clear that transnational consortia and networks are a key way forward in research and delivering new and improved therapeutic care. Not surprisingly funding and organisation aspects vary from country to country (see Fig. 13.2).

	Steering	Source of funding	Centres of expertise	Gene identification	National register
Germany 2013	State + patient organisation (ASCHE)	State + patient organisation (ASCHE)	36 centres working with 8 research centres + 10 centres for NDD	RD-Connect programme (EU funding 2018–2022): register relating to -> research Biobanks and the creation of an EU platform	Se-Atlas: 8000 genes CORD-MI project €160 million invested between 2016 et 2021
Spain 2009	State	State	19 centres of expertise Spain UDP consortium	The Human Genetic Area (AGH) for diagnosed diseases. SpainUDP for undiagnosed diseases	SpainRDR Funding from the State / Regions and collaboration with private partners
France 2004	State	State	400 reference centres for rare diseases (CRMRs); 27 National Rare Disease Health Networks (FSMRs)	France Genome 2025 programme High-throughput platform	Deployment of the BaMaRa register
United Kingdom 2012	State	State	76 centres Emphasis on patient care and empowerment	13 centres, involving 85 hospitals Target 2023: sequencing of 50,000 genes	-
Canada 2015	State: Canadian Organization for Rare Diseases (CORD)	Genome Canada, funded by federal government, the provinces and manufacturers	20 mother and child research centres	6 genomic centres Care4Rare, international, transdisciplinary consortium, with 21 sites	PhenomeCentral: national register with international scope
USA 1983	State: NIH	State	Network of 20 consortia, with 350 sites in the United States and 22 worldwide	Undiagnosed Diseases Network (2015), with 12 sites	Data Management and Coordinating Center (DMCC)
Japan 1972	State	State	34 clinical investigation centres 4 analysis centres	Consortium for the Initiative on Rare and Undiagnosed Diseases (IRUD)	RADDAR platform connected to international platforms

Fig. 13.2 International approaches to rare disease research funding. (From Cortial et al. [16])

Patient Support Groups

The impact of patient support groups and charities cannot be overestimated. Not only do they raise large sums for research, but they also provide multiple means of support and information to families, and their engagement has driven up standards of care. These groups are too numerous to mention but include Muscular Dystrophy Campaign, Cure SMA, Cure Congenital Muscular Dystrophy (CDC) and the ALS Association. Patients have been increasingly involved in setting research priorities and trial design, and the use of patient reported outcome measures (PROMS) has proved to be a major step forward.

Holistic Medical Care Pathways in NMD

The evolution of care practices and pathways in NMD is an interwoven story dating back many years. Often championed by key individuals, supportive care for many years, if not centuries, has progressed from increased diagnostic rigour to specific interventions that have changed the natural history such as ventilatory support (invasive and non-invasive), secretion clearance practices and comprehensive care for cardiac involvement, bone health, swallowing, nutritional care and active symptom management, as described in previous chapters. This has led to increases in survival, e.g. from death in mid-teens in DMD to survival to a median age of around 30 years, with many individuals surviving to middle age, as seen in Fig. 13.3. Children with many neuromuscular disorders who previously did not live to adult age are now transitioning to adult care [17].

On top of this, new therapeutic approaches are having a further significant impact on outcomes with the introduction of new therapies, gene editing and gene therapy as indicated earlier. We are so far in the foothills of those revolutions.

Standards of Care

International standards of care have undoubtedly been improved and harmonised by the development of consensus statements and guidelines [18–23], and as time passes and the research base grows, these are increasingly evidence-based. While national guidelines exist, many standards of care protocols are now drawn up by international teams meaning that variations in care globally will be reduced. It is true however that not all guidelines are straightforward to implement, and funding limitations, especially in middle- and low-income countries, plus the human factors described below, may play a part in the persistence of variations in care.

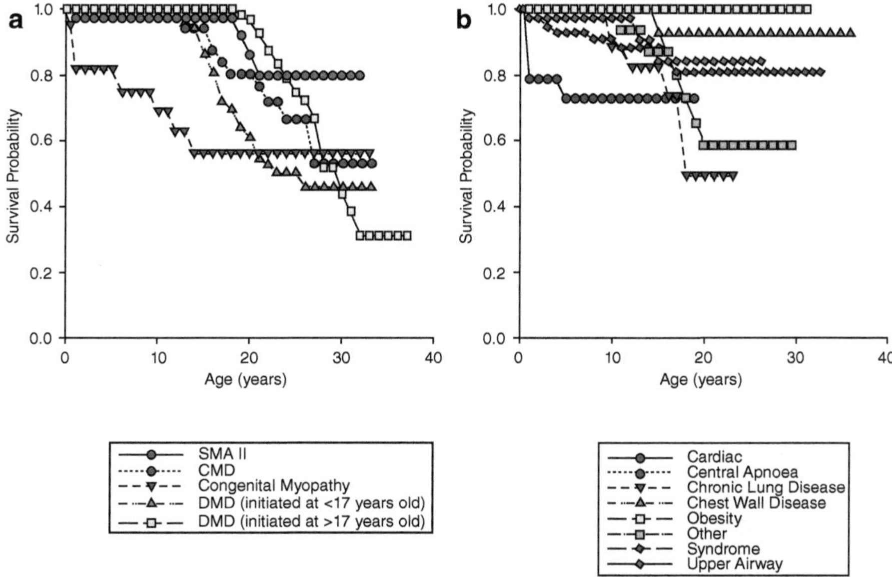

Fig. 13.3 Survival probabilities of patients with neuromuscular disease who start non-invasive ventilation in childhood (<17 years). (**a**) shows children with neuromuscular diseases using non-invasive ventilation, compared to (**b**) children with non-neuromuscular conditions using non-invasive ventilation. (Adapted from Chatwin et al. [17])

Delivery of Care

As described above, inevitably there are global differences in the *delivery* of care related to a range of factors, historical and cultural organisation of healthcare facilities and funding models. Many of the new therapies are expensive, resulting in inequitable access to these. While generalisations are often unhelpful, there is a focus on care of the patient with severe dependency needs in the home in Europe, while there are more long-term facilities for such individuals in countries such as the USA and Japan. The proportion of patients receiving non-invasive ventilation versus invasive (tracheotomy) ventilation also varies, and this is particularly pronounced in ALS, probably related to historical and cultural factors.

International Comparisons in Home Mechanical Ventilation in NMD

Home mechanical ventilation (HMV) is increasingly applied and is a major part of care in patients with NMD causing respiratory insufficiency. Toussaint et al. [24] have recently carried out an international review of the organisation and delivery of

HMV internationally in people with NMD. They showed considerable variation in the provision of HMV across countries and even between different regions within countries. Figure 13.4 shows the most recent estimates of national prevalence of HMV in 24 countries across Europe, North America, South America and Asia. This ranges from 1.2 to 47 per 100,000 population, with an average of about 7.3/100,000, although this figure may be an underestimate. As a rule of thumb, the authors suggest about 10% of NMD patients will require HMV, and within this group, about 60% use nocturnal support, 20% some daytime and nocturnal ventilation and around 20% require 24-h ventilatory support. This makes HMV in NMD a highly specialised treatment. Regionally the authors found prevalences varying between 0.4 and 15.5 in nine territories of Canada, 1.2 and 4.0 in the 16 regions of Poland and between 4.5 and 13.00 in the eight states and territories of Australia. This constitutes a considerable variation despite the fact that these countries, by and large, have health systems that are homogenous. Explanatory factors for these regional discrepancies include prescribing patterns that differ according the HMV centre location, size and experience. Also, the enthusiasm of clinicians and health teams in the HMV speciality area can play a significant part in the development of services. Dybwik et al. [25] examined the reasons for variation in the prevalence of HMV in Norway and showed that there were differences in attitudes between, say, pulmonologists and neurologists, but a dominant finding was that a driving force for the development of services was 'wise enthusiasm' among experienced medical team leaders. This embraced the components of 'high competence' (for which an adequate throughput of patients is required); 'spreading competence', i.e. building experience and teaching others; and multidisciplinary collaboration, the latter being important in ethical decisions. In several decades ago, Bach et al. [26] had shown that recommendations for ventilator use in muscular dystrophy patients were influenced by clinical directors' estimates of the quality of life that might result from the intervention, despite the fact the clinical directors underestimated the quality of life of those individuals. These attitudes have evolved over time by being informed by outcome studies including the impact of HMV on health-related quality of life and standards of care guidelines. But some vestiges persist, for example, with respect to the use of HMV in ALS or the use of tracheotomy versus non-invasive ventilatory support.

On balance it seems that 'wise enthusiasm' among clinical leaders (who are not equally distributed geographically) in part explains regional variations in the availability of HMV services and that attitudes can still affect the uptake of clinical guidance nationally and internationally.

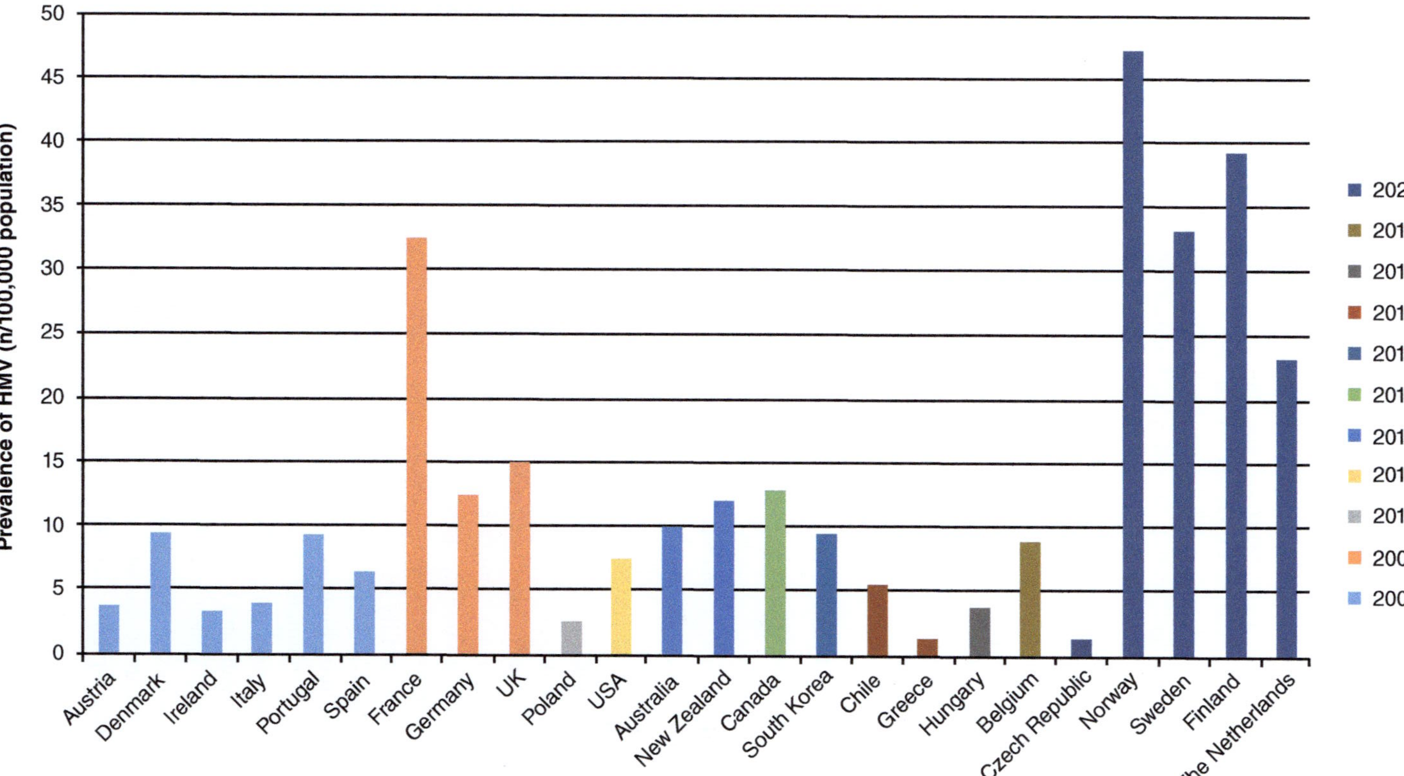

Fig. 13.4   Most recent estimates of the prevalence of home mechanical ventilation internationally. (From Toussaint et al. [24])

Relationship Between the Prevalence of HMV and National Wealth

A positive correlation between the prevalence of HMV and gross domestic product (GDP) of countries is to be expected, and indeed this is broadly true for GDP and the human development index (HDI) which is a compound measure of the life expectancy, level of education and the standard of living of a country. These positive correlations were indeed seen in the study of Toussaint et al. [24], but interestingly there was substantial variation in the prevalence of HMV among countries with higher rather than lower indices, showing financial resources are not the only determinant. Importantly while many HMV programmes in Northern Europe and North America started their programmes with predominantly NMD patients (often dating from the poliomyelitis epidemics) and these numbers have grown due to new treatment approaches, the biggest growth in HMV use is now in patients with obesity hypoventilation syndrome and COPD.

New Modes of Care Delivery: Remote Care and Telemonitoring

Over the last decade, it has become increasingly possible to monitor people on home ventilation in the home, and this process was disseminated widely during the COVID-19 pandemic. Whether HMV devices are portable bilevel ventilators or life support machines, many manufacturers now have monitoring platforms in which data transfer to the monitoring centre is affected, and changes to settings can be made. Adherence monitoring, measurement of leaks from the interface, adequacy of ventilation and fine-tuning of settings to solve problems can be achieved remotely. Indeed, for some NMD conditions, the whole care pathway can be delivered in the patient's home, from remote sleep study to home set-up of ventilator and then subsequent telemonitoring. Clearly this is most effective in relatively stable patients and with the availability of an outreach team. Positive outcomes, for example, in patients with ALS, are recorded where hospital admissions and ER visits plus costs may be reduced with high levels of patient satisfaction. For those in whom travel to the hospital is problematic, this can be a great boon, and virtual delivery of care is likely to be seen increasingly. There are limitations in that it is difficult to compare directly home-based and hospital-based pathways; also data reliability, security and accuracy can be a concern, and additional monitoring devices may be required to get a measure of oximetry, transcutaneous CO_2, and sleep efficacy [27]. Furthermore, reimbursement can be inconsistent. Nonetheless remote care is a valuable complement to centre/hospital-based NMD programmes.

International Impact of COVID-19 in NMD

A telling measure of the provision of a clinical service is what happens when it is challenged by an outside shock, such as COVID-19. Worldwide care for patients with chronic disorders was disrupted with an early expectation that many patients with NMD would succumb. In fact, many NMD patients especially those with respiratory insufficiency shielded at home and were early recipients of the SARS-CoV-2 vaccine. Other than a small subgroup receiving immunosuppression, e.g. myasthenia gravis patients and children with DMD receiving prednisolone, individuals with NMD usually have normal immune responses and so are not more likely to be infected with a virus. However, if they are infected, the consequence of that infection may be worse than those without that risk factor. Global studies have shown relatively reassuring results as to the impact of COVID-19 in the NMD population. An international registry recruiting patients from Europe, the USA, India, South Africa and Namibia gathered data on COVID-19 infection in 328 NMD patients from May 2020 to December 2021 [28], the largest diagnostic groups comprising myopathies (40.6%), neuropathy (31.8%), neuromuscular junction disorders (20%) and anterior horn cell disease (7.6%). Of these patients 55.5% did not require hospitalisation, 8.6% were hospitalised without the need for supplemental oxygen, 28.9% were hospitalised and required oxygen therapy or ventilation and 7% died. The majority (62.9%) fully recovered, and some recovered with reported sequelae, although it is not clear how long these persisted. Risk factors for hospitalisation were older age, obesity, ethnicity other than white race/ethnicity, moderate or severe functional disability and glucocorticoid therapy at the time of diagnosis of COVID-19. Respiratory dysfunction was also a risk factor, which was defined by the co-presence of chronic obstructive pulmonary disease, asthma, interstitial lung disease, restrictive lung disease and tracheotomy. Male patients tended to be more severely affected by COVID-19 infection, but this was not significant and offset by a larger number of affected female patients with myasthenia gravis. Overall comorbidity burden with conditions such as obesity and hypertension was associated with increased odds of a worse outcome, just as in the general population. On the topic of myasthenia gravis (MG), compared to a population-matched Canadian cohort, people with MG showed increased risk of hospitalisation (HR 2.48 95% CI 1.61–3.79) and death (2.22 95% CI 1.17–3.78) pre-vaccination, but high SARS-Cov-2 vaccine update, no evidence of exacerbation of myasthenia post vaccination and reduced risk of COVID-19 infection after and negligible admissions post vaccination [29].

In a nationwide French registry study [30] of NMD patients with COVID-19 which collected data in the first wave in 2020, in 48% the severity of COVID-19 was low, it was moderate requiring hospitalisation in 28%, and 15% of patients required ICU admission. Here too, known risk factors of diabetes, hypertension and severe functional impairment were associated with more unfavourable outcomes. In this cohort steroid therapy in MG patients did not affect outcome, but this may be related to the dose, dose timing and degree of immunosuppression. Respiratory failure was not a predictive factor either, and this was present on over a third of patients at baseline.

In the general population age was a major risk factor for adverse outcome from COVID-19 with children less severely affected. As in the adult group, there have been a series of small cohort studies observing outcomes in children with NMD. A registry study [31] of 29 children with NMD in Spain, including predominantly those with SM1&2 and DMD, showed almost 90% of cases were asymptomatic or mild and 10% as moderate. All three patients hospitalised had SMA 1, two required an increase in hours using NIV, but all recovered. The authors concluded that young age as a protective factor in COVID-19 infection trumps reduced respiratory reserve and weak cough.

While results from the literature are still accumulating, a take-home message broadly is that the outcome of COVID-19 in NMD is not as severe as initially predicted at the start of the pandemic, and risks factors such as the comorbidities of obesity, diabetes and age may outweigh problems such as respiratory insufficiency, although marked functional impairment and immunosuppression carry higher risk. To be sure shielding, particularly in the first wave of the pandemic, played an important part in reducing the spread of infection. This social exclusion came at some psychosocial cost [32], although NMD patients are often extremely resourceful. A Danish paediatric study [33] showed the considerable impact of the pandemic on routine clinic appointments, research studies, interventional therapies and adjuncts such as physiotherapy. The authors also found that the individual's or families' anxiety related to perceived risk of COVID-19 infection and potential adverse outcome was markedly overestimated, compared to the actual risk which was often low.

References

1. Carey IM, Banchoff E, Nirmalanathan N, Harris T, DeWilde S, Chaudhry UAR, Cook DG. Prevalence and incidence of neuromuscular conditions in the UK between 2000 and 2019. A retrospective study using primary data. PLoS One. 2021;16:e0261983.
2. Theadom A, Rodrigues M, Roxburgh R, Balalla S, Higgins C, Bhattacharjee R, Jones K, Krishnamurthi R, Feigin V. Prevalence of muscular dystrophies: a systematic literature review. Neuroepidemiology. 2014;43:259–68.
3. Mah JK, Korngut L, Fiest KM, Dykeman J, Day LJ, Pringsheim T, Jette N. A systematic review and meta-analysis on the epidemiology of the muscular dystrophies. Can J Neurol. 2016;43:163–77.
4. Crisafulli S, Sultana J, Fontana A, Salvo F, Messina S, Trifiro G. Global epidemiology of Duchenne muscular dystrophy: an updated systematic review and meta-analysis. Orphanet J Rare Dis. 2020;15:141.
5. Marin B, Boumediene F, Logroscino G, Couratier P, Babron M-C, Leutenegger AL, Copetti M, Preux P-M, Beghi E. Variation in worldwide incidence of amyotrophic lateral sclerosis: a meta-analysis. Int J Epidemiol. 2017;46:57–74.
6. Mehta P, Raymond J, Punjani R, Larson T, Han M, Bove F, Horton DK. Incidence of amyotrophic lateral sclerosis in the United States, 2014–2016. Amyotroph Lateral Scler Frontotemporal Degener. 2022;23:378–82.

7. Logroscino G, Piccininni M. Amyotrophic lateral sclerosis descriptive epidemiology: the origin of geographic difference. Neuroepidemiology. 2019;52:93–103.

8. Pliner HA, Mann DM, Traynor BJ. Searching for Grendel: origin and global spread of the C9ORF72 repeat expansion. Acta Neuropathol. 2014;127:391–6.

9. Kirschner JK, Lee SW. Burden of neuromuscular conditions. In: The burden of musculoskeletal diseases in the United States. 4th ed. United States Bone and Joint Initiative; 2015.

10. Larkindale JYW, Hogan PF, Simon CJ, Zhang Y, Jain A, et al. Cost of illness for neuromuscular diseases in the United States. Muscle Nerve. 2013;49:431–8.

11. Understanding Neuromuscular Disease Care. Current state and future prospects. IQVIA Institute Report 2018; Oct 30.

12. Landfeldt E, Lindgren P, Bell CF, Schmitt C, Guglieri M, Straub V, Lochmuller H, Bushby K. The burden of Duchenne muscular dystrophy. Neurology. 2014;83:529–36.

13. Klug C, Schreiber-Katz O, Thiele S, Schorling E, Zowe J, Reilich P, Walter MC, Nagels KH. Disease burden of spinal muscular atrophy in Germany. Orphanet J Rare Dis. 2016;11:58.

14. Dean R, Jensen I, Cyr P, Miller B, Maru B, Sproule DM, Feltner DE, Wiesner T, Malone DC, et al. An updated cost-utility model for onasemnogene abeparvovec (Zolgensma) in spinal muscular atrophy type 1 patients and comparison with evaluation by the Institute for Clinical and Effectiveness Review (ICER). J Market Access Health Policy. 2021;9:1889841.

15. Weidlich D, Servais L, Kausar I, Howells R, Bischof M. Cost-effectiveness of newborn screening for spinal muscular atrophy in England. Neurol Ther. 2023;12:1205–20.

16. Cortial L, Nguyen C, Julkowska D, Cocqueel-Tiran F, Moliner AM, Blin O, Trentesaux V. Managing rare diseases: examples of national approaches in Europe, North America and East Asia. Rare Dis Orphan Drugs J. 2022;1:10.

17. Chatwin M, Tan LB, Bush A, Rosenthal M, Simonds AK. Long term non-invasive ventilation in children: impact on survival and transition to adult care. PLoS One. 2015;10:e0125839. https://doi.org/10.1371/journal.pone.0125839.

18. Duong T, Krosschell KJ, James MK, Nelson L, Alfaro LN, Eichinger K, Mazzone E, et al. Consensus guidelines for improving quality of assessment and training for neuromuscular diseases. Front Genet. 2021;12:735936.

19. Narayan S, Pietrusz A, Allen J, DiMarco M, Docherty K, Emery N, et al. Adult North Star Network (ANSN): consensus document for therapists working with adults with Duchenne muscular dystrophy (DMD)—therapy guidelines. J Neuromusc Dis. 2022;9:365–81.

20. Birnkrant DJ, Panitch HB, Benditt JO, Boitrano LJ, Carter ER, Cwik VA, et al. American College of Chest Physicians consensus statement on the respiratory and related management of patients with Duchenne muscular dystrophy undergoing anesthesia or sedation. Chest. 2007;132:1977–86.

21. American Thoracic Society Consensus Statement. Respiratory care of the patient with Duchenne muscular dystrophy. Am J Respir Crit Care Med. 2004;170:456–65.

22. Finkel RS, Mercuri E, Meyer OH, Simonds AK, Schroth MK, Graham RJ, et al. Diagnosis and management of spinal muscular atrophy: part 2: pulmonary and acute care; medications, supplements and immunizations; other organs systems; and ethics. Neuromuscul Disord. 2018;28:197–207.

23. Bushby K, Finkel R, Birnkrant DJ, Case LE, Clemens PR, Cripe L, et al. Diagnosis and management of Duchenne muscular dystrophy, part 2: implementation of multidisciplinary care. Lancet Neurol. 2010;9:177–89.

24. Toussaint M, Wijkstra PJ, McKim D, Benditt J, Winck JC, Nasilowski J, Borel J-C. Building a home ventilation programme: population, equipment, delivery and cost. Thorax. 2022;77:1140–8.

25. Dybwik K, Tollali T, Nielsen EW, Brinchmann BS. Why does the provision of home mechanical ventilation vary so widely? Chronic Resp Dis. 2010;7:67–73.

26. Bach JR. Standards of care in muscular dystrophy association clinics. J Neuro Rehab. 1992;6:67–73.

27. Ackrivo J, Elman L, Hansen-Flaschen J. Telemonitoring for home-assisted ventilation: a narrative review. Ann Am Thorac Soc. 2021;18:1761–72.
28. Pizzamiglio C, Pitceathly RD, Lunn MP, Brady S, De Marchi F, Glana L, Heckmann JM, et al. Factors associated with the severity of Covid-19 outcomes in people with neuromuscular diseases: data from the International Neuromuscular Covid-19 Registry. Eur J Neurol. 2023;30:399–412.
29. Alcantara M, Koh M, Park AL, Bril V, Barnett C. Outcomes of COVID-19 infection and vaccination among individuals with myasthenia gravis. JAMA Netw Open. 2023;6:e239834.
30. Pisella LI, Fernandes S, Sole G, Stojkovic T, Tard C, Chanson J-B, Bouhour F, et al. A multicentre cross-sectional French study of the impact of COVID-19 on neuromuscular diseases. Orphanet J Rare Dis. 2021;16:450.
31. Natera-de Benito D, Aguilera-Albesa S, Costa-Comellas L, Garcia-Romero M, Miranda-Herrero MC, Olives JR, et al. COVID-19 in children with neuromuscular disorders. J Neurol. 2021;268:3081–5.
32. Spurr L, Tan H-L, Wakeman R, Chatwin M, Hughes Z, Simonds A. Psychosocial impact of COVID-19 pandemic and shielding in adults and children with early-onset neuromuscular and neurological disorders and their families: a mixed-methods study. BMJ Open. 2022;12:e055430.
33. Handberg C, Werlauff U, Hojberg A-L, Knudsen LF. Impact of the Covid-19 pandemic on biopsychosocial health and quality of life among Danish children and adults with neuromuscular diseases (NMD)—patient reported outcomes from a national survey. PLoS One. 2021;16:e0253715.

Chapter 14
Palliative Care and End-of-Life Decision-Making for People with Neuromuscular Disease

Alpa Uchil and Lora L. Clawson

Introduction

Palliative care is defined by the WHO as the "prevention and relief of suffering" in all aspects of physical, psychological, social, and spiritual domains [1]. Fundamentally, by way of relieving suffering, the main purpose of palliative care is to improve the quality of life of patients, families, and caregivers facing a severe health experience. Palliative care is frequently utilized for terminal conditions. A terminal health experience or life-debilitating disease defines any disease with "high risk of mortality, negatively impacts the quality of life and daily function, and/or is burdensome in symptoms, treatments, or caregiver stress" [2]. Neuromuscular diseases, the focus of this chapter, clearly are life-debilitating diseases, although disease progression varies across etiologies. While there is abundant literature regarding palliative care in amyotrophic lateral sclerosis (ALS), less attention has been given to palliative care in other neuromuscular diseases [3]. In this chapter, we will provide a brief overview of palliative care, including its benefits, essential communication skills, and a decision-making model, and then focus on palliative care across the spectrum of neuromuscular diseases. We will also discuss the differences between palliative care and hospice care and the role of hospice care in end-of-life decision-making.

A. Uchil (✉)
Department of Neurology, Johns Hopkins University School of Medicine, Johns Hopkins School of Nursing, Baltimore, MD, USA
e-mail: apalich2@jhmi.edu

L. L. Clawson
Department of Neurology, Johns Hopkins University School of Medicine, Baltimore, MD, USA
e-mail: lclawson@jhmi.edu

© The Author(s), under exclusive license to Springer Nature Switzerland AG 2024
N. Lechtzin (ed.), *Pulmonary Complications of Neuromuscular Disease*, Respiratory Medicine, https://doi.org/10.1007/978-3-031-65335-3_14

Overview of Palliative Care

Globally, the need for palliative care is significant, as only 12% of that need is currently being met and this need is expected to double by 2060 [4]. Even in countries with rich resources, not all patients with terminal conditions are aware of, or have access to, palliative care services [5]. Some reasons for these barriers include a lack of awareness by healthcare providers, patients, and caregivers, misconceptions about the purpose of palliative care services, inadequate policies, limited resources, lack of training, and regulations on controlled palliative medicines [6]. As with access to healthcare in general, other barriers include geographic location and financial capabilities.

A common misconception is that palliative care is only for the dying and should be initiated when a patient reaches the end stage of disease progression. Rather, palliative care is a model of care appropriate for any patient suffering from intractable symptoms or pain from a serious illness, at any stage during the course of the condition. Palliative care is needed at all levels of primary, secondary, and tertiary settings [4] because it aims to mitigate the physical, psychological, social, and spiritual impact of disease through the continuum of the patient's experience from diagnosis to death. Palliative care is most beneficial earlier in the course of the illness, in addition to other therapies recommended by the medical team, to provide support to patients and caregivers [4]. There is evidence showing that delays in initiating palliative care services can result in poor disease management, increased suffering, and increased need for hospitalizations [2]. Conversely, evidence shows the benefits of palliative care in improving pain, enhancing decision-making, and decreasing healthcare costs [7].

Additionally, palliative care can be provided in concert with standard treatment options for terminal conditions. For example, in our experience in providing care for individuals with ALS, palliative care is discussed in addition to recent pharmacologic advancements, rehabilitation therapies, and symptom management which target the slowing of ALS progression. This provides collaboration, communication, and effective facilitation between the patient, family, and all members of the healthcare provider team in approaching all available treatment options. Given the impact of ALS on patients and caregivers, this combined approach can be comforting for patients as it lessens the perception that life has come to an end and thus consequently improves the quality of life.

The ideal structure for an interdisciplinary model of palliative care delivery has been defined by the National Consensus Project for Quality Palliative Care. This aspirational model includes eight domains [2] (see Table 14.1):

1. Structure and processes of care: The interdisciplinary team (IDT) includes physicians, nurses, chaplains, social workers, and pharmacists. Each team member has defined elements of assessment and care planning.
2. Physical: Assessment and treatment of symptoms and care planning emphasize patient-directed and family-directed holistic care.

Table 14.1 Domains of quality palliative care

Domain	
1. Structure and process of care	5. Spiritual
2. Physical	6. Cultural
3. Psychological and psychiatric	7. End of life
4. Social	8. Ethical and legal

Ref: [2]

3. Psychological and psychiatric: Psychological and psychiatric care needs are addressed in the context of serious illness.
4. Social: Patient and family social support needs are assessed, and a plan is developed to address these needs.
5. Spiritual: Spiritual, religious, and existential needs, including the importance of screening for unmet needs, are identified, and a plan is developed to address these needs as well.
6. Cultural: The cultural context that influences both the way in which care is delivered and the experience of care by patients and families from the time of diagnosis through death and bereavement is reflected in all aspects of care planning.
7. End of life: Symptoms and situations that focus on the final days and weeks of life are contemplated.
8. Ethical and legal: Advance care planning, surrogate decision-making, and regulatory and legal considerations, focusing on ethical imperatives and processes to support patient autonomy, are implemented.

To implement this consensus model of palliative care, cultural sensitivity, rapport, and empathy are essential. Culturally sensitive care is an approach to healthcare delivery that recognizes and respects the unique cultural background of each patient. It acknowledges the impact of culture on a person's beliefs, values, customs, and lifestyle. Cultural sensitivity is broadly recognized as the awareness by the healthcare provider of the various attitudes and beliefs of people in cross-cultural settings. This awareness informs knowledge and skills to work well with, to respond effectively, and be supportive of patients from all cultures. Cultural sensitivity is not solely the acceptance of cultural differences, but rather a transformational process that allows individuals to acknowledge interdependence and align with a group other than their own. Culturally proficient healthcare, in particular, makes use of a patient's language and culture as tools to improve outcomes for that individual. Culturally and linguistically appropriate services, broadly defined as care and services that are respectful of and responsive to the cultural and linguistic needs of all individuals, hold the promise to reduce these health outcome disparities. Such services are the hallmark of culturally proficient healthcare delivery for an increasingly diverse population.

Establishing a solid rapport between patients, caregivers, and knowledgeable professionals, ensuring access to information, and coordinating all aspects of care are essential in the delivery of palliative care. Both patients and families require ongoing information regarding diagnosis, disease progression, and the possible outcomes of medical treatments (both prospective treatment successes and failures), as well as potential or impending death. It is imperative that patients and their families feel free to ask questions throughout the disease trajectory. Empathic communication on the part of the healthcare team facilitates an open and authentic exchange with patients and families. An empathetic approach helps patients and their families focus on topics of utmost importance to them. Empathy can be a tool used by the members of the healthcare team to maintain emotional equilibrium and remain focused on the needs of patients and families.

In most instances, patients want to participate in decision-making for care and treatment, including end-of-life decisions. The basis for patient participation is open communication, positive patient-provider relationships, a favorable environment, and mutual information. The healthcare professional is responsible for ensuring successful patient participation. Open communication and consensus throughout the care planning experience can reduce disagreements and conflicts between patients and caregivers [8].

One approach to help healthcare professionals with clinical decision-making is using the Jonsen, Siegler, and Winsdale model, which takes into account the four aspects of medical indications, patient preferences, quality of life, and contextual features [9].

Diagnosis determines treatment, and the choices of treatments made available to patients play a major role in decision-making. Identifying goals of care, answering questions, and explaining interventions are important for good decision-making. Patient preferences must be considered after ensuring they have understood available treatment options. However, healthcare professionals must be aware that patients' decisions are based on their values, preferences, context, and goals of care. Additionally, there are other factors in any clinical situation that influence optimum decision-making. These include factors like family, society, relationships, finances, legal, insurance, and the institution where the patient is at the time of the decisions [9].

The patient should be at the center of all decision-making. Decision-making is an evolving process and, while grounded in the philosophy of care, can change rapidly depending on a multiplicity of factors. Ethical dilemmas occur even when providers try to adhere to the four guiding medical ethical principles of respect for autonomy, beneficence, non-maleficence, and justice. Reflective practice by providers is important for personal development as well as for the profession [10]. More work is needed to investigate the perspectives of patients to understand how best to facilitate and optimize self-determination in healthcare planning [11].

Overview of Neuromuscular Diseases

Neuromuscular diseases (NMDs) involve injury or dysfunction of peripheral nerves or muscle. This may include the motor neurons and sensory neurons, muscle, or the neuromuscular junction [12]. Manifestations of NMDs vary across etiologies and can range from mild to life-threatening. Disease progression also varies across etiologies, ranging from slow gradual decline, rapid progressive decline, and slow decline alternating with periods of rapid progression. Although there are pharmacologic interventions to slow disease progression in many NMDs, there is no curative treatment for most; thus symptom management is a mainstay addressing disease manifestations, such as muscle cramping and pain, fatigue, dysphagia, and respiratory difficulties. NMDs like Duchenne muscular dystrophy (DMD), spinal muscular atrophy (SMA), muscular dystrophies, Pompe's disease, amyotrophic lateral sclerosis (ALS), and primary lateral sclerosis (PLS) often cause death due to respiratory and cardiac failure and benefit from palliative care referral. However, there is limited data on palliative care use and its benefits in these diseases [3].

Involvement of parents and/or legal guardians is required in the palliative care process of those with SMA, DMD, myotonic dystrophy, and Pompe's disease given onset in infancy and childhood. In these NMDs, palliative care management involves parents and legal guardians until the affected individual reaches age 18 years.

Specific Areas to Be Addressed and Interventions

Respiratory Management

Most individuals with NMD die of respiratory failure. The end-stage management of respiratory failure in NMD can be fragmented and fraught with distress on the part of the patient and family members if there is progression in breathing difficulties. The outcome can be optimized by placing the focus on patient education about expected disease progression, symptom management and relief, and involving patients and families in decision-making along the way.

Studies have found that in ALS, noninvasive ventilation (NIV) can increase life expectancy and improve quality of life despite continual disease progression and physical decline. However, in patients with severe bulbar insufficiency, NIV use is challenging making clinical management difficult. Nocturnal NIV use as a treatment for respiratory failure in patients with NMD has helped people attain a longer life expectancy, and the use of NIV in children with DMD has allowed them to live into adulthood [13]. In some instances, individuals with ALS may elect to pursue tracheostomy. This level of care requires 24/7 care in the home setting or care in a facility that provides care to individuals who require mechanical ventilation. This heightened level of care can impose added physical and emotional care burdens to families as well as financial burdens [13]. Even with tracheostomy and mechanical ventilator support, disease progression continues, and patients will often die from pneumonia or other sequelae of chronic disease. Individuals who have tracheostomy and mechanical ventilator support may choose to withdraw life support and die peacefully at home under hospice care. Patient and family support in these decisions is critical. Most often this takes the form of early and ongoing communication, providing educational material, explaining disease progression, and expected outcomes of various treatment decisions. It is important to keep the patient at the center of all decision-making discussions.

Nutrition and Hydration

Bulbar function is compromised in many NMDs, affecting chewing and swallowing mechanisms. A gastrostomy feeding tube or nasogastric feeding tube may be required during the disease course to sustain nutrition and hydration. A comprehensive assessment by a speech and language pathologist provides a treatment plan with options of swallowing techniques, texture changes, and swallowing strategies helpful in facilitating safe and effective swallowing. Early discussions about patient's wishes regarding a feeding tube can help gain insights into their goals, as well as provide an opportunity to discuss the benefits and burdens of enteral nutrition [14]. Factors influencing the timing and safe placement of the gastrostomy include weight loss, and pulmonary function, especially in ALS and DMD. A pulmonary consult and pulmonary function testing should be performed prior to gastrostomy placement to secure a successful outcome. Education on the benefits of a gastrostomy tube, explaining the procedure, expected side effects, and post-operative care, prepares the patient and family for what to expect. Having the tube provides access to nutrition, hydration, and medication administration as the disease progresses.

Pain

Musculoskeletal pain and neuropathic pain are commonly reported by individuals with NMD. A multidisciplinary approach is required to manage pain while promoting function and providing coping strategies, including stretching exercises, range of motion exercises, proper positioning, and relieving areas of pressure from immobility. Simple analgesia should be the first course of treatment, but if this doesn't work, low-dose opioids or neuropathic pain medications, such as gabapentin, are beneficial for short-term use [14]. During the end of life, if the patient is unable to tolerate oral intake, pain medicines can be given via gastrostomy tube, topical or subcutaneous routes [14]. It is important for prescribers to provide education to family or caregivers on administering and monitoring opioids in addition to having Narcan available during this end-of-life stage.

Fatigue

Fatigue is common in NMD and can compromise quality of life. Many factors contribute to the management of fatigue, including sleep, diet, and exercise. Assessment and management with the multidisciplinary team to provide a plan of care to treat these factors are essential. Rehabilitation specialists can provide recommendations for bed modifications; nutritionists can provide counseling to optimize nutrition; and physical and occupational therapists can provide instruction on energy conservation and proper exercise routines. In Clawson et al. [15], three types of exercises were studied—resistance using weights, endurance using pedal bike, or ALS standard-of-care stretching/range-of-motion exercises. The study found all three forms of exercise were safe to perform and tolerated without any adverse effects.

Depression and Anxiety

Individuals diagnosed with NMD may experience anxiety and depression. This may be related to the impact of disease on functioning and social interactions, or it may be part of the pathology as seen with somnolence and apathy in myotonic dystrophy [14]. There is a higher prevalence of depression and anxiety in individuals with DMD or BMD compared to the general population [16]. Ongoing assessment and appropriate treatment, including referral to psychiatry and formal counseling, and treatment with antidepressant and antianxiety medications should be part of the care plan as indicated. Education of parents or caregivers on how to detect depression or anxiety is important for a timely referral to a specialist as this can improve quality of life [16].

Communication

Open communication with patients and families throughout the disease course is essential. Education, assessment of patients' disease progression, and medical updates should be ongoing with the medical care team. It is vital that the goals of care are mutually agreed upon and explicit. Equally important is to recognize that the task of coordinated care falls upon all members of the team caring for a patient with NMD [14]. As bulbar function deteriorates in many NMDs, assessment by the multidisciplinary team speech and language pathologist for an adaptive/alternative communication device, such as magic slate, smartphone applications, and sophisticated eye gaze systems, is indicated. Implementation of these communication devices can facilitate patients' expression of their desired plan of care. For an individual with communication impairment, Augmentative and Alternative Communication (AAC) includes no-technology, low-technology, and high-technology options and can optimize function and provide a method for the individual to participate in decision-making [17].

Advance Care Planning

Early and ongoing discussions with patients and families regarding diagnostic evaluation, medical treatment options, and end-of-life care planning are important communications throughout the disease course. While early discussions allow the patient to be a part of the decision-making process, ongoing discussions provide opportunities for patients to explore options, understand the benefits and burdens of options, and actively participate in their end-of-life planning [14]. Discussions evolve in progressive NMD and include decisions surrounding initiating or terminating NIV, tracheostomy and long-term ventilation, gastrostomy tube, and/or disease-modifying medications. Reviewing patients' wishes routinely allows patients to change or modify their choices with their treatment experiences over the disease course.

Discussing death and long-term care decisions with young adults with life-limiting illnesses is particularly challenging and requires a sensitive approach, developmentally appropriate discussions, and coordinated efforts by all members of the healthcare team [14]. As with adults, planning care for young adults needs to evolve as the patient's needs and understanding evolve over the course of the illness.

End-of-life decision-making in pediatric patients is challenging and sometimes controversial given that autonomy is determined by capacity, and children with NMD may not be in the state to understand or consent, defaulting the decision-making to parents and the medical team. While decision-making in pediatric patients takes into account similar factors as those in adults and young adults (that of social, cultural, religious, legal, and economic factors), the role of media has been increasingly influencing this process [18].

Palliative care in pediatric patients needs to be comprehensive as it takes into account the physical, psychological, social, and spiritual aspects to ensure the highest possible quality of life for the child and the family throughout the bereavement period which includes time from diagnosis to time after the death of the child [19]. Advance care planning process has the potential to inform patients and family members about future shared decisions. In a cognitively impaired patient, this early planning process proves to be especially beneficial when the patient reaches a point of not being able to cognitively participate [14]. Involving these patients to the extent of their ability should be encouraged.

Surrogate Decision-Making

Ideally, patients have created a durable power of attorney for healthcare. If a patient did not do this, state statutes specify which individuals can serve as surrogates; a current spouse typically is the first choice in many states. Healthcare providers may want to provide surrogates in advance care planning discussions prior to decision-making, allow discussions of surrogate stressors during decision-making, and designate the surrogate decision-maker to communicate information about the patient's current condition, prognosis, and treatment options and any updates to patient condition changes.

Ethical Considerations

The four universal ethical principles are autonomy, beneficence, non-maleficence, and justice. We focus on autonomy as it impacts decision-making. Autonomy is defined as the patient's right to determine and decide what kind of medical care they want and have those decisions respected. Healthcare providers are ethically required to respect patient's decisions, even for patients who are unable to decide. One way to respect patient's wishes is to utilize advance directives which include living wills, healthcare proxies, and "do not resuscitate" DNR orders [20].

It has been argued that living wills are not useful as implemented in the Terri Schiavo and Barbara Howe supreme court cases and that appointing a healthcare proxy is better [21]. In 1990, a young Terri Schiavo was left unconscious and unable to communicate after a cardiac arrest. As Terri didn't have written advance directives, the court appointed her husband, Michael, as her legal guardian to make decisions regarding her care. Terri's healthcare team confirmed her irreversible persistent vegetative state. She was kept alive through artificial nutrition and hydration by a feeding tube. In 1998, Michael asked the court to have the feeding tube withdrawn, but Terri's parents fought the petition. The legal battle of opposing end-of-life decision-making between Michael and the parents continued for several years leading to the feeding tube being removed and re-inserted two times. Finally in 2005, the tube was removed for the third and final time on March 18, and Terri died on March 31. In 1991, Barbara Howe was diagnosed with ALS, which progressed over the next few years until 2003 when she became completely paralyzed, breathing with a ventilator, and unable to communicate. While Howe knew what ALS prognosis meant, she made it very clear to her doctors that she wanted to be kept alive as long as she could enjoy her family. When the hospital's end-of-life committee recommended that she be allowed to die, Howe's daughter Carvitt who was the legally designated healthcare proxy insisted on life support. This legal battle of opposing decisions went on for 2 years before the daughter agreed to the hospital's recommendation to withdraw ventilation and allow Howe to die [21].

In both cases, a legal representative was making decisions for the patient. For healthcare providers, respecting the patient's autonomy is only possible if the competent patient has prepared advance directives for a time in the future or in the event the patient becomes unable to make decisions and provides them to their healthcare provider. Even with early planning, however, there are limitations because people change their minds and the definition of "terminal" varies from state to state [21].

A healthcare proxy is chosen by the patient to legally speak on their behalf should the patient be unable to make or communicate a decision. Usually, a proxy is a person who the patient trusts deeply to honor their wishes and knows the patient's preferences based on prior discussions about medical decision-making. Healthcare proxies can make decisions about treatment, procedures, and life support [20].

Patients always have the right to determine what treatment they want, what treatment they want to refuse, and what treatments they want to stop (e.g., life support). In the event that the patient has lost the ability to do so, the priorities of decision-making follow the sequence of advance directives if the patient has prepared them, healthcare proxy if no advance directives, family members if no proxy, and healthcare team if the family is unable or unwilling to decide [20]. Most institutions have legal support for formal consultations available for healthcare teams in this legal situation.

Psychological and Spiritual Support

Psychological support of the individual with NMD is critical. Most patients want to remain in their homes with familiar surroundings and family members. It is important that this occurs with caregiver support and the physical and emotional support of an experienced multidisciplinary care team, including home hospice care. Relieving symptoms of distress and fear of dying may require antianxiety and opioid medications.

Spiritual care is an important part of palliative care. Having a terminal illness often leads people to think about their lives in new ways, and their spiritual needs may change. All health and social care professionals can help explore the patient's spiritual needs and identify when someone might need more support.

Spirituality means different things to different people. For example, it can be about searching for meaning and purpose in life. Or it can mean finding the best relationship with ourselves, others, society, or nature. For some people spirituality might involve religion, but it's not the same as religious beliefs. Spiritual issues can affect everyone—people do not need to be religious to have spiritual needs. Spiritual needs are different for everyone and can change over time. These can include the need for meaning, purpose, and value in life; for love; to feel a sense of belonging; or to feel hope, peace, and gratitude. Spiritual needs are connected to physical, social, and emotional needs.

Spiritual needs may change when someone is diagnosed with a terminal illness. Patients may feel a sudden strong need to repair a broken relationship or deal with unfinished business. Patients may process thoughts about death, loss, and grief in different ways. Patients and those important to them may need support to make sense of the situation. Some patients will want to reflect on the meaning of life. Spiritual practice, including religion, may become important. Also, there may be spiritual or religious needs related to funeral arrangements.

End of Life and Hospice

A subtype of palliative care service is hospice care which focuses on end-of-life care for patients with a life expectancy of 6 months or less (Fig. 14.1). Hospice focuses on pain control, anxiety and agitation related to end-of-life distress, and caregiver's well-being.

Similar to palliative care, the model of care for hospice services includes coordinated and interdisciplinary care provided to terminally ill patients, their families, and caregivers in all domains of physical, psychosocial, and spiritual needs and in all care settings including the patient's home [22].

The components of hospice referral and care systems include an attending physician who clinically manages patient care and symptoms, registered nurse, certified home health aide, social worker, spiritual counselor, and mental health counselor as needed [2].

Once admitted under hospice care, the patient stays on service until they choose to be discharged, they choose to pursue disease modifying treatment, or the physician decides to discharge patient from services [22].

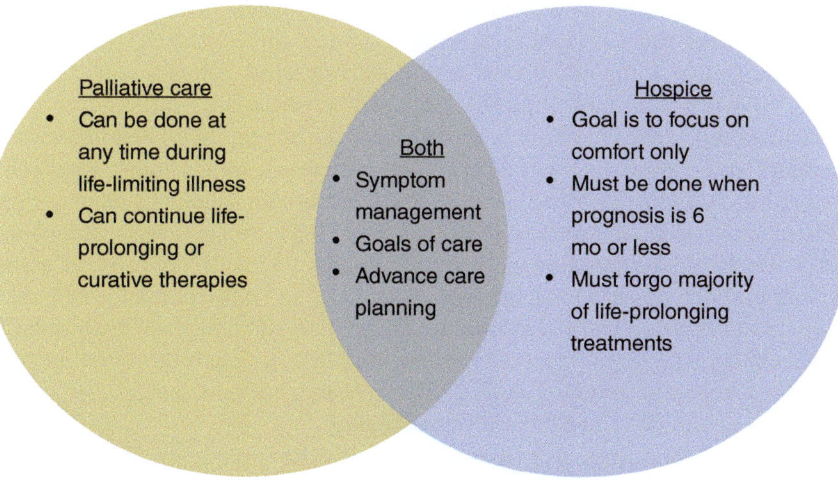

Fig. 14.1 Similarities and differences of hospice and palliative care [2]

Some discussion facets that can help patients and families decide to pursue palliative or hospice services include focus on comfort care and quality of life, decision to pursue curative and long-term treatments, decrease in functional status in the setting a terminal condition like ALS, prognosis, change in abilities to perform activities of daily living, decline in functional capabilities, frequent emergency room visits and hospitalizations, and increasing caregiver burden and distress [22].

End-of-Life Decision-Making

Many cultures tend to focus on life not death. A discussion about end of life is not a popular dinner table conversation. Life-altering decisions are usually forced when a loved one is diagnosed with an incurable disorder or a terminal illness.

For patients with ALS, discussion about life-sustaining measures starts at the first visit in most multidisciplinary ALS clinics. Given that most patients will die within 3–5 years of ALS diagnosis, discussions about clinical care and day-to-day management occur early, usually at the first visit to clinic. Advance directives are brought up, but the discussion may not go beyond providing the patient and family with an educational packet, given their need to adapt to the news of diagnosis. At the follow-up visits, advance directives and end-of-life discussions are ongoing, and decisions take shape with information and education through open communication.

Most patients are not ready to talk about death or what the experience is going to be as ALS progresses. Most patients are also not ready to appoint a guardian or a healthy proxy to make decisions until a situation that demands decision-making arises. Waiting to make decisions until an emergency occurs can cause challenges for patients, families, and healthcare providers.

Some of the topics where difficulty in decision-making is seen include cardiopulmonary resuscitation (CPR), mechanical ventilation, artificial nutrition and hydration, and/or withholding treatment [20]. For some patients with a terminal illness, CPR is not desired, a decision that can be particularly difficult for a loved one witnessing a cardiopulmonary arrest. Mechanical ventilation can be viewed as a support for a patient having respiratory insufficiency, rather than a treatment to prolong life. Assistive ventilation can be used to decrease a patient's anxiety related to breathlessness and to promote comfort. One of the most challenging decisions in end-of-life care is artificial nutrition and hydration. While many medical associations support that this is a form of comfort care meeting basic human needs, the US Supreme Court stated in 1990 that artificial nutrition and hydration are similar to a life-sustaining intervention and not for comfort [20]. Decisions surrounding patient choices such as discontinuing feeding or respiratory support are another situation that can be emotionally and ethically challenging.

For a healthcare provider managing this sensitive experience, communication that is centered on patient's autonomy and is family-oriented is crucial [20]. There is little systematic research to date on end-of-life care in neuromuscular patients. It seems what worries patients most is a lack of autonomy over the circumstances of their dying, such as powerlessness over decisions about medical treatments, including those that prolong life. In an article by Clark [23], the fear of death is replaced by the fear of dying.

Advance directives including a living will and power of attorney for healthcare, as well as DNR directives, should be utilized to expand specific discussions and explanations of possible complicated medical outcomes affecting a patient's quality of life. Ideally, these discussions by healthcare providers would take place shortly after the time of diagnosis, with perspective from the patient as to what choice they might make rather than waiting for a time when emotional and physical reserves may be low.

While many patients welcome the opportunity to participate in decision-making and communicate these views to their family and medical team, hurried hospital room and/or clinic visits can lead to misunderstandings and miscommunications on the part of the healthcare provider. Patients value highly the chance to discuss symptom management, anticipated disease progression and complications, and how this will affect the rest of their lives, in addition to open discussion on the topic of DNR and how they might die if the treatments are not successful.

After a diagnosis, patients usually hope for a cure. However, they also hope for a lack of pain, lucidity, a good quality of life, and a healthcare team that is committed to being with them throughout the care process. While the terminal nature of the condition needs to be confronted, hope can be directed to the quality of life and positive aspects of the here and now [24].

Further observations from families, patients, and healthcare providers on what constitutes a good death include pain and symptom management, clear decision-making, preparation for death, sense of completion, contributing to others, and affirmation as a whole person. Healthcare providers on the other hand see a good death as providing sufficient pain and symptom relief. Patients and families characterize a "bad death" as the inability to plan ahead, inability to manage their personal affairs, inability to decrease family burden, or having inadequate time to say goodbye to their loved ones [24].

Patients require ongoing and frequent communication from their healthcare providers in terms of information about disease diagnosis, the course of their disease, its evolving management, why treatments may be of value at strategic points in the disease course and not others, and how the individual will be supported both physically and emotionally throughout the course of their illness. The amount of information will vary from patient to patient and from family to family and probably will change over time. The relationship the healthcare provider has with the patient and family, ongoing patient education, and their clinical judgment play key roles in patient and family communications.

References

1. World Health Organization. Integrating palliative care and symptom relief into primary health care: a WHO guide for planners, implementers and managers. 2018. https://www.who.int/publications/i/item/integrating-palliative-care-and-symptom-relief-into-primary-health-care. Accessed 25 May 2023.
2. Tatum PE, Mills SS. Hospice and palliative care: an overview. Med Clin North Am. 2020;104(3):359–73. https://doi.org/10.1016/j.mcna.2020.01.001.
3. de Visser M, Oliver DJ. Palliative care in neuromuscular diseases. Curr Opin Neurol. 2017;30(6):686–91. https://doi.org/10.1097/WCO.
4. World Health Organization. Quality health services and palliative care: practical approaches and resources to support policy, strategy and practice. 2021. https://www.who.int/publications/i/item/9789240035164. Accessed 25 May 2023.
5. Hawley P. Barriers to access to palliative care. Palliat Care. 2017;10:1178224216688887. https://doi.org/10.1177/1178224216688887.
6. World Health Organization. Palliative care: key facts. 2020. https://www.who.int/news-room/fact-sheets/detail/palliative-care. Accessed 26 Jun 2023
7. Lalani N, Cai Y. Palliative care for rural growth and wellbeing: identifying perceived barriers and facilitators in access to palliative care in rural Indiana, USA. BMC Palliat Care. 2022;21:25. https://doi.org/10.1186/s12904-022-00913-8.
8. Symmons SM, Ryan K, Aoun SM, et al. Decision-making in palliative care: patient and family caregiver concordance and discordance—systematic review and narrative synthesis. BMJ Support Palliat Care. 2022;13:374. https://doi.org/10.1136/bmjspcare-2022-003525. PMID: 35318213.
9. Mahon M. Clinical decision making in palliative care and end of life care. Nurs Clin N Am. 2010;45(3):345–62. https://doi.org/10.1016/j.cnur.2010.03.002.
10. Birchall M. Decision-making in palliative care: a reflective case study. Contemp Nurse. 2005;19(1–2):253–63. https://doi.org/10.5172/conu.19.1-2.253.
11. Kuosmanen L, Hupli M, Ahtiluoto S, et al. Patient participation in shared decision-making in palliative care—an integrative review. J Clin Nurs. 2021;30:3415–28. https://doi.org/10.1111/jocn.15866.
12. Morrison BM. Neuromuscular diseases. Semin Neurol. 2016;36(5):409–18. https://doi.org/10.1055/s-0036-1586263.
13. Simonds AK. Living and dying with respiratory failure: facilitating decision making. Review series: ethical issues surrounding lung disease. Chron Respir Dis. 2004;1(1):56–9. https://doi.org/10.1191/1479972304cd014rs. PMID: 16281669.
14. Elverson J, Evans H, Dewhurst F. Palliation, end of life care and ventilation withdrawal in neuromuscular disorders. Chron Respir Dis. 2023;20:1–11. https://doi.org/10.1177/14799731231175911. PMID: 37199317; PMCID: PMC10201157.
15. Clawson LL, Cudkowicz M, Krivickas L, et al. A randomized controlled trial of resistance and endurance exercise in amyotrophic lateral sclerosis. Amyotroph Lateral Scler Frontotemporal Degener. 2018;19(3–4):250–8. https://doi.org/10.1080/21678421.2017.1404108.
16. Pascual-Morena C, Cavero-Redondo I, Reina-Gutiérrez S, et al. Prevalence of neuropsychiatric disorders in Duchenne and Becker muscular dystrophies: a systematic review and meta-analysis. Arch Phys Med Rehabil. 2022;103(12):2444–53. https://doi.org/10.1016/j.apmr.2022.05.015.
17. Brownlee A, Palovcak M. The role of augmentative communication devices in the medical management of ALS. NeuroRehabilitation. 2007;22(6):445–50. PMID: 18198430.
18. Drake M, Cox P. Ethics: end-of-life decision-making in a pediatric patient with SMA type 2: the influence of the media. Neurology. 2012;78(23):e143–5. https://doi.org/10.1212/WNL.0b013e318258f835.

19. Chabrol B, Desguerre I. Ethical aspects in the care of a child with infantile spinal muscular atrophy (SMA). Arch Pediatr. 2020;27(7S):7S50–3. https://doi.org/10.1016/S0929-693X(20)30278-5.
20. Akdeniz M, Yardimci B, Kavukcu E. Ethical considerations at the end-of-life care. SAGE Open Med. 2021;9:1–9. https://doi.org/10.1177/20503121211000918.
21. Jost K. Right to die. CQ Researcher. Document ID: cqresrre2005051300. 2005. https://library.cqpress.com/scc/document.php?id=cqresrre2005051300. Accessed 4 Aug 2023.
22. Daly FN, Ramanathan U. Chapter 13—End-of-life and hospice care for neurologic illness. Handb Clin Neurol. 2022;190:195–215. https://doi.org/10.1016/B978-0-323-85029-2.00006-3.
23. Clark J. Patient centred death. BMJ. 2003;327(7408):174–5. https://doi.org/10.1136/bmj.327.7408.174. PMID: 12881232; PMCID: PMC1126561.
24. Steinhauser KE, Clipp EC, McNeilly M, et al. In search of a good death: observations of patients, families, and providers. Ann Intern Med. 2000;132(10):825–32. https://doi.org/10.7326/0003-4819-132-10-200005160-00011. PMID: 10819707.

Index

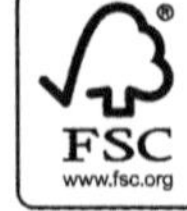

MIX
Papier aus verantwortungsvollen Quellen
Paper from responsible sources
FSC® C105338

If you have any concerns about our products,
you can contact us on
ProductSafety@springernature.com

In case Publisher is established outside the EU,
the EU authorized representative is:
Springer Nature Customer Service Center GmbH
Europaplatz 3, 69115 Heidelberg, Germany

Printed by Libri Plureos GmbH
in Hamburg, Germany